Nursing Innovation and Quality Improvement

Nursing Innovation and Quality Improvement

Guest Editor

Ashley Shepherd

MDPI

Basel • Beijing • Wuhan • Barcelona • Belgrade • Novi Sad • Cluj • Manchester

Guest Editor
Ashley Shepherd
Faculty of Health Sciences
and Sport
University of Stirling
Stirling
UK

Editorial Office
MDPI AG
Grosspeteranlage 5
4052 Basel, Switzerland

This is a reprint of the Special Issue, published open access by the journal *Nursing Reports* (ISSN 2039-4403), freely accessible at: https://www.mdpi.com/journal/nursrep/special_issues/9055N223K7.

For citation purposes, cite each article independently as indicated on the article page online and as indicated below:

Lastname, A.A.; Lastname, B.B. Article Title. *Journal Name* **Year**, *Volume Number*, Page Range.

ISBN 978-3-7258-6656-4 (Hbk)
ISBN 978-3-7258-6657-1 (PDF)
https://doi.org/10.3390/books978-3-7258-6657-1

Contents

About the Editor

Ashley Shepherd

Ashley Shepherd is a senior nursing academic at University of Stirling, where she holds a strategic leadership role within the Faculty of Health Sciences and Sport. She has established an internationally recognised programme of research focused on advancing evidence-based nursing practice, improving patient safety, and strengthening workforce capability across health systems. Her work is widely published in high-impact peer-reviewed journals and demonstrates a strong citation performance, reflecting the reach and influence of her scholarship within the global nursing community.

Ashley Shepherd has secured competitive research funding and has led multidisciplinary collaborations that bridge academia, policy, and frontline clinical practice. Her research is characterised by methodological rigour and a clear translational impact, informing service development and contributing to national and international policy discourse. She has supervised numerous doctoral candidates to completion, mentored early-career academics, and played a significant role in building research capacity within nursing and allied health professions.

In addition to her substantive role in Scotland, she holds an Honorary Associate Professor appointment with the University of Pennsylvania School of Nursing, further reflecting the international standing of her work and enabling global research collaboration. In her senior management capacity, she provides strategic oversight for research development, academic quality, and international engagement. She is committed to fostering a high-performing, inclusive academic culture that promotes innovation, leadership, and professional growth. Through sustained research excellence, high citation impact, and strong institutional leadership, Professor Shepherd continues to advance the discipline of nursing and contribute to improved health outcomes across diverse populations.

nursing reports

MDPI

Article

Experiences of Newly Qualified Nurses' Engagement with Quality Improvement in Practice: A Qualitative Follow-Up Study

Lorraine Armstrong *, Ashley Shepherd and Fiona Harris

Faculty of Health Sciences, University of Stirling, Stirling FK9 4LA, UK; ashley.shepherd@stir.ac.uk (A.S.); fiona.harris@stir.ac.uk (F.H.)

* Correspondence: lorraine.armstrong@stir.ac.uk

Abstract: Background: Nurse education plays an essential role in preparing future nurses to engage with quality improvement (QI) initiatives in their organisations and improve patient care. However, frontline nurses continue to report that a lack of QI knowledge hinders their abilities to engage in improvement work. In the UK, student nurses are now trained in QI within their degree to enable them to contribute to improvements once qualified. Objectives: This qualitative follow-up study investigated the sustainability of QI engagement in nurses who undertook QI training and a QI project during their degree and explored the factors influencing their engagement in QI once qualified. Methods: This paper followed the COREQ criteria to report upon 10 semi-structured interviews undertaken with registered nurses and focuses on their experiences of QI engagement post-registration. The data were investigated using an inductive thematic analysis and Nvivo 14. Findings: Five themes emerged: transition to a newly qualified nurse, QI knowledge decline, influencing factors (hierarchy, leadership, COVID-19 pandemic, data access and location), and skill transferability. Conclusions: This study showed that qualified nurses can sustain their QI knowledge and remain engaged with QI where they experience positive QI leadership and were exposed to ongoing QI activity in their preceptorship year. However, a lack of QI opportunities and a culture which does not consider QI a responsibility of new nurses is seen to hinder engagement. Educational institutions and practice partners require careful collaboration to assess and develop ongoing QI learning activities that support new nurses to engage in QI.

Keywords: quality improvement; nursing students; degree-level education; practice; qualitative analysis; follow-up; nurses; engagement; lived experience

1. Introduction

There is a drive in the UK (United Kingdom) and internationally to increase quality and service improvement content within nursing degree programmes to prepare future nurses to improve health and care services. This initiative is in response to professional standards set out by the Nursing and Midwifery Council (NMC) who make safety and quality of care an explicit proficiency to achieve [1]. To help inform faculties on how to develop and evaluate quality improvement (QI) curricular content in their programmes, a collection of research reviews and international primary research articles have focused on exploring QI in degree level nurse education [2–6]. This evidence confirms that student nurses learn to contribute to systematic change through practice-based QI projects and there is compelling evidence to suggest this pedagogical approach, in the right context, can foster QI-related behaviour change [7].

In 2016, a Scottish university in partnership with their local health board serving a population of around 300,000, facilitated a QI practice-based educational assessment called the QI Practicum. The development phase and QI intervention are described elsewhere [8] and detailed in Table 1.

Nurs. Rep. **2024**, *14*, 2990–3006. https://doi.org/10.3390/nursrep14040218 https://www.mdpi.com/journal/nursrep

Table 1. The QI Practicum curriculum content [8].

Semester	IHI Open School Courses	Teaching
1.		1. Person/patient-centred care 2. Introduction to the concept of quality in healthcare 3. Example of quality initiatives in action—Scottish Patient Safety Programme.
2.	QI101 Fundamentals of Improvement PS100 Introduction to Patient Safety PS101 Fundamentals of Patient Safety	1. QI Questions in MCQ exam 2. Evidence-based learning
3.	PS102 Human Factors and Safety PS103 Teamwork and Communication Q102 The Model for Improvement: Your Engine for Change	1. Evidence-informed practice 2. Quality improvement model
4.	QI103 Measuring for Improvement QI104 Putting it All Together: How QI Works in Real Health Care Settings	1. Improvement and Safety 2. QI questions in MCQ exam 3. Practice-based assignment—Care Partnerships, Care Study
5.	QI106 Level 100 Tools	1. Tools for quality improvement
6.	PS 104 Root Cause and System Analysis PS105 Communicating with patients after Adverse Event	1. Decision-making 2. Evidence for practice 3. Resources for Practicum online
7.	PS106 Introduction to the Culture of Safety L101 So you want to be a Leader in Health Care	1. Podcasts 2 2. Introduction to Practicum 3. Practicum: essential skills workshop 4. Preparing to work at SCQF level 10 5. Practicum assignment Q&A 6. Resilience workshop
8.		1. Collaborative improvement project (Practicum) 2. Practice events 3. Online/email/telephone/interview/workshop support 4. Reading week

The QI Practicum was designed to enable student nurses to gain practical experience of QI during an 8-week placement and identify and test changes to improve an area of practice using an established QI model. Powell et al. [9] report that the five most common improvement models used in healthcare are total quality management or continuous quality improvement, business process reengineering, lean thinking, six sigma, and IHI's rapid cycle change, also referred to as PDSA cycles. In the QI Practicum, students were taught about PDSA cycles as part of the model for improvement through seminars, e-learning modules, webinars, and podcasts [10].

This model suited the students' level of education and offered a 'bottom-up' approach for them to find problems and test low risk solutions in practice [10]. In line with other studies, the students used QI tools during their projects which included process mapping, pareto charts, driver diagrams, run charts, cause/effect diagrams, and bar graphs [8,11,12]. Students completed QI projects in pre-operative assessment, community health centres, hospitals, hospices, nursing homes, the emergency department, and acute care. Areas they focused on to improve included oral care, handover communication, the inclusion of patients' carers, adherence with personal protective equipment, reducing pressure damage and creating dementia friendly environments. A previous teaching evaluation of the QI Practicum concluded that where students engaged in QI in the practice setting there was a transformation from panic and an ignorance of QI to a state of appreciation of and commitment to using QI methods in the future [8].

Following their three-year degree programme, students registered as newly qualified nurses (NQNs) with the UK NMC [13]. Some NQNs secured posts locally in their health boards or private organisations, others returned to their home countries to practice, and some worked in different health boards or practiced internationally. To develop into confident and capable registered practitioners, those who remained in Scotland undertook a national development programme called Flying Start within their first 12 months [14]. This transition programme is designed to combine individual learning with support in the workplace to help NQNs gather evidence and demonstrate that they are upholding professional standards. Thereafter, they join frontline nurses in building evidence portfolios to support their professional development and prepare for a revalidation process every three years to maintain their NMC registration. Despite professional standards making safety and quality of care an explicit proficiency to achieve, there is consensus that a knowledge gap remains as to whether student nurses who received degree level QI education continue to be engaged in QI once qualified. This study therefore aimed to explore the sustainability of QI engagement in post-registration nurses and identify the factors influencing their engagement.

1.1. QI Education

The international literature offers various definitions of QI. Batalden and Davidoff [15] present a holistic overview of QI and propose it is 'the combined and unceasing efforts of everyone—healthcare professionals, patients and their families, researchers, payers, planners, and educators—to make the changes that will lead to better patient outcomes (health), better system performance (care) and better professional development (learning)'. Cepero [16], on the other hand, defines the method as a practical and concise approach that involves 'a cyclical process designed to evaluate workflow and clinical indicators or outcomes'. It is reasonable to suggest that QI is in fact an umbrella term that encompasses multiple systematic 'change methods' to support improvement and better outcomes for patients and services [10,17].

The UK pre-registration nursing workforce is expected to initiate improvements and demonstrate QI competence prior to registration [13]. Over the years, student nurses have been taught QI concepts such as improvement methods, the model for improvement, quality indicator measures, plan–do–study–act (PDSA) cycles, root cause analysis, systems thinking, interprofessional learning, clinical governance, data, human factors, and evidence-based practice [8,11,18]. Approaches to teaching QI have ranged from inviting QI experts to talk with students to involving them in clinical audit and completing QI projects [5]. The latter pedagogical approach is known to foster experiential learning and supports student nurses to apply the theoretical concepts in the real world and develop their QI competencies [2]. By teaching QI this way, it is suggested that organisations benefit from student nurses who can offer added capacity and support to implement improvement projects [19]. Student nurses also gain a sense of belonging in situations where they contribute to policy and protocol changes in real-time while learning from the interprofessional team [3].

However, QI education is complex and comprises components relating to the faculty, the learner, the practice setting, the professional team, the patient, and the QI endeavour. The practice settings in which nurses work are equally complex and involve the physical space, psychosocial and interaction factors, and organizational culture [20,21]. The interrelationships occurring between these factors is what makes it difficult to identify causality between QI educational assessments and nurses' future engagement with QI. However, many studies have attempted to explore nurses' QI engagement.

1.2. QI Nurse Engagement

There has been a shortage of attempts to define QI engagement in the nursing literature. For the purpose of this paper, we defined nurse engagement in QI as undertaking QI training after qualifying, involvement in QI initiatives, or applying QI methods/tools to projects in the practice setting.

A systematic review finds that studies reporting on the engagement of nurses in QI have been published for almost 20 years [22]. The findings of these studies show that where nurses engage in QI, improvements have been seen in patient outcomes relating to falls (23%), blood stream infections (70%), and pressure damage (66%) as well as job satisfaction for nurses and reduced staff sickness. A substantial proportion of the healthcare workforce is made up of frontline staff nurses who are ideally placed to identify opportunities for improvement. However, a recent survey (n = 409) showed that this population perceived themselves to have low levels of preparedness in quality and safety and showed that two thirds of frontline nurses were not currently involved in any QI or patient safety initiatives [23]. These findings are consistent with the results determined by a 'QI in practice tool', which aimed to determine nurses' QI engagement (n = 681). The findings showed that a third of nurses were unsure whether their unit had conducted QI and less than 50% reported taking part in QI [24].

A recent qualitative study which explored nurses' QI engagement emphasised that leadership influence on QI culture such as creating buy-in, supporting a just culture, and working in partnership with frontline nurses is essential [25]. Nurse leadership involvement has been known to influence the success of QI for over two decades and they currently remain the most engaged subgroup of nurses in QI [23,24,26]. A nurse leaders' role in engaging frontline nurses is crucial to overcome the added organisational barriers that nurses face such as time pressures, lack of QI expertise, siloed departments, and access to prompt data [25]. These barriers are unlikely to be overcome if nurses are not adequately trained in the foundations of QI. Given that only 33% of early career nurse managers felt prepared by their employers to use QI data analysis tools, the workforce cannot rely upon leaders alone to increase the levels of frontline nurses' engagement with QI [27]. Earlier research concludes that there is value in determining whether nurses who completed QI training and a QI project during their degree programme remain engaged with QI as qualified practitioners [6,8,22,23]. So, this was the aim of our study.

1.3. Context

The study reported in this paper includes the second and final phase of a longitudinal evaluation of the QI Practicum.

The first phase was undertaken between 2016–2018 with the purpose of exploring what contextual factors influenced students' QI learning experiences in the practice setting. Ethnographic methodology was employed to capture the students' complex and everyday lived experiences within the cultural context of their practice placements. Data collection included 84 h of participant observations with 30 adult field student nurses across nine clinical practice settings within an acute hospital. Fieldwork occurred over two months using informal interviewing, in-depth interviews, focus groups, and documentary analysis. This methodology enabled new insights into QI in nursing education where previous studies' designs such as pre-/post-surveys or self-reported data have limited understanding [2]. Discussing the findings from phase one is outside of the scope of this paper. However, in sum, student nurses' QI learning experiences were influenced by sixteen contextual factors grouped into five themes: practice learning environment, organisational culture, leadership, data for improvement, the assignment, and the student nurse. These factors were experienced as facilitators or barriers, depending on the students' practice setting. Further, the inter-relationship of contextual factors differed between students and influenced the level on which they engaged in their QI Practicums, ranging from no engagement to engaging in organisational projects. The findings are significant in that they provide new perspectives of undertaking QI education in practice for pre-registration nurses and can inform academic and practice partners who are integrating and/or supporting QI education. Phase two of the study is now reported.

The second and final phase of the evaluation, which is reported in this paper, involved follow-up interviews with the same study participants once they qualified as registered nurses. The purpose was to determine if they had remained engaged with QI as qualified nurses and determine what the factors were influencing their engagement.

2. Methods

2.1. Design

Phase two of the study used qualitative semi-structured follow-up interviews, and an inductive thematic analysis [28]. Qualitative research is described as 'an approach for exploring and understanding the meaning individuals or groups ascribe to a social or human problem' (p. 4) [29]. We considered this design to be the most appropriate to explore phenomena not yet thoroughly researched, such as newly qualified nurses' long-term engagement with QI. Corben and Strauss [30] refer to qualitative research as dynamic, and we believe this fits with the principles that underpin improving complex and fluid healthcare. The literature has previously criticised designs using pre-/post-surveys and self-reported data in QI educational evaluations [2]. However, our study does not use qualitative interviewing in isolation to explore nurses' QI experiences. Instead, semi-structured interviews are used to supplement a larger ethnographic evaluation. Due to the disparity in nurses' work locations in phase two, a multi-site ethnography was not appropriate. To ensure explicit and comprehensive reporting, we applied the consolidated criteria for reporting qualitative research (COREQ) checklist [31].

2.2. Research Team

The research team consisted of three females. The lead researcher was a nurse and PhD candidate who held positions during the first and second phase of the evaluation as a clinical academic whose focus was on QI and then a lecturer in nursing (LA). The two supervisory team members included a Professor of Nursing with QI subject expertise (AS) and a non-clinical Professor of Social Anthropology (FH) without QI knowledge but had extensive qualitative training and experience. While the research team were resident at the same university, none of the research team were involved in delivering teaching or marking the QI Practicum for the participants involved in this study.

2.3. Participants

As the intention of this study was to follow up on previous participants who had undertaken the QI Practicum to determine their engagement with QI once qualified; a purposive sample was used initially. Participants (n = 30) were approached through their email addresses and/or telephone numbers provided during the first phase of the evaluation; however, some contact details were no longer valid. Where responses were not received, a second attempt to contact participants was made and a message left on their voicemail. A final attempt to reach participants was made through searching public social media pages where contact was made through their private messaging option. A total of 17 participants responded and received follow-up study information sheets by email. They were given seven days to have queries answered and decide whether to take part in the study. Although our original ethics approval permitted us to make contact with participants in a follow-up study, and participants had consented to be contacted at any time, we re-established consent before interviews took place. Consent was recorded verbally at the start of each interview. Overall, seven participants decided not take part in an interview due to being on maternity leave (n = 3), expressing a lack of time through work commitments (n = 2), or did not attend the interview (n = 2). Participants were contacted again to reschedule where they did not attend but no reply was received by the research team. Therefore, the inclusion of participants in the study was reduced to a convenience sample (n = 10).

The mean age of participants was 38 (range 29–47) and the group consisted of 8 females and 2 males. Included in the sample were front-line staff nurses (n = 6), senior staff nurses (charges $n = 3$), and a former staff nurse who had recently left the profession (n = 1). The sample reflected the variety of engagement witnessed during their QI Practicums. Study sample characteristics can be found in Table 2. While we acknowledge that demographic characteristics can influence nurses' attitudes towards QI, such as salary and working in private or public service [32], the analysis of such was outside of the scope of this study and was not included.

Table 2. Characteristics of study sample.

	Gender	Age	Current Designation/Employment	Engagement in QI Once Qualified	QI Practicum Location as a Student Nurse	Contextual Factors Influencing Engagement in QI Practicum
Participant A	Female	47	Staff Nurse Acute Medicine	Reported involvement in QI initiatives	Medicine	Confidence to articulate ideas and persistence to obtain early manager buy-in facilitated engagement.
Participant B	Female	29	Senior Staff Nurse Community	Reported involvement in QI initiatives	Medicine	Supportive QI culture and knowledgeable mentors encouraged and facilitated QI engagement.
Participant C	Male	32	Senior Staff Nurse Acute Medicine	Reported involvement in QI initiatives	Surgical	Knowledgeable senior charge and positive change culture permitted autonomy to engage in QI.
Participant D	Female	36	Staff Nurse Community	Reported involvement in QI initiatives and application of QI methods/tools	Surgical	Knowledgeable senior charge and positive change culture permitted autonomy to engage in QI.
Participant E	Female	47	Senior Staff Nurse Community	Reported involvement in QI initiatives	Rehabilitation	Jaded mentors' attitudes and senior leadership changes reduced ability to engage in QI activity.
Participant F	Female	32	Staff Nurse Acute Medicine	No involvement	Medicine	Hierarchy meant that staff did not perceive students' QI projects as important; in turn, this reduced student's engagement.
Participant G	Female	29	Staff Nurse Acute Medicine	No involvement	Telephone Support	Too many student projects going on simultaneously which reduced support to engage in QI.
Participant H	Male	34	Staff Nurse Acute Medicine	No involvement	Medicine	Active QI culture made it difficult to find a QI project to engage in as 'everything was already being done'.
Participant I	Female	32	Staff Nurse Acute Medicine	No involvement	Medicine	Familiarity of placement and positive growth mindset enhanced QI engagement.
Participant J	Female	35	Former Staff Nurse Left the Profession	No involvement	Medicine	Practicalities of large complex environment posed challenges to timely engagement.

2.4. Data Collection

Data collection was undertaken between February and April 2024 by the lead researcher (L.A.). To enable objectivity during data collection, a second member of the supervisory team was present at the start of data collection to oversee the conduct of the first few interviews and to be able to contribute to refining future iterations of the interview schedule (F.H.). A combination of face-to face interviews online through Microsoft Teams (n = 5) and telephone interviews (n = 5) were undertaken. A semi-structured qualitative interview guide was designed and informed by the analysis of contextual factors influencing students' engagement in the QI Practicum during the first phase of the evaluation. A key focus of the follow-up interviews was to explore whether QI knowledge had been sustained and to explore the nuances involved with QI engagement once qualified and within nurses' current practice. Given the timeframe between the first and second phase of the evaluation, strategies to mitigate potential participant recall were undertaken. A preliminary meeting was held before each interview where the researcher provided a summary of the QI practicum and an account of the individuals' reported experiences of their QI engagement at that time. Participants were given an opportunity to reflect and ask questions before they participated in the interview. The interview guide was piloted with one nurse initially and thereafter reviewed by the research team through regular discussion. The interview guide was adjusted accordingly to reflect the analysis during phase one, address the current study aims and account for any new and emerging ideas (Supplementary Materials File S1). Interviews lasted approximately 30 min and were audio-recorded and automatically transcribed using Microsoft Teams (https://www.microsoft.com/en-us/microsoft-teams, accessed on 1 February 2024). Recurring themes were identified with no new data emerging following eight interviews. Two further interviews were conducted to help validate findings. The lead researcher (L.A.) reviewed all transcripts for accuracy of text and corrected anomalies produced by Microsoft Teams. Each supervisory member of the team cross-checked 10 percent of transcriptions for accuracy (F.H./A.S.).

2.5. Qualitative Analysis

Our thematic analysis of interview transcripts was guided by Corbin and Strauss' analytic strategies [30] and managed through Nvivo qualitative data analysis (CDAS), version 14.23.0 (Lumivero, Denver, CO, USA). To become acquainted with the data, transcripts were read in-depth by the lead researcher (L.A.). The supervisory team each read twenty percent of the transcripts (A.S./F.H.). Initial themes were identified in advance using the coding framework generated within the first phase of the evaluation to search for similarities and differences in the data relating to factors influencing nurses' QI engagement once qualified (Supplementary Materials File S2). This original coding framework from phase 1 had been developed and validated by all of the research team (L.A., A.S., and F.H.). To remain open to new ideas and themes within the data, interview scripts were coded individually, firstly by the lead researcher (L.A.). To mitigate bias, each member of the supervisory team thereafter coded twenty percent of the transcripts to check for inter-rater reliability. New codes and ideas were explored by the researcher team during a debriefing session where probing questions emerged from QI and non-QI perspectives to justify new and emerging ideas. A constant comparison approach between participants' experiences was then undertaken until no new codes were identified. Themes and subthemes were reviewed and finalised by the lead researcher (L.A.) and agreed by the research team [30].

2.6. Ethical Considerations

The University of Stirling Research Ethics Committee (SREC) approved the study on the 7 December 2015 (Ref: SREC 15/16—Paper No. 40). The research study was underpinned by the principles within the Data Protection Act [33] and conducted per the University of Stirling Code of Good Research Practice and NHS (National Health Service) Code of Confidentiality [34].

3. Results

3.1. Transition to Newly Qualified Nurse

The QI Practicum had intended to equip the next generation of nurses with the QI knowledge and skills required by the NMC. Some NQNs reported placing a value on undertaking QI and included their skills and experiences in their job applications and curriculum vitae (CVs). Some had drawn upon their QI experience during job interviews, which led to one NQN being offered a job in the ward she had completed her QI project in:

> *'I put that in my CV and then discussed it at length with the Charge Nurse at my interview, because she obviously helped me implement it. We kept it running in the ward and when I started there, I used it for my flying start and became one of the link nurses for QI.'* (Interview D)

Other NQNs did not contemplate adding QI skills to their CVs or job applications. Further, these nurses reported that managers in their preceptorship year asked them to focus on learning the basic fundamental skills of a NQN for at least 6–8 months prior to increasing their responsibilities. This manager advice aligned to students' beliefs that QI felt like an unnecessary extra as well as being an unsuitable time to be involved during their first year:

> *'Immediately after I qualified my first goal was to actually get more experience because you don't really know anything. So, my first goal was to learn my skills, and just be enough. I don't think my focus was on improvement.'* (Interview A)

3.2. QI Knowledge Decline

Beyond preceptorship, the nurses discussed QI-related behaviours but demonstrated less knowledge. They spoke of writing reflective accounts about QI during their NMC revalidation and being involved in improving admissions paperwork, enhancing patient transition to short stay wards, and creating sustainable healthcare delivery through single-use medication cups. Despite associating their behaviours with improvement, the nurses admitted to using a less formal QI process:

> *'The basics of QI are straightforward, you do it without thinking about it—it's just that I've not necessarily used all the diagrams and everything, there were no charts that we used.'* (Interview E)

> *'I have engaged in improvement, but not in a proper assessed way you know, it doesn't go through a process, but it's just me wanting to work better to improve.'* (Interview A)

Although nurses were taught the model for improvement during their degree, their recall of QI knowledge and terminology during interviews was vague. They admitted revisiting old coursework prior to their interview to remind themselves of the QI process. A 'use it or lose it' attitude towards QI was evident as nurses reported losing some their learning:

> *'I had to look back over my practicum before we started this chat. Looking back in practice, it's not something I've come across, or think about daily. To get involved, I would need to study again for more knowledge, and then maybe some of this stuff would come back to me.'* (Interview G)

3.3. Influencing Factors

3.3.1. Hierarchy

After qualifying, some of the participants claimed they had no exposure to QI activity. One nurse stated that QI was undertaken by management or staff working towards promotion and often in their own time. A hierarchy often deterred nurses from engaging in QI:

> *'It was mostly higher up that were initiating the changes—one of my colleagues tried quality improvement stuff, but she got a lot of push back by higher up management, so you need to jump these barriers all the time.'* (Interview H)

This hierarchical exposure to QI was validated as one nurse, now in a senior post, spoke of only just then receiving exposure to the information needed to engage with QI. This nurse reported having full autonomy and greater insight into how the organisation functioned, now that they were more involved and keener to advance their services:

> *'It's quite good to be accepting of change. In my previous post, I feel like I didn't have the opportunity for QI, whereas I feel now that I'm in a senior role, I feel like I can take a step back and identify ideas that I want to change and make improvements.'* (Interview C)

3.3.2. Leadership

The nurses were able to draw upon their QI educational experience as a student to identify factors they believed influenced their current QI engagement. Regardless of being a preceptor or senior staff nurse, those engaged with QI further reported the experience of supportive leadership during their QI Practicums:

> *'I was very lucky, our SCN at the time was just so up for QI and so positive and transparent with data. I felt so supported and felt that I had control over doing QI projects when I became a registered nurse.'* (Interview D)

While this transformational leadership style influenced nurses' engagement in QI, others experienced a more laissez-faire leadership style which produced opposite effects. Nurses without greater line-management input perceived that they lacked the permission to initiate change, and without clear direction, nurses did not see the point engaging in QI. One nurse requested that clearer expectations from management around the nurses' role in QI was needed:

> *'There is a real lack of management expectations—but you need authority from them to go and do QI, you need like a recognised person to say go and do it. If you do it yourself, it's more difficult.'* (Interview H)

Despite the leadership style demonstrated by nurse managers, there was a recognition by new nurses that staff in all roles were under constant time pressures, which meant committing to QI was difficult; this included management:

> *'I would like to take forward my QI project, but we are not given the time for that, I'm not blaming my manager, she's under so much pressure on every part. It doesn't seem to matter what level of the system that you're actually at, everybody is struggling to make things their priority.'* (Interview A)

3.3.3. COVID-19 Pandemic

The COVID-19 pandemic was referred to by many nurses as a reason they did not participate in QI, even where they had retained QI knowledge or experienced supportive leadership. One nurse reported that their QI project involving the interprofessional team was put on hold to deal with the core requirements of working in the pandemic. While this nurse reported getting involved in QI again as services returned to normal, others emphasised that the lasting effects of COVID-19 had been 'hellish' and 'chaotic'. This experience had resulted in burnout for some nurses and hindered their engagement in QI:

> *'The aftermath of COVID was actually worse, the atmosphere is just totally different, and it's been a really hard year, and I haven't got a break. Everyone is just done. Even if you see people trying to improve something, a lot of people just aren't interested.'* (Interview F)

Burnout from the COVID-19 pandemic was reported to come from caring for sicker patients and managing the ever-changing demands placed upon them throughout this time. As a result, nurses reported having to psychologically prioritise their families over their work and do only what was necessary in practice before going home. However, there was an indication that while COVID-19 no longer posed the same set of challenges, its lasting effects, such as a lack of engagement in QI, had continued:

'COVID has a lot to say about forgetting about QI for me. It's also been a good excuse for people not returning to some key principles that we should be focused on.' (Interview A)

3.3.4. Data Access

When nurses were asked if they could access the information needed to identify areas for improvement, some demonstrated negativity towards statistics. For instance, nurses who had progressed into senior positions reported feeling confident when asking for the necessary data, but those remaining at the frontline admitted to not knowing where to retrieve it and associated data with negative performance:

'We don't get like statistics on things as a staff nurse unless it's something negative. You know, you kind of get your audits for things, where we are told where we need to improve. I wouldn't know where to start in terms of getting access to other data though.' (Interview H)

Some of the participants asserted that despite being qualified nurses, their experience of needing permission to access data through gatekeepers remained similar to their experience as a student during the QI Practicum. Consequently, nurses lacked the necessary information needed to engage in QI and so they did not try. Contrastingly, other nurses retrieved data with ease which was attributed to having login credentials for online health systems where they could explore problems. These nurses were able to demonstrate their retained QI knowledge and positive attitudes round the importance of data:

'It wasn't a problem for us to collect data as registered nurses, our manager was open about it, you know, just being honest, it's good to have that transparency, we knew exactly where we were. You could actually implement changes because you know the data was accurate. I know others in the hospital struggle, so I don't know if that's just because of where we were.' (Interview D)

3.3.5. Location

The nurses had developed their QI learning as students during the QI Practicum in the same acute hospital setting. As nurses they were drawing upon their experiences of QI engagement from acute and community settings across different regions in Scotland:

'So, when I moved from one health board to another, I was a charge nurse and really keen to implement a lot of changes. But, when I got there, I experienced a lot of barriers and there was more politics in that hospital than in my last one.' (Interview D)

The practice setting in which nurses worked was a key influence on QI engagement. Despite displaying positive individual characteristics such as embracing challenges, having an intrinsic value to do better, upholding a passion for nursing, and practicing a growth mindset, if the location did not exude a positive QI culture, engagement was difficult:

'Location and the staff you work with has a lot to do with QI—it really depends on where you are, some health boards are very clique and hierarchical.' (Interview B)

3.4. Transferrable Skills

There was evidence that nurses transferred their QI knowledge and skills inside and outside of the healthcare environment. One nurse who had substantial experience of supporting QI spoke of drawing upon their expertise in a new post. In their annual professional development plan, they had objectives to create a 'QI link nurse' role and mentor others:

'Just before I went on maternity leave, I had my annual review and I agreed to go back and develop a role in QI, I would love to be able to do that again. I love where I work, and they are big on QI.' (Interview D)

Moving beyond the healthcare environment, one nurse described their engagement with their son's school improvement agenda to enhance the learning experience of young people in primary education. They had transferred QI knowledge and skills learned during their degree to benefit the wider community:

> *'I'm engaging a lot more with the community and have found a lot of purpose improving well-being. QI can be used in all areas, and I'm engaged with the school for example to develop a community garden initiative. For me, I would work in the community for health improvement, but I don't see a lot of opportunities for that.'* (Interview A)

Lastly, despite the challenges faced, most nurses agreed that QI was a transferable skill, if nurses remained engaged. They saw the importance of QI as a taught component to continue within degree level nurse education and identified its value in raising awareness of change and ensuring the future generation of nurses continue to improve and grow.

4. Discussion

Preregistration nurses in the UK will inevitably encounter QI education within their nursing degree and there has never been a more critical time to have frontline nurses demonstrate competence in healthcare and service improvements. Our study, the first follow-up study of its kind, set out to investigate if registered nurses who completed a practice-based QI project in the final year of their degree remained engaged with QI once qualified. While this generation of new nurses educated in QI can create and foster a culture of improvement in practice, our study which presents a snapshot of this phenomena, suggests that much work is still needed to support this agenda.

NQNs entered the profession with different views on the value of receiving QI training and undertaking a QI project in practice. The unique position that students were exposed to by receiving QI training was emphasised to them regularly during their degree. Some students capitalised on this QI training as an attribute to enhance their employment prospects. However, the analysis showed that some employers and NQNs did not regard QI as an essential skill to attain early in their professional career. This perception may have been influenced at the time by the Flying Start Programme, which new nurses undertook to support their preceptorship year, as it made no reference to QI standards. In 2019, this transition programme was refreshed to reflect the ever-changing needs of the environments in which NQNs work. NQNs are now required to reflect upon and attain evidence linked to quality and service improvement [14]. Therefore, healthcare employers will be compelled to support NQNs and provide opportunities for them to engage in QI activities. This responsibility has implications for practice leaders who will need to reassess their own nursing team's QI involvement and consequently plan suitable QI-related learning activities for new nurses to evidence their QI competences. Further, as NQN enter the profession and become accountable for their learning, they need to actively seek out QI-related opportunities to become involved. In the past five years, the increased momentum of QI nurse educational research has emerged due to the QI alignment between faculties and professional nursing standards [2–6]. Given this shift, there are now greater opportunities to investigate the views of NQNs in the current context in order to determine what value they place on their QI education and their role within it during their preceptorship year. The requirements of healthcare employers to support NQNs to engage with QI activities will need to be understood to enable effective strategies to be put in place. We recommend that research is prioritised in this area to ensure that we can foster and benefit from these nurses' QI knowledge.

There is now a professional requirement and desire from practice partners to have new nurses enter the profession with sufficient knowledge of improvement theories and tools [13,35]. The nurses in our study were uniquely positioned to enter the profession with QI training and knowledge. Faculties had selected an experiential learning approach in practice to tutor students about QI due to its ability to enhance QI knowledge [2]. However, the findings showed that educational efforts to develop nurses' QI knowledge were reversed where a lack of engagement opportunities in QI activity existed. Nurses' lack of knowledge is one of the most often reported barriers to engagement in QI [25,27,36]. As such, greater alignment between academic and practice partners will be essential to create an infrastructure that builds upon new nurses' QI capabilities and supports their ongoing professional development [35,37]. Practice education facilitators could be central in this role given their oversight of nurses' learning needs and their contribution to developing regular practice training updates. Their role in evaluating what current opportunities exist for new nurses to engage in QI could be useful to inform future educational pathways. Fostering engagement in QI activities for new nurses can create future QI leaders and change agents, as was shown in our study through the specialist roles nurses adopted, such as the QI link nurse. Capacity building in this way could be a solution to increase the QI knowledge of future front-line early career nurse managers, of whom only 30% reported feeling prepared to undertake QI [27]. Further, nurse leaders and nurses report wanting to learn together through workshops and drop-in seminars, and seek to partner together to work on QI projects [36]. Learning through QI academies, of which there is evidence in UK health boards, could enable such QI partnerships to be developed [38]. Future research studies should examine the feasibility of new nurses and leaders partnering together in QI activities and determine how QI academies might help in sustaining new nurses' QI knowledge after they enter the profession.

This study highlighted and found that QI was considered by nurses as a progressive responsibility undertaken as their roles advanced. This view exposed a culture in which QI was not considered an everyday nursing role. Hierarchy in organisations is often reported by nurses as a barrier that prevents them engaging in QI activity [25,36]. Our findings suggest that nurses brought ideas for change forward but did not feel like their managers listened. A potential reason for this lack of consultation may be due to nurse leaders facing their own hierarchical barriers such as disproportional funding for QI projects between disciplines and lack of physician buy-in, which can take several months of persuasion [25,36]. A lack of autonomy and ability to speak up to challenge leaders was discussed by some of the nurses in our study. This skill is necessary to enable nurses to advocate for change and improve patient care and services. Thus, further investigation into the personal attributes of nurses and how they influence QI engagement is needed. Further, future research that investigates how the power dynamics between disciplines impact nurses' engagement in QI will be necessary to develop strategies that enable nurses at all levels to have a voice which reinforces the values and behaviours that underpin high-quality care.

Our findings showed that where nurse leaders modelled positive QI values and behaviours during nurses' degree, nurses reported sustained engagement in QI. Leadership has been significantly associated with the success of QI and attributed to high-functioning teams [26]. Nurses believe leaders are highly influential in encouraging engagement in QI where they adopt transformational leadership styles through creating buy-in, supporting a just culture, and working in partnership with more junior staff [36]. In contrast, our study showed that where co-operation between nurses and leaders was based upon a laissez-faire approach to QI activities, it led to unclear expectations about QI roles. This confusion hindered active engagement and mirrors findings found within other studies [39]. Leadership influence in QI appears to begin during students' degree and has potential to affect engagement in QI once qualified. Therefore, leaders involved with QI will need to assess and reflect upon their own leadership styles when supporting new nurses and students undertaking QI. Students were distributed to one of the many practice settings to undertake their QI project, and thus students' exposure to a leader who modelled positive QI values and behaviours was serendipitous. Students would benefit from undertaking QI activities across a range of settings to optimise their chances of working in a culture conducive to QI and increase the likelihood of engaging in QI once qualified. These changes would have implications for how QI is taught in educational programmes, because curriculum developers will need to redesign their modular content to include more frequent experiential learning opportunities for students to engage in QI.

During the COVID-19 pandemic, opportunities for rapid improvements and catalysing change efforts were at the forefront of all health professionals' practice. For the nurses in our study, however, it was a stressful period during which QI activity was postponed and no engagement in QI was reported. These findings should be interpreted with caution though, as nurses referred to COVID-19 being used as a cover-up to justify why engagement in QI had not resumed post-COVID. The emotional stress that nurses faced could have also potentially skewed their memories during such events.

Using data to monitor performance is the cornerstone of improving patient care and services. Student nurses are expected to acquire knowledge of data before qualifying and during their degree; students collected, analysed, and displayed data using run charts for the QI Practicum [13]. Earlier studies report that students have lacked information about where to collect data; perceived data to be tedious, uninteresting, boring, or non-educational and irrelevant; and 60% of student in a survey replied they had not collected any data using fishbone diagrams or process maps during their QI projects [12,18]. If students' QI learning experiences influence their engagement in QI once qualified, then faculty need to ensure effective QI learning activities around data are developed. The qualified nurses in our study reported only having access to data in QI roles or in senior positions. This outcome aligns to a survey in which nurse leaders were more likely to report access to data as a facilitator of engagement in QI than clinical nurses [40]. However, data must be used to generate open and transparent conversations about improvements between leaders and nurses if a culture of psychological safety is to be developed. Scrutiny of our analysis instead reveals that nurses developed a negative association with data (or statistics) and had a fear of wrongdoing. These findings show that efforts in education and practice should focus on developing positive attitude and beliefs around data if QI engagement is to be increased.

Nurses in our study displayed positive beliefs and attitudes about QI and had a will to improve patient care. Despite these best intentions, they asserted that QI engagement was decided upon by the location in which they worked. This finding is unsurprising given the contextual nature upon which QI depends for success [26]. Location encompasses many interacting contextual factors that influence engagement in QI, such as leadership, mentorship, data, culture, and hierarchy [36,40]. While understanding these facilitators and barriers are useful in figuring out new nurses' engagement in QI, research should go beyond qualitative and quantitative methods to employ a realist methodology which answers 'what works, for whom and in what circumstances?' [41]. Developing rich case studies to explore 'why' these facilitators and barriers exist in different contexts will help in recommending future QI engagement strategies for nurses. Phase one of the study revealed that students' locations presented associated challenges for not engaging with their QI Practicums, namely in regard to familiarity and size of the setting, shift type and patterns, balancing workloads, and the presence of QI expertise. While nurses in our study did not discuss these factors in depth, they could be key to planning effective engagement in QI for new nurses and thus warrant further investigation.

Lastly, a surprising finding relating to the transferability of nurses QI skills was identified. While some nurses transferred their QI knowledge and skills to new nursing roles, others applied them to real-world issues outside of healthcare, such as early years education. These findings coincide with attempts seen to optimise QI education and improve wider societal concerns. In undergraduate medical education, the SusQI education framework links concepts of sustainable healthcare with QI methods [42], and in New Zealand, nurse education aligns cultural agendas to the QI curriculum to improve equity and inclusion of the Māori culture [6]. These findings highlight the potential reach of QI education and the possibility of exploring QI projects being applied to and within different contexts. There are reports of students being more motivated and engaged in QI where there is a shared vision or personal preference in the QI topic being undertaken [43]. While the need for small QI projects in the practice setting still exists, the global demands and responsibilities placed upon us are now greater than ever before. As a result, educational faculties may wish to consider more innovative and engaging pedagogical approaches to teach nurses QI methodology.

5. Study Limitations

While this study has generated important findings about nurses' engagement with QI following QI training within their degree, the sample is limited to one university programme in central Scotland, and the findings should be seen within this context. Despite the small sample allowing us to explore what supports or impedes QI practice post-registration, our findings cannot be generalised to other fields of nursing such as mental health, children, or learning disability due to the different contexts in which nurses practice. A large-scale survey would be needed to determine how representative the findings are in Scotland. In QI research, it is understood that while an intervention works in one setting, it may not work in another due to the complexity of the inter-related contextual factors present. Similar can be said about our own follow-up findings; however, because our findings mirror those established in the wider QI education [2], they serve as a starting point to further explore the factors influencing new nurses' engagement in QI.

Future research may wish to address a key limitation of this study. Firstly, an extended period occurred between students qualifying and follow-up interviews being conducted. Recruitment was planned for the first quarter of 2020 but postponed due to non-COVID-19-related research being temporarily ceased. This delay may have resulted in recruiting only 10 participants from the original sample of 30, due to invalid contact details, student nurses no longer seeing the relevance of taking part in the research or the attrition of nurses leaving the profession following the COVID-19 pandemic [44]. While there was also a potential for selection bias, such as nurses who were more involved in QI agreeing to be interviewed, our participants included nurses not involved in QI and those no longer in the profession. Consistent with other qualitative studies, our sample was sufficient within the parameters of our defined aims, and we reached data saturation before the end of the data collection period [45]. Secondly, the extended period potentially affected the reliability of nurses' recall during the earlier years, which included transitioning to a newly qualified nurse and the preceptorship year. Thus, the cognisance of the accuracy of nurses' lived experiences should be accounted for when interpreting the findings. For instance, it may have resulted in events being over- or under-reported or heightened states during the pandemic leading to distorted nurses' memories. Triangulation during data collection should be considered in future research follow-up studies to mitigate recall bias. This could be achieved through regular entries about nurses' QI engagement in a participant reflective diary. This could have potentially allowed our findings to be explored in greater depth and strengthened our findings. Given the similarity and consistency of participants' interview responses in line with the wider literature, we are confident the findings present a trustworthy and valid depiction of how nurses engage with QI in practice following their degree education.

6. Conclusions

Qualified nurses have the potential to become agents of future change and sustain their knowledge and engagement in QI following the completion of a QI project during their degree. However, the juxtaposition in supporting new nurses to become engaged in QI activity will need to be carefully considered between educational institutions and practice partners. To foster QI engagement in new nurses, multiple QI learning opportunities made available during pre-registration degree programmes should be developed and continued through ongoing professional development and in collaboration with nurse leaders in practice, who can reflect upon their own leadership styles and organisational culture. The role that practice education facilitators play in identifying suitable QI learning opportunities could enable more innovative pedagogical approaches in QI to be developed within nursing programmes. Lastly, the greater exploration of the influencing factors affecting new nurses' engagement in QI could be enhanced by investigating a larger sample using realist evaluation methodology.

Supplementary Materials: The following supporting information can be downloaded at: https://www.mdpi.com/article/10.3390/nursrep14040218/s1. File S1: Interview Questions Follow Up Phase; File S2: Phase 1 Ethnographic Coding.

Author Contributions: Conceptualization, L.A. and A.S.; methodology, L.A., F.H. and A.S.; software, L.A.; validation, L.A., A.S. and F.H.; formal analysis, L.A. investigation, L.A.; resources, L.A. and A.S.; data curation, L.A. and F.H.; writing—original draft preparation, L.A.; writing—review and editing, L.A., A.S. and F.H.; supervision, A.S. and F.H.; project administration, L.A. All authors have read and agreed to the published version of the manuscript.

Funding: This research received no external funding.

Institutional Review Board Statement: The study was conducted in accordance with the Declaration of Helsinki and approved by the Ethics Committee of University of Stirling on 7 December 2015 (code: SREC 15/16—Paper No.40—Version 1).

Informed Consent Statement: Informed consent was obtained from all subjects involved in the study to publish this paper.

Data Availability Statement: Ethics permission does not allow data sharing of interview data.

Public Involvement Statement: No public involvement in any aspect of this research.

Guidelines and Standards Statement: This manuscript was drafted against the COREQ 32-item Checklist for Qualitative Research [31].

Use of Artificial Intelligence: AI or AI-assisted tools were not used in drafting any aspect of this manuscript.

Acknowledgments: We would like to thank the participants in the study who provided their time and experience as student nurses and as qualified nurses.

Conflicts of Interest: The authors declare no conflicts of interest.

References

1. Nursing and Midwifery Council. *Standards for Pre-Registration Nursing Programmes;* NMC: London, UK, 2019.
2. Armstrong, L.; Shepherd, A.; Harris, F. An evaluation of approaches used to teach quality improvement to pre-registration healthcare professionals: An integrative review. *Int. J. Nurs. Stud.* **2017**, *73*, 70–84. [CrossRef] [PubMed]
3. Kirby, K.F.; Good, B. From education to practice: Incorporating quality improvement projects into a baccalaureate nursing curriculum. *AORN J.* **2020**, *111*, 527–535. [CrossRef] [PubMed]
4. Strand, K.; Tveit, B. Planning and implementing quality improvement projects in clinical practice: Third-year nursing students' learning experiences. *J. Clin. Nurs.* **2020**, *29*, 4769–4783. [CrossRef] [PubMed]
5. Mak, V.; Brand, G.; Morphet, J. Partnering with healthcare organisations to teach pre-registration health professions students about quality improvement: A systematic review. *J. Clin. Nurs.* **2023**, *32*, 3219–3232. [CrossRef] [PubMed]
6. Honeyfield, J.; Sims, D.; Proverbs, A. Teaching Quality Improvement in Pre-Registration Nursing Education: Changing Thinking, Changing Practice. In Proceedings of the ITP Research Symposium, 25–26 November 2020; ePress, Unitec, Te Pukenga: Auckland, New Zealand, 2020; pp. 108–120. [CrossRef]
7. Lucas, B.; Nacer, H. *The Habits of An Improver: Thinking about Learning for Improvement in Healthcare;* Health Foundation: London, UK, 2015.
8. James, B.; Beattie, M.; Shepherd, A.; Armstrong, L.; Wilkinson, J. Time, fear and transformation: Student nurses' experiences of doing a practicum (quality improvement project) in practice. *Nurse Educ. Pract.* **2016**, *19*, 70–78. [CrossRef]
9. Powell, A.E.; Rushmer, R.; Davies, H.T.O. *A systematic Narrative Review of Quality Improvement Models in Health Care;* NHS Quality Improvement Scotland: Edinburgh, UK, 2009.
10. Langley, G.J.; Moen, R.D.; Nolan, K.M.; Nolan, T.W.; Norman, C.L.; Provost, L.P. *The Improvement Guide: A Practical Approach to Enhancing Organizational Performance;* John Wiley & Sons: Hoboken, NJ, USA, 2009.
11. Baillie, L.; Bromley, B.; Walker, M.; Jones, R.; Mhlanga, F. Implementing service improvement projects within pre-registration nursing education: A multi-method case study evaluation. *Nurse Educ. Pract.* **2014**, *14*, 62–68. [CrossRef]
12. Trent, P.; Dolansky, M.A.; DeBrew, J.K.; Petty, G.M. RN-to-BSN students' quality improvement knowledge, skills, confidence, and systems thinking. *J. Nurs. Educ.* **2017**, *56*, 737–740. [CrossRef]
13. Nursing and Midwifery Council. *The Code: Professional Standards of Practice and Behaviour for Nurses, Midwives and Nursing Associates;* NMC: London, UK, 2018.
14. Flying Start NHS. *The Definitive Guide to the Programme;* NHS Education Scotland: Edinburgh, UK, 2017.

15. Batalden, P.B.; Davidoff, F. What is "quality improvement" and how can it transform healthcare? *BMJ Qual. Saf.* **2007**, *16*, 2–3. [CrossRef]
16. Cepero, J. Differences among quality improvement, evidence-based practice, and research. *J. Neurosci. Nurs.* **2011**, *43*, 230–232. [CrossRef]
17. Backhouse, A.; Ogunlayi, F. Quality improvement into practice. *BMJ* **2020**, *368*, m865. [CrossRef] [PubMed]
18. Skledar, S.J.; McKaveney, T.P. A method for teaching continuous quality improvement to student pharmacists through a practical application project. *Curr. Pharm. Teach. Learn.* **2009**, *1*, 79–86. [CrossRef]
19. VanGraafeiland, B.; Sloand, E.; Silbert-Flagg, J.; Gleason, K.; Himmelfarb, C.D. Academic-clinical service partnerships are innovative strategies to advance patient safety competence and leadership in prelicensure nursing students. *Nurs. Outlook* **2019**, *67*, 49–53. [CrossRef] [PubMed]
20. Flott, E.A.; Linden, L. The clinical learning environment in nursing education: A concept analysis. *J. Adv. Nurs.* **2016**, *72*, 501–513. [CrossRef]
21. Armstrong, L.; Shepherd, A.; Harris, F. Adapting improvement education to context: Smallscale projects or diverse and reflective portfolios? In Proceedings of the International Forum on Quality and Safety in Healthcare, London, UK, 10–12 April 2024; ExCeL: London, UK, 2024.
22. Robinson, J.; Gelling, L. Nurses+ QI= better hospital performance? A critical review of the literature. *Nurs. Manag.* **2019**, *26*, 22–28. [CrossRef] [PubMed]
23. Gallen, A.; Kodate, N.; Casey, D. How do nurses and midwives perceive their preparedness for quality improvement and patient safety in practice? A cross-sectional national study in Ireland. *Nurse Educ. Today* **2019**, *76*, 125–130. [CrossRef] [PubMed]
24. Tschannen, D.; Alexander, C.; Taylor, S.; Tovar, E.G.; Ghosh, B.; Zellefrow, C.; Milner, K.A. Quality improvement engagement and competence: A comparison between frontline nurses and nurse leaders. *Nurs. Outlook* **2021**, *69*, 836–847. [CrossRef]
25. Alexander, C.C.; Tschannen, D.; Hays, D.; Clouse, M.; Zellefrow, C.; Amer, K.S.; Milner, K.A. An integrative review of the barriers and facilitators to nurse engagement in quality improvement in the clinical practice setting. *J. Nurs. Care Qual.* **2022**, *37*, 94–100. [CrossRef]
26. Kaplan, H.C.; Brady, P.W.; Dritz, M.C.; Hooper, D.K.; Linam, W.M.; Froehle, C.M.; Margolis, P. The influence of context on quality improvement success in health care: A systematic review of the literature. *Milbank Q.* **2010**, *88*, 500–559. [CrossRef]
27. Djukic, M.; Kovner, C.T.; Brewer, C.S.; Fatehi, F.; Jun, J. Educational gaps and solutions for early-career nurse managers' education and participation in quality improvement. *J. Nurs. Adm.* **2015**, *45*, 206–211. [CrossRef]
28. Denzin, N.K.; Lincoln, Y.S. Introduction. The discipline and practice of qualitative research. In *The Sage Handbook of Qualitative Research*; Denzin, N.K., Lincoln, Y.S., Eds.; SAGE Publications: Thousand Oaks, CA, USA, 2005; pp. 1–32.
29. Creswell, J.W. *Research Design: Qualitative, Quantitative and Mixed Methods Approaches*; Sage: Thousand Oaks, CA, USA, 2014.
30. Corbin, J.D.; Strauss, A. *Basics of Qualitative Research: Techniques and Procedures for Developing Grounded Theory*; Sage Publications: Thousand Oaks, CA, USA, 2015.
31. Tong, A.; Sainsbury, P.; Craig, J. Consolidated criteria for reporting qualitative research (COREQ): A 32-item checklist for interviews and focus groups. *Int. J. Qual. Health Care* **2007**, *19*, 349–357. [CrossRef]
32. Adolfo, C.; Albougami, A.; Roque, M.; Almazan, J. Nurses' attitudes toward quality improvement in hospitals: Implications for nursing management systems. *Nurs. Pract. Today* **2021**, *8*, 206–215. [CrossRef]
33. The Data Protection Act 2018, c. 12. Available online: https://www.legislation.gov.uk/ukpga/2018/12/contents (accessed on 7 October 2024).
34. Scottish Government Records Management: Health and Social Care Code of Practice (SCOTLAND). 2020. Available online: https://www.informationgovernance.scot.nhs.uk/wp-content/uploads/2020/06/SG-HSC-Scotland-Records-Management-Code-of-Practice-2020-v20200602.pdf (accessed on 7 October 2024).
35. McComb, S.A.; Kirkpatrick, J.M. Infusing systems and quality improvement throughout an undergraduate nursing curriculum. *J. Nurs. Educ.* **2017**, *56*, 752–757. [CrossRef] [PubMed]
36. Alexander, C.; Tschannen, D.; Argetsinger, D.; Hakim, H.; Milner, K.A. A qualitative study on barriers and facilitators of quality improvement engagement by frontline nurses and leaders. *J. Nurs. Manag.* **2022**, *30*, 694–701. [CrossRef] [PubMed]
37. Armstrong, L.; Moir, C.; Taylor, P. How, and under what contexts, do academic–practice partnerships collaborate to implement healthcare improvement education into preregistration nursing curriculums: A realist review protocol. *BMJ Open* **2023**, *13*, e077784. [CrossRef] [PubMed]
38. NHS Forth Valley Quality Improvement Academy: 6-month Progress Report May–Dec 2023 Unpublished.
39. Elizalde, J.; Lumibao, J.; Lizarondo, L. Barriers and facilitators to health professionals' engagement in quality improvement initiatives: A mixed-methods systematic review. *Int. J. Qual. Health Care* **2024**, *36*, mzae041. [CrossRef] [PubMed]
40. Blok, A.C.; Alexander, C.C.; Tschannen, D.; Milner, K.A. Quality improvement engagement: Barriers and facilitators. *Nurs. Manag.* **2022**, *53*, 16–24. [CrossRef]
41. Pawson, R. *The Science of Evaluation: A Realist Manifesto*; Sage Publication: Leeds, UK, 2013.
42. Spooner, R.; Stanford, V.; Parslow-Williams, S.; Mortimer, F.; Leedham-Green, K. "Concrete ways we can make a difference": A multi-centre, multi-professional evaluation of sustainability in quality improvement education. *Med. Teach.* **2022**, *44*, 1116–1124. [CrossRef] [PubMed]

43. Clery, P.; d'Arch Smith, S.; Marsden, O.; Leedham-Green, K. Sustainability in quality improvement (SusQI): A case-study in undergraduate medical education. *BMC Med. Educ.* **2021**, *21*, 425. [CrossRef]
44. See, E.C.W.; Koh, S.S.L.; Baladram, S.; Shorey, S. Role transition of newly graduated nurses from nursing students to registered nurses: A qualitative systematic review. *Nurse Educ. Today* **2023**, *121*, 105702. [CrossRef]
45. Hennink, M.; Kaiser, B.N. Sample sizes for saturation in qualitative research: A systematic review of empirical tests. *Soc. Sci. Med.* **2022**, *292*, 114523. [CrossRef]

nursing reports

MDPI

Article

A Pilot Study to Create a Culture of Innovation and Quality: Focus on a Nursing Association, Credentialing Center, and Foundation

Marcela Cámpoli [1,*], Tanya Mulvey [1], Olivia Lemberger [2], Hannah Person [1], Kasey Bellegarde-Armstrong [3] and Oriana Beaudet [2]

1 Institute for Nursing Research and Quality Management, American Nurses Enterprise, 8403 Colesville Road, Suite 500, Silver Spring, MD 20910, USA; tanya.mulvey@ana.org (T.M.); hannah.person@ana.org (H.P.)
2 Innovation Department, American Nurses Enterprise, 8403 Colesville Road, Suite 500, Silver Spring, MD 20910, USA; olivia.lemberger@ana.org (O.L.); oriana.beaudet@ana.org (O.B.)
3 Formerly American Nurses Enterprise, 8403 Colesville Road, Suite 500, Silver Spring, MD 20910, USA; kbellegardearmstrong@hcwh.org
* Correspondence: marcela.campoli@ana.org

Abstract: Background/Objectives: In today's rapidly evolving healthcare landscape, fostering a culture of innovation and continuous improvement is essential—especially within a nursing association that leads individual and organizational credentialing. **Methods**: Colleagues from the American Nurses Enterprise (ANE) Innovation Department and the Institute for Nursing Research and Quality Management collaborated to develop the *Culture of Innovation and Quality Model*™. This process involved conducting a literature review, developing a survey instrument, and administering a pilot pre-survey to ANE employees to collect baseline data. Future research will include a comparison with a post-survey after interventions aimed at strengthening the culture of innovation and quality. **Results**: The results of the pilot pre-survey were high overall and guided the team in identifying areas with the greatest opportunities for improvement. Based on these findings, interventions are being developed that will be implemented at ANE to enhance the practice of and promote the synergy between innovation and quality. **Conclusions**: Achieving and sustaining high-quality standards of care and advancing the professional development of nurses requires a culture where staff feel safe and have opportunities to create, innovate, improve, and learn. This will help promote an environment where people thrive while ensuring that the nursing profession and practice remain cutting-edge and aligned with emerging technologies and evolving healthcare complexities. The *Culture of Innovation and Quality Model*™ may provide a blueprint for organizations who seek to advance innovation and quality knowledge, engagement, and practices and assist their employees in providing better service to colleagues, partners, and customers while adapting to the evolving healthcare environment.

Keywords: innovation; quality management; continuous improvement; nursing; healthcare; organizational culture; credentialing; association; assessment; leadership

1. Introduction

Today's fast-paced and complex work environment requires an organizational culture that embraces new ideas and strives for excellence. Burgeoning factors such as the coronavirus pandemic, artificial intelligence, including political and social shifts have necessitated new approaches for organizational innovation and experimentation, and created an imperative for capacity building, timely knowledge sharing, and organizational prioritization of research and practice [1]. Healthcare organizations that actively practice innovation through nurturing new ideas, scanning and planning for change, centering people and their needs, and being unafraid to take risks are well-equipped to respond nimbly to complex challenges and navigate uncertainty with strategic, future-focused action. At the same time, organizations that embody a spirit of continuous improvement, implementing processes and systems to meet quality standards and customer expectations, set the bar for standards of excellence in delivering high-quality, cutting-edge products and services.

Increasingly, organizations are recognizing the synergistic relationship of innovation and quality, seeking opportunities to connect these complimentary concepts in high-performing work cultures. The methods of innovation and quality share multiple similarities that when implemented together may provide deeper understanding of customer needs [2] and enhance the impact of national associations. Both innovation and quality approaches embrace a culture of inquiry and learning, prioritize customer/user needs, and employ methods to produce data-driven and novel work. Cultures that integrate innovation and quality create opportunities for idea generation which may drive standards for excellence and provide transparency around the evolving nature of healthcare.

Cultures that support innovation, wellness, and evidence-based practices have demonstrated significant positive correlations with provider well-being, mental and physical health, and job satisfaction [3]. Leadership support has been routinely identified as crucial for the successful implementation and long-term sustainability of innovation and quality endeavors. Research exploring organizational culture and knowledge management in the high-technology industry found that supportive and participative leaders were more likely to increase the efficiency of knowledge management practices leading to enhanced innovation capabilities [4]. Oftentimes innovation and quality initiatives are considered from a top-down (leadership to staff) approach [5]. However, to successfully achieve a culture of innovation and quality, all staff need the knowledge, resources, and support to lead and engage in innovation and quality practices. A thriving innovation and quality culture necessitates a shift in which employees view the tasks that are routinely associated with innovation and quality practices to become second nature and infused into daily work [6].

Nursing associations play a crucial role in addressing health challenges by reimagining healthcare ecosystems, improving access to high-quality care, and promoting the advancement of nursing through research and evidence-based practices. Nurses and nursing allies serve as key advocates, co-designers and co-collaborators in the creation of high-performing healthcare cultures that prioritize teamwork, innovation, and a commitment to quality and excellence in patient care. In 2024, colleagues from the American Nurses Enterprise (ANE) Innovation Department and Institute for Nursing Research and Quality Management came together to collaborate on an initiative to promote and foster an organizational culture of innovation and quality. This initiative directly supports the ANE 2024 strategic plan goal of *enabling operational excellence with an objective to deliver data-driven and customer focused excellence through enhanced and agile technology and innovation.* It also aligns with the successful ISO 9001:2015 [7] quality management certification of the American Nurses Credentialing Center (ANCC), one of ANE's three core entities. The team designed a study for which a new organizational innovation and quality assessment was developed to support data-driven decisions. The goal of this study is to measure the effectiveness of interventions designed to promote a thriving culture of innovation and quality practices. This initiative is particularly significant, as research on fostering a culture of innovation and quality in the workplace remains limited, with neither a standardized survey nor comprehensive data on the impact of combined innovation and quality initiatives published to date. Building off existing organizational strengths may be an approach to advance innovation and quality synergies. As Nowak [8] stated, "quality and innovation processes are interlinked and should not be treated separately." Studies have shown that innovation and quality approaches should not be viewed separately, disputing the misunderstanding that to achieve innovation, quality must be discarded. Integrated approaches researched by Zeng and colleagues [9] found that quality management provided a foundation for innovation to occur.

When collaborating across organizations, it is imperative to incorporate shared definitions to ensure a mutual understanding of the application and incorporation of concepts. One of the initial steps of the collaborative journey was to examine multiple definitions of innovation and quality. This process required multiple meetings with protected time for in-depth conversations on the meanings, overlap, and shared understanding of how these definitions could be used synergistically. This study used Lachman and colleagues' [10] definition of *innovation*: "the application of creativity or problem solving that results in a widely adopted strategy, product, or service that meets a need in a new and different way" and the ISO 9001:2015 [7] definition of *quality:* "The totality of features and characteristics of a product or service that bear on its ability to satisfy stated or implied needs." Further study is needed to identify the overlapping areas that highlight the desired balance between quality standardization and the need for novel innovative approaches.

The *Culture of Innovation and Quality Model*™ was adapted based on the National Association of County and City Health Officials (NACCHO) Version 2.0 2018 Roadmap to a Culture of Quality [6]. The concept in [Figure 1] represents the synergistic components of innovation and quality that were used in designing the pilot pre-survey questionnaire. The pilot pre-survey highlighted six key domains that collectively foster a culture of innovation and quality: staff empowerment, teamwork and collaboration, leadership, customer focus, infrastructure, and continuous improvement. Synergistic methods to support a thriving culture of innovation and quality practices include finding ways to use new tools and strategies; creative problem solving to meet customer needs; developing, redesigning, or implementing work processes; collaborative brainstorming with colleagues; and looking for ways to improve operational efficiency, effectiveness, and quality of work.

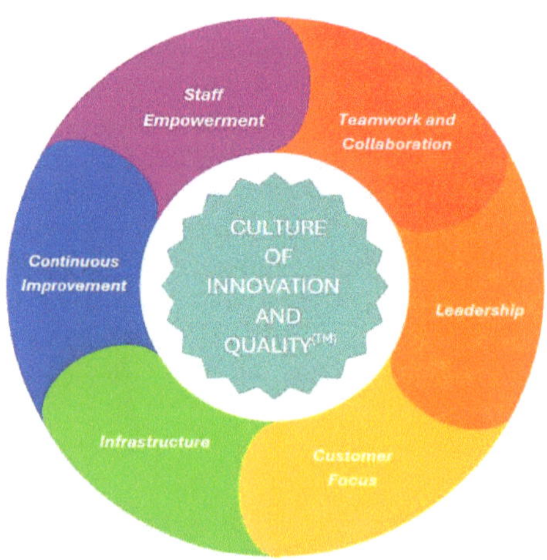

Figure 1. *Culture of Innovation and Quality Model*™.

2. Materials and Methods

This descriptive, pre-post pilot study on the culture of innovation and quality at a non-profit nursing association surveyed a population of full- and part-time employees of the ANE. The study received exempt determination from an IRB. The objectives of the study were to quantitively summarize: (1) pre-intervention baseline attitudes toward innovation and quality knowledge, engagement, and practices; (2) post-intervention measures of employee attitudes toward innovation and quality knowledge, engagement and practices after one year of innovation and quality education and guidance compared to baseline levels of knowledge, engagement and practices; and (3) employee perceptions of changes in innovation and quality knowledge, engagement, and practices during the year. This article is only focused on the study design and administration of the pilot pre-survey related to objective one because the study is still ongoing.

The research team was formed from a collaboration between the ANE Innovation Department and the Institute for Nursing Research and Quality Management. First, a literature review was conducted on the intersections between innovation and quality to develop background information and identify gaps in the literature. Additionally, these sources were used to inform definitions for innovation and quality, and to find synergistic frameworks and theories bridging these concepts. Because no framework or survey instrument was found that combined the assessment of these two concepts, the research team developed the *Culture of Innovation and Quality Model*™, which was adapted from NACCHO's Roadmap to a Culture of Quality [6], and then created a new instrument based on this model.

The research team designed the survey instrument to have two questions to assess each of the six components of the model, repeated separately for innovation and quality. Additional questions were included to measure perceptions of overall level of innovation and quality within the organization. Feedback on question wording and face validity was gathered from the internal ANE Scholarly Collaborative workgroup. After further revisions, the instrument was pilot tested by an internal group of volunteer employees from various departments. Further revisions were made to the instrument based on pre-survey pilot testing and internal stakeholder feedback. The survey introduction explained the scope of the study and stated the purpose of the initiative was "to support and promote a thriving culture of innovation and quality practices" at the organization. Participants were informed that the survey was anonymous and results would only be reported in aggregate. Consent to participate and confirmation that respondents were 21 years old or older was obtained via a survey question. Upon providing consent, participants were given definitions of innovation and quality with examples of activities related to innovation and quality. This was done to ensure understanding of these concepts and to enhance response validity. The initial questions asked employees to rate their level of knowledge and engagement in activities related to innovation and quality over the past year. Next, employees indicated their level of agreement with two innovation and two quality statements for each of the six components of the *Culture of Innovation and Quality Model*™: staff empowerment, teamwork and collaboration, leadership, customer focus, infrastructure, and continuous improvement. Then employees rated their perception of the current level of innovation and quality at the organization and indicated how familiar they were with innovation and quality resources provided by the organization. The survey concluded with an open-ended question to collect feedback or suggestions on implementing innovation and quality across the organization. Demographics were collected on entity, tenure with the organization, and management versus non-management position to examine representation of respondents and to compare differences between these groups. The ANE includes three distinct entities: a professional association, a credentialing center, and a foundation. The credentialing center is ISO 9001:2015 certified for quality management. For an overview of the complete survey outline, see Appendix A.

The researchers used various survey design methods in an effort to improve data quality and reduce potential bias. To prevent order effects, the six components were presented to participants in random order; however, the innovation statement always preceded the quality question to avoid respondent confusion. Separate items were used to measure innovation and quality so participants could respond about one concept at a time and to measure innovation and quality independently. The 4-point scale ranged from strongly disagree to strongly agree. A midpoint option was not included due to the difficulty of interpretation for both respondents and researchers and to strongly encourage respondents to provide evaluative responses based on their own experiences and perceptions wherever possible. The scale also included an unsure option with a required open-ended text field to understand why respondents may have difficulty rating particular statements. The unsure option was visually offset to separate it from the 4-point scale.

The survey administration was planned carefully to ensure leadership buy-in and promotion, awareness from all staff, and to coordinate with other internal survey efforts. One week prior to fielding the survey, a pre-notification message was included in the weekly newsletter emailed to all ANE employees as well as posted to the organization's intranet homepage. Personalized survey invitations were emailed to employees through the organization's survey platform, Alchemer Survey (July 2024, Alchemer, Louisville, CO, USA). The survey remained open for two weeks with up to two reminder emails sent to those who had not yet completed the survey.

Analysis of the pilot pre-survey included frequencies for employment demographics and each survey question, crosstabs reporting results for each question by management/non-management and entity using Chi-square to test for statistically significant differences in agreement vs. disagreement at a level of $p \leq 0.10$. Additionally, t-tests were conducted for the knowledge and frequency of engagement in activities questions, comparing management status and entity. For all analyses, unsure responses were excluded. Qualitative responses underwent a thematic analysis to report key findings.

3. Results

The survey results have two main purposes: first to collect baseline and post-intervention data on employee knowledge, engagement, and practices related to innovation and quality that can be used to measure the effectiveness and impact of interventions one year later, and second, to inform the interventions based on gaps and qualitative feedback identified in baseline data. The results section will only discuss key pilot pre-survey findings for each of the six components of the *Culture of Innovation and Quality Model*™, as well as describe planned interventions.

The pilot pre-survey was sent to all 324 regular full- and part-time ANE employees and received 131 valid responses for a 40% response rate. Responses were considered valid if they answered any of the non-demographic questions. The responses to the pre-survey were 40% from credentialing center employees, 57% from association employees, and 4% from foundation employees. Thirty-seven percent of respondents were in a management position. The tenure of employment with ANE of respondents was: 26% up to 2 years, 27% 2 to 5 years, 47% more than 5 years. In examining demographic results, respondents were representative of employees for entity of employment and management/non-management position. For tenure, those who had been with ANE for more than 5 years were overrepresented (47% vs. 36%).

Qualitative analysis was conducted for narrative responses, which included 21 responses to the question collecting feedback or suggestions on implementing innovation and quality across the organization, 13 comments on the questions about resources, and 42 responses to the open-ended unsure options. Five broad themes were identified from these responses. Themes included Data Integration, Learning & Education, Culture, Change Adoption, and Leadership. The identified themes and responses provided deep insight and informed the planned study interventions and dissemination strategies (see Table 1).

Table 1. Planned Study Interventions and Dissemination.

Presentations to American Nurses Enterprise Leadership, Employees, Scholarly Collaborative
External Presentations (International/National Nursing Conferences, Webinar, ANE Research Advisory Council)
Internal dissemination of Infographic with Summary of Key Findings
Educational Offerings (Sip, Learn, and Grow, Elevating the Enterprise Modules)
Office Hours
Ongoing Communication (Intranet, Newsletter)

The survey highlighted six key domains that collectively foster a culture of innovation and quality. Figure 2 displays the innovation and quality composite percent agreement scores for each domain. Employees reported strong results across all areas, with customer focus rated highest and infrastructure identified as the greatest opportunity for growth. While closely aligned, quality consistently outperformed innovation and respondents from the entity that routinely engaged with ISO 9001:2015 quality management standards had statistically significantly higher perception ratings of quality compared to the other areas of the organization (overall quality rating question: $t(111) = -3.636$, $p < 0.001$; domain-specific quality questions: Chi-square $p < 0.10$ for all but one quality question). Additionally, management respondents indicated higher knowledge (innovation: 2.45 vs. 2.11, quality: 2.56 vs. 2.29) and frequency of engagement (innovation: 2.67 vs. 1.63, quality: 3.19 vs. 2.31) in innovation (knowledge: $t(111) = 3.385$, $p = 0.001$; frequency: $t(111) = 5.194$, $p < 0.001$) and quality (knowledge: $t(109) = 2.423$, $p = 0.017$; frequency: $t(111) = 3.681$, $p < 0.001$) than non-management respondents.

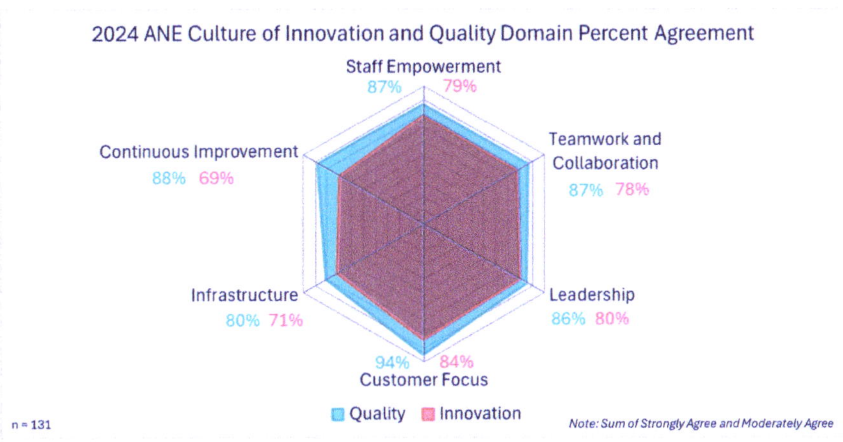

Figure 2. Pilot pre-survey domain composite percent agreement scores.

3.1. Staff Empowerment

Respondents reported high levels of engagement and opportunities to engage in both innovation (79%) and quality (87%). Self-reported engagement opportunities for quality were higher for management (95%) compared with non-management (82%) employees (X^2 (1, N = 113) = 4.207, p = 0.04). Interventions will include hybrid "Sip, Learn, and Grow" sessions open to all employees to share key survey findings, provide education on available resources, and to engage employees in discussions on how they are implementing innovation and quality in their work, challenges and barriers, and sharing ideas to further promote the culture across the organization.

3.2. Teamwork and Collaboration

Respondents similarly reported high levels of teamwork and collaboration for innovation (78%) and quality (87%). Survey results found that respondents reported higher levels of collaboration within departments than across multiple departments. Despite these findings, the organization has many examples of cross-department collaboration, including committees, workgroups, meetings, events, initiatives, and projects. This suggests that the opportunities to work across teams may be unbalanced and dependent upon factors such as department, level, and role. Another factor that may be impacting teamwork and collaboration is that nearly all employees have been working remotely while the headquarters was being moved to a new location. It will be interesting to see how the new office space, designed to promote collaboration, may impact these opportunities. Interventions related to teamwork and collaboration will include education on the benefits of working together and sharing strategies to create opportunities to collaborate on innovation and quality to advance organizational strategic goals, improve efficiency, effectiveness and have greater impact on advancing our vision "A healthy world through the power of nursing."

3.3. Leadership

The research team had support from executive leadership to lead this initiative and study with the goal of promoting a thriving culture of innovation and quality across the organization. To demonstrate this support to all employees, survey communications were sent from a chief officer. In the survey results, most respondents felt they had management support to engage in innovation and quality activities. Composite scores of leadership support were high for innovation (80%) and quality (86%). At the same time, qualitative results included suggestions to ensure leadership support for employees to feel empowered to participate in both innovation and quality activities. Interventions will include presenting results and recommendations to leadership, so that they are aware of opportunities for improvement. After this survey was given, organization leadership provided multiple educational opportunities around broader examples of innovation, which all received very high attendance from employees.

3.4. Customer Focus

Customer focus was the strongest area for the organization, with the highest results for both innovation (84%) and quality (94%). This shows that the organization has a very strong culture in valuing and meeting customer needs. Interventions will include education about how quality management contributes to customer satisfaction and sharing tools and resources for implementing quality based on customer requirements. Examples include collecting customer feedback, tracking trends, and considering customer requirements in the process of innovation and continuous improvement.

3.5. Infrastructure

Results found that most respondents had self-created or drafted performance goals that included activities related to innovation and quality. Somewhat fewer respondents agreed that the organization dedicated resources to support engagement in innovation and quality activities. Overall, 71% of respondents agreed with these statements for innovation and 80% for quality. Additionally, employees were more familiar with resources for quality (58%) compared with innovation (43%); however, there was variation in the level of awareness with specific types of resources for both innovation and quality. Therefore, interventions around infrastructure will focus mostly on increased education, promotion, and communication about resources. Opportunities to provide additional resources will also be explored in discussions with employees in the "Sip, Learn, and Grow" sessions. These planned intervention sessions will be developed based on qualitative survey feedback that requested educational offerings to be scheduled to avoid meal times (e.g., lunch and learns). While resources are currently available on organizational intranet and external webpages, the research team will work to improve the organization, cross-promotion, and awareness of these resources.

3.6. Continuous Improvement

While results for continuous improvement were strong in the area of quality (88%), the greatest opportunity for growth was identified in innovation (69%). This included following documented work processes and adopting lessons learned into work processes. Survey questions in this domain received the highest numbers of unsure responses, with qualitative responses indicating a lack of awareness of documented work processes. Interventions will include education on strategies and tools for documenting work processes and adopting lessons learned. While many resources are currently available for both innovation and quality as it relates to continuous improvement, greater awareness and implementation is needed.

4. Discussion

The pilot pre-survey served as an initial assessment to guide understanding of the strengths and opportunities for improvement of ANE employees related to innovation and quality based on the *Culture of Innovation and Quality Model*™. Cultures of innovation and quality may differ across an organization. Not surprisingly, our findings indicated that respondents from the entity that routinely engages with ISO 9001:2015 quality management standards had statistically significantly higher perception ratings for quality compared to the other areas of the organization. This helps to inform effective and efficient use of interventions to make a larger impact toward the goal of promoting quality across the entire organization. Pilot study findings revealed that there was more collaboration in innovation and quality activities within departments than between departments. This indicates that intentional focus on innovation and quality practices that occur across departments will be necessary to improve cross-department collaboration and knowledge sharing to facilitate the breakdown of siloed approaches. This approach may aid in creating a shift in which innovation and quality practices become more routine and infused into employees' daily work practices.

Pilot pre-survey results showed less familiarity of employees with innovation compared to quality. The majority of employees were unfamiliar with innovation resources, work processes, and formal procedures despite reporting having opportunities to engage in innovation. The American Nurses Association Innovation Accelerator Study revealed the importance of fostering and maintaining a learning community for the further development of innovative knowledge [11]. Innovation and quality development require safe learning environments where employees can share ideas, ask questions, acknowledge mistakes, and reflect on their development journey. Increasing awareness of existing resources and providing more opportunities for learning engagement may address the barrier of visibility and familiarity and provide needed transparency on ways to actively translate innovation and quality knowledge into daily activities.

A valuable lesson learned from this initiative is that innovation and quality initiatives may be improved with the use of shared models and tools such as the RASCI model (responsible, accountable, support, consulted, informed). The research team used the RASCI model as a project management tool to clarify the roles and responsibilities throughout this endeavor. This model was pivotal in aiding task completion, shared decision making, time management, and the successful completion of deliverables. For the successful advancement of collaborative initiatives across organizations, increased communication around the use of shared models and tools is essential.

Limitations to this study include that the post-survey portion of this study has not yet been completed. This manuscript reflects a high-level overview of pilot pre-survey findings that will inform the interventions. The high-level findings reflect the need to protect the confidentiality of organizational data. Further research is also needed to validate the survey instrument.

Next steps of this study include interventions related to pilot pre-survey findings. An infographic was created to share pilot pre-survey results, highlight opportunities for growth, and provide internal links to innovation and quality resources. The conceptual *Culture of Innovation and Quality Model*™ will be used to guide our interventions for the various domains including staff empowerment and infrastructure (Sip Learn and Grow sessions), teamwork and collaboration (educational offerings), leadership (pilot pre-survey results presentation), customer focus and continuous improvement (sharing innovation and quality tools, office hours). Intervention strategies will need to move from an understanding of the facts of innovation and quality to a deeper understanding of how innovation and quality practices when employed synergistically can lead to a thriving culture, achieving more than one approach could accomplish independently. Dissemination opportunities such as presentations and webinars will be conducted both nationally and internationally. A post-intervention survey will be used to measure ANE employees' attitudes toward, knowledge of, and engagement in innovation and quality, as well as familiarity with innovation and quality education and guidance compared to the initial level of innovation and quality knowledge, engagement, and practices. The research team intends to publish additional articles and share further findings on the effectiveness of the interventions after the completion of the post-intervention survey.

5. Conclusions

A central tenet of the journey as co-collaborators at the ANE has focused on the exploration and amplification of innovation and quality synergies that can be used to galvanize a thriving organizational culture. Sustainability efforts to promote standards of care and professional development require a culture of innovation and quality where staff feel safe and have opportunities to create, collaborate, and learn. The *Culture of Innovation and Quality Model*™ may provide a blueprint for organizations who seek to advance innovation and quality knowledge, engagement, and practices and assist their employees in providing better service to colleagues, partners, and customers while adapting to the evolving healthcare environment. Continued emphasis on the synergistic and complementary approaches to innovation and quality practices requires collective support and further research to propel healthcare environments towards a flourishing future. These synergies may illuminate the underlying factors that make meaningful engagement in innovation and quality practices a sustained reality.

Author Contributions: Conceptualization, M.C., T.M., O.L., H.P., K.B.-A. and O.B.; methodology, M.C., T.M., O.L., H.P., K.B.-A. and O.B.; formal analysis, H.P. and O.L.; investigation, T.M., O.L., H.P. and K.B.-A.; writing—original draft preparation, T.M. and O.L.; writing—review and editing, M.C., T.M., O.L., H.P., K.B.-A. and O.B.; visualization, H.P. and K.B.-A.; supervision, M.C. and O.B.; project administration, O.L. and T.M. All authors have read and agreed to the published version of the manuscript.

Funding: This research received no external funding.

Institutional Review Board Statement: Ethical review and approval were waived for this study since using the Department of Health and Human Services regulations found at 45 CFR 46.104(d)(2), the Institutional Review Board determined that this research project is exempt from Institutional Review Board oversight.

Informed Consent Statement: Informed consent was obtained from all subjects involved in the study.

Data Availability Statement: The datasets presented in this article are not readily available because the study is ongoing and the information is proprietary to the American Nurses Enterprise.

Public Involvement Statement: No public involvement in any aspect of this research.

Guidelines and Standards Statement: This manuscript was drafted against the Revised Standards for Quality Improvement Reporting Excellence (SQUIRE 2.0).

Use of Artificial Intelligence: AI or AI-assisted tools were not used in drafting any aspect of this manuscript.

Conflicts of Interest: The authors declare no conflicts of interest.

Appendix A

Survey questionnaire outline:

1. Introduction
    a. Consent question
    b. Innovation and quality definitions and examples
2. Knowledge
    a. Rating question of knowledge about innovation
    b. Rating question of knowledge about quality
3. Frequency
    a. Rating question of frequency of engagement in innovation
    b. Rating question of frequency of engagement in quality
4. Randomized domain sections:
    a. Staff Empowerment
        i. Agreement question 1 for innovation
        ii. Agreement question 1 for quality
        iii. Agreement question 2 for innovation
        iv. Agreement question 2 for quality
    b. Teamwork and Collaboration
        i. Agreement question 1 for innovation
        ii. Agreement question 1 for quality
        iii. Agreement question 2 for innovation

      iv. Agreement question 2 for quality
   c. Leadership
      i. Agreement question 1 for innovation
      ii. Agreement question 1 for quality
      iii. Agreement question 2 for innovation
      iv. Agreement question 2 for quality
   d. Customer Focus
      i. Agreement question 1 for innovation
      ii. Agreement question 1 for quality
      iii. Agreement question 2 for innovation
      iv. Agreement question 2 for quality
   e. Infrastructure
      i. Agreement question 1 for innovation
      ii. Agreement question 1 for quality
      iii. Agreement question 2 for innovation
      iv. Agreement question 2 for quality
   f. Continuous Improvement
      i. Agreement question 1 for innovation
      ii. Agreement question 1 for quality
      iii. Agreement question 2 for innovation
      iv. Agreement question 2 for quality
5. Overall
   a. Rating question for level of innovation
   b. Rating question for level of quality
6. Resources
   a. Rating question for familiarity of resources for innovation
   b. Rating question for familiarity of resources for quality
7. Open-ended feedback or suggestions question
8. Demographics

References

1. Edmondson, A.C.; Bransby, D.P. Psychological safety comes of age: Observed themes in an established literature. *Annu. Rev. Organ. Psychol. Organ. Behav.* **2023**, *10*, 55–78. [CrossRef]
2. Crowe, B.; Gaulton, J.S.; Minor, N.; Asch, D.A.; Eyet, J.; Rainosek, E.; Flint, K.; Joo, J.; Chambers, C.; Bright, S.; et al. To improve quality, leverage design. *BMJ Qual. Saf.* **2022**, *31*, 70–74. [CrossRef] [PubMed]
3. O'Hara, S.; Melnyk, B.M.; Hsieh, A.P.; Helsabeck, N.P.; Giuliano, K.K.; Vital, C. Innovation, Wellness, and EBP Cultures Are Associated With Less Burnout, Better Mental Health, and Higher Job Satisfaction in Nurses and the Healthcare Workforce. *Worldviews Evid.-Based Nurs.* **2025**, *22*, e70012. [CrossRef] [PubMed]
4. Lam, L.; Nguyen, P.; Le, N.; Tran, K. The Relation among Organizational Culture, Knowledge Management, and Innovation Capability: Its Implication for Open Innovation. *J. Open Innov. Technol. Mark. Complex.* **2021**, *7*, 66. [CrossRef]
5. Bababekov, Y.J.; Stapleton, S.M.; Hashimoto, D.A.; Witkowski, E.R.; Haynes, A.B.; Goldstein, A.M.; Mullen, J.T.; Isselbacher, E.M.; Lillemoe, K.D.; Chang, D.C. Open innovation facilitates department-wide engagement in quality improvement: Experience from the Massachusetts General Hospital. *Surg. Endosc.* **2021**, *35*, 5441–5449. [CrossRef] [PubMed]
6. National Association of County and City Health Officials. Organizational Culture of Quality Self-Assessment Tool: Staff Version. 2018. Available online: https://qiroadmap.org/assessment (accessed on 24 June 2024).
7. *ISO 9001:2015*; Quality Management Systems—Requirements. International Organization for Standards: Vernier, Switzerland, 2015.
8. Nowak, A. Strategic relationship between quality management and product innovation. *Mid-Atl. J. Bus.* **1997**, *33*, 119–135.

9. Zeng, J.; Phan, C.A.; Matsui, Y. The impact of hard and soft quality management on quality and innovation performance: An empirical study. *Int. J. Prod. Econ.* **2015**, *162*, 216–226. [CrossRef]
10. Lachman, V.D.; Glasgow, M.E.S.; Donnelly, G.F. Teaching innovation. *Nurs. Adm. Q.* **2006**, *33*, 205–211. [CrossRef] [PubMed]
11. Lemberger, O.; Beaudet, O.; Bellegarde, K. The ANA Innovation Accelerator: Galvanizing the Future of Nursing. *OJIN Online J. Issues Nurs.* **2025**, *30*, 1. [CrossRef]

nursing reports

MDPI

Article

Simulated Practice Learning Experience in a Virtual Environment: An Innovative Pedagogical Approach to Practice Learning for Nursing Students

Sharon Faulds * and Anne Taylor

Faculty of Health Sciences and Sport, University of Stirling, Stirling FK9 4LA, UK; a.d.taylor@stir.ac.uk
* Correspondence: sharon.faulds@stir.ac.uk

Abstract: Background/Objectives: The use of simulated learning as a teaching approach has been used and embedded in nursing theoretical curriculum for many years. There is a wealth of evidence to support the positive impact simulated learning or simulated-based education can have on the student experience, developing skill competency and enhancing patient outcomes. However, the evidence on the use of simulation as a replacement for clinical practice learning in undergraduate nursing education is limited. In response to the challenges posed by the COVID-19 pandemic, the authors introduced virtual simulated practice learning experiences (SPLE) for a cohort of year one pre-registration adult and mental health nursing students. The SPLE project aimed to assess the effectiveness of simulated practice learning as a viable alternative to traditional clinical practice learning and to explore student satisfaction with the new practice learning experience approach. **Methods:** All year one student nurses attending the four simulated practice learning experience (SPLE) weeks were invited to participate and complete a generated questionnaire within the virtual practice environment on their final day of each SPLE week. The questionnaire employed a mix of both quantitative and qualitative questions across key areas to evaluate the effectiveness of the SPLE and explore student satisfaction with their overall practice learning experience. **Results**: A total of 216 students participated in the simulated practice learning weeks across the spring semester in 2023 with a response rate of 98–100% across all four SPLE weeks. Students reported an overall satisfaction score of 88%, highlighting their preparedness and positive feedback on the organisation, delivery, and content of the SPLE. Qualitative analysis revealed key themes, including the development of transferable skills and personal growth, the value of peer learning, the benefits of a virtual environment, and appreciation of service user and healthcare professional input. Students reported significant personal growth, improved communication skills, and a deeper understanding of holistic care through interactive and collaborative learning experiences. **Conclusions:** This evaluation underscores the innovative potential of simulated practice learning to enhance nursing practice education, emphasising the importance of integrating emerging technologies and diverse pedagogical approaches. The findings suggest that SPLEs can effectively prepare nursing students for the complexities of clinical practice while addressing the evolving demands of healthcare. Future research should focus on longitudinal studies to assess the sustained impact of simulated learning on clinical experiences and professional development.

Keywords: innovation; pedagogy; simulated practice learning experience; virtual practice learning; student nurse; practice placement; virtual learning; nursing education; online learning

1. Introduction

Innovation is not just about new technologies or methodologies but also about adopting a mindset that encourages creativity, problem-solving, and the implementation of new ideas in nurse education and in clinical practice [1]. The COVID-19 pandemic and ongoing NHS service re-design has forced many nurse educators to be innovative and creative to maintain practice learning placements for student nurses, with many United Kingdom Higher Education Institutions (HEI) adopting virtual or simulated practice learning experiences [2]. This novel and unique approach to practice learning provided pre-registration nursing students with a means to fulfilling the required Nursing and Midwifery Council (NMC) practice hours allowing them to successfully complete their nursing programme on time, attain registration, and furthermore join the much-needed nursing workforce.

Background

In the United Kingdom, the Nursing and Midwifery Council [3] plays a crucial role in setting and maintaining the standards for undergraduate nursing education and practice. To ensure high-quality care, the NMC expects nursing students to effectively integrate theory into their direct practice learning, accruing 2300 hours during their nursing programme for registration. Due to the significant effect of COVID-19 on practice learning, in 2021, the NMC approved the continued use of the COVID-19 recovery standards permitting HEIs to deliver 300 to 600 hours of practice learning using a range of new and innovative practice simulation methods. Simulated practice learning, defined by the NMC, is practice learning that meets requirements set out in the NMC standards around practice learning, in particular the requirements contained within the standards for pre-registration nursing programmes and the standards for student supervision and assessment [4]. Any approaches or methods adopted for practice learning through the development of simulated practice learning experiences (SPLEs) must align with the desired practice learning outcomes and contribute to the student being able to demonstrate safe and effective practice [2].

The use of simulated learning as a teaching approach has been used and embedded in nursing theoretical curriculum for many years. There is a wealth of evidence to support the positive impact simulated learning or simulated-based education can have on the student experience, developing skill competency and enhancing patient outcomes [5–7]. The use of simulated or virtual learning aims to provide nursing students with an authentic and immersive learning environment, enabling the application of theoretical knowledge to practical scenarios [8]. This experiential learning approach allows students to develop their critical thinking skills and bridge the gap between theory and practice; however, it is critical that the learning environment is authentic and is representative of real-life situations to promote fidelity and authentic learning for the students [6]. The change to the NMC standards in 2021 allowed HEIs in the UK to consider how they could replicate the learning from the theoretical training of nursing students into the practice learning context and accrue direct practice hours.

Research into the use of simulation as a replacement for clinical practice learning in undergraduate nursing education is limited [9]. By scoping the literature, it is evident the value that virtual or simulated practice learning can have on students from across a range of health professions. Pit et al. [10] emphasises, from a medical student's perspective, how virtual practice learning allows the students interest in healthcare technology to grow, which stems from its increasing conventional relevance and its invaluable role in their future careers. This view is reinforced by studies from West [11] and Mian and Khan [12] who emphasise the importance of integrating digital technologies into medical education. They argue that this is not only a necessary response in light of the COVID-19 pandemic but also a critical foundation for future educational practises in healthcare. Inman et al. [13]

highlight the effectiveness of technology in facilitating reflective sessions and supervision, promoting flexibility, efficient time management, and, moreover, access to a wider team of supervisors. The use of virtual or digital technologies is regarded as essential for enhancing learning and upholding professional standards and students should expect to be involved in simulation to prepare them for working in clinical environments increasingly using technology. Medical students appreciated the exposure to a broad range of virtual clinics, diverse clinicians, and peers, thereby significantly enhancing their practice learning capacity [14], with Peart et al. [15] demonstrating that virtual practice learning offers unique opportunities for students, fostering flexibility and lateral thinking. However, there are also legitimate concerns and challenges associated with this mode of learning reported in the literature. Triemstra et al. [16] reports that in-person practice learning offers many more benefits than virtual practice learning in terms of collaborative practice, professional identity formation, and the accumulation of clinical knowledge and judgement. This consensus is shared by Hammond et al. [17], emphasising that patient contact is essential for developing context-specific communication skills and the irreplaceable nature of face-to-face learning experiences. Furthermore, Walker and Stapleton [18] report that no medical student preferred virtual learning, citing reduced opportunities for meaningful patient contact and less engaging experiences, with Franklin et al. [19] finding that medical students felt inadequately prepared for practice, leading to concerns about future career prospects. A recent scoping review carried out by Amankwaa et al. [20] presents a wealth of evidence on the impact on the use of virtual and simulated approaches adopted by nurse educators in HEIs during the COVID-19 pandemic. They highlight the negative impact on nursing student mental health and well-being [21], the effects of blended learning [22], and the challenges of online learning [23]. The authors describe how some HEIs adopted simulated or virtual approaches to clinical placements using simulated skills sessions, experiential case studies and tele-health technology, noting the many benefits of these approaches in the delivery of innovations in a range of clinical environments. However, they note the lack of studies that demonstrate the long-term effectiveness and sustainability of virtual practice learning as we move away from the pandemic. This paper will describe and present the evaluation from the first run of a novel simulated practice learning experience project, showing its effectiveness on practice learning and satisfaction with year one pre-registration nursing students.

2. Materials and Methods

2.1. Design and Context of the SPLE Weeks

To maximise the opportunity that the NMC had provided, the project team reviewed clinical learning environments that students typically had limited or no access to during their nurse training or where placement capacity post-pandemic had significantly reduced. In response, the team designed the four-week SPLE to address these gaps, ensuring students gained exposure to crucial areas of practice—see Figure 1. Historically, adult and mental health student nurses in maternity care placements would have two weeks observing and shadowing a range of midwives across various clinical settings, learning about their role. To reflect this observational experience, a maternity SPLE week was developed, allowing the students to follow a fictional couple's pregnancy journey from ante-natal to post-natal care, gaining a unique insight into the clinical needs and care of a pregnant woman and her family. Currently only, a small number of mental health students gain access to direct practice placements in the field of learning disability nursing. The project team had a unique opportunity to develop an SPLE to immerse all students, providing them with the opportunity to engage with key healthcare professionals and individuals with learning disabilities, gaining insights into real-life challenges and care needs in a way that was previously inaccessible. A child health SPLE week was developed which provided a unique and innovative opportunity for students to gain exposure to caring for individuals from birth through to adolescence, an experience that had previously been limited due to the shortage of child health practice placements. Finally, a community care SPLE week was developed that offered a solution to the post-pandemic challenge of limited placement opportunities within district nursing community teams for the students. All students during this SPLE week learned how district nursing teams assess, discuss, and plan compassionate, dignified care for patients, an essential skill for future nurses and engaged in activities such as completing referral forms, practising assessments, and learning procedural skills like using syringe drivers.

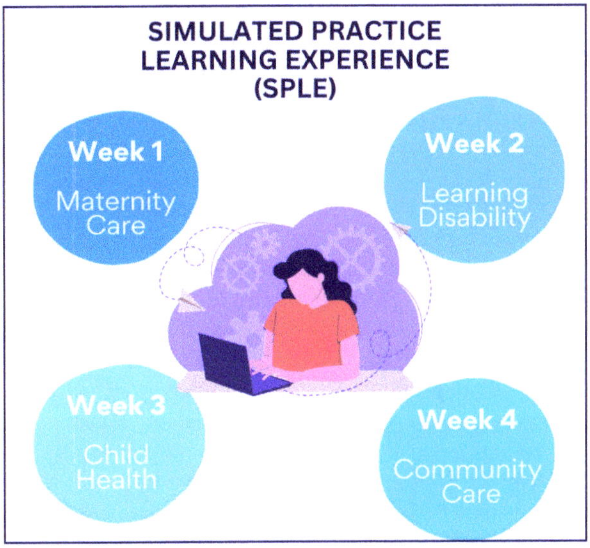

Figure 1. Simulated practice learning experience (SPLE) 4-week design.

Each SPLE week was aligned with the desired practice learning outcomes for year one students and mapped to key platforms and proficiencies, ensuring the student was able to demonstrate safe and effective practice through engaging in key activities and assessment. Scenarios and case studies for each of the SPLE weeks were drawn from real clinical experiences and carefully aligned with the NMC Standards of Proficiency for Registered Nurses [24], ensuring an authentic and immersive learning environment. These scenarios allowed students to follow a cohesive and engaging narrative that spanned various aspects of holistic care across the four SPLE weeks. In the maternity week, students followed the fictional couple's pregnancy journey, from giving birth to a healthy baby to experiencing the birth and care of a child with a learning disability during the learning disability week. The child health week expanded on this narrative by exploring the role of the health visitor in supporting a family with both a healthy child and a child with mental health or complex needs. Finally, the community care week introduced a neighbour of the fictional couple who required ongoing support from district nursing teams, further emphasising the continuum of care, from birth to death, across the four SPLE weeks. These various learning experiences allowed students to consolidate their clinical learning in a safe and supportive virtual environment.

Canvas by Instructure, the universities web-based learning management system, was utilised to host the SPLE required educational materials, blending technology with pedagogy to create an immersive and interactive learning environment [25]. Beyond its conventional use, Canvas was strategically operated to host all SPLE-required educational materials, ensuring seamless access to weekly programmes, daily itineraries, Microsoft Teams links for live clinical sessions, weblinks, quizzes, and multimedia content such as videos and podcasts. This approach transformed Canvas into a dynamic, central hub for students, enabling a cohesive and integrated learning experience. The Information Technology team played a crucial role in customising Canvas to support the unique needs of the SPLE weeks and supporting the facilitation of each week, significantly contributing to the smooth operation of the IT platform. The platform's user-friendly interface and comprehensive toolset made it an ideal choice for delivering the SPLE's content, demonstrating a forward-thinking approach to practice learning delivery in a virtual environment [26].

Thinglink (Version K12) was embedded and utilised in three out of the four SPLE weeks to provide an authentic clinical learning environment. Thinglink is a digital platform that creates visual interactive tools which allow users to turn any image or video into an interactive and visual learning experience [27]. Its interface is user friendly, intuitive, and incorporates immersive reader, which supports accessible and inclusive learning. The Thinglink platform permits the user to upload a base image and then add a selection of icon tags, which, once clicked, can provide links to additional text, images, audio/media files, or links to websites or documents. These icon tags can be selected in various symbol formats or colours and placed anywhere within the base image [28]. The final product is a flexible and navigable resource with multiple media sources linked together in a logical manner.

As the SPLE was required to meet the standards for student supervision and assessment (SSSA) [29], a practice "virtual induction" was conducted on the first morning of each SPLE week to familiarise the students with the Canvas virtual practice environment. The students completed bespoke SPLE pre-practice activities to ensure they all had access to the digital and online resources they would need and furthermore were informed via the virtual induction how to access support available to them in case of any issues. This session guided students through activities to ensure their devices were suitably prepared to accommodate the technical requirements of the SPLE, such as testing software compatibility and internet connectivity. This comprehensive preparation aimed to equip students with the necessary knowledge and confidence to navigate the SPLE successfully.

Daily debriefs played a pivotal role in enriching the simulated practice learning experience by promoting reflection, collaboration, and knowledge consolidation among the students during and at the end of each day. Utilising Microsoft Teams, these debrief sessions brought together a diverse learning community in the virtual environment, enabling students to share their experiences, receive real-time feedback from lecturers and clinicians, and engage with service users in a supportive and interactive setting.

A structured approach to engagement and assessment was implemented through the Canvas platform to support the students in demonstrating their learning. This was crucial in meeting the standards for student supervision and assessment [29] and ensuring that all practice hours were monitored and accounted for in line with NMC requirements. To ensure attendance and participation were accurately tracked, students were required to demonstrate their attendance at the beginning, middle, and end of each day through Microsoft Teams calls, with registers taken to cross-check their hours. This structured attendance system not only supported accountability but also helped maintain engagement throughout the day. Additionally, at the end of each day, students completed an online quiz or activity specifically designed to assess their understanding of that day's learning materials, further ensuring that their knowledge and skills aligned to the expected learning outcomes. Upon completing the mandatory end-of-day activity, the students then generated and downloaded a certificate as evidence of their engagement and knowledge. These certificates (five per week) were then uploaded to a dedicated section within their electronic

Practice Assessment Document (ePAD). Once reviewed by the students' nominated practice supervisor, who was a clinician involved in the specific SPLE week or a member of staff from the SPLE team, the allocated practice hours for that day (maximum 6 hours per SPLE day) were awarded. This method of assessment not only kept students actively engaged but also provided a clear and documented way to track their learning progress and practice hours, ensuring a systematic process was in place to meet NMC governance.

2.2. Study Design and Methodology

The objective of this project evaluation was to establish the effectiveness of the SPLE and to explore student satisfaction with their simulated practice learning experience.

An evaluation questionnaire was used to gather a more comprehensive understanding of the effectiveness of the SPLE and the students' experiences and perceptions of the SPLE weeks. The questionnaire, which integrated both qualitative and quantitative questions, offered a thorough understanding of the SPLE project's impact, implementation, and context. It allowed the ability for the project team to compare the findings from the questionnaire, thereby enhancing the validity and reliability of the project evaluation. Additionally, using a mix of questions during the evaluation allowed for explanations that might be overlooked by quantitative data alone, providing a more holistic perspective on the novel SPLE project [30].

Fitzpatrick et al. [31] describe project evaluation as a systematic methodology used to assess the effectiveness, efficiency, and impact of a given project. It involves the collection and analysis of both qualitative and quantitative data to measure outcomes against predefined objectives and goals. To collect the data in this project, an evaluation questionnaire was designed and embedded into Canvas. The questionnaire consisted of 16 questions that aimed to assess key aspects of the students' overall experience, learning, and activities, and their perception of the virtual practice learning environment. The student evaluation questionnaire was categorised into key questions relating to the specific SPLE content, information, and use of technology, and a shortened version of the validated NHS Education for Scotland [32] Student Practice Learning Experience Feedback form was included, which is the standard practice placement evaluation that is completed by all students across all practice placements. By completing the evaluation questionnaire, students enabled the project team to capture valuable insights into their learning and engagement during the SPLE and identify ways to enhance and improve the SPLE weeks in future iterations. Eleven of the questions were quantitative in design to provide numerical data that could be analysed statistically to identify trends and patterns. The responses on the questionnaire were generated using the quiz function embedded within Canvas platform using the Likert scale of strongly agree; agree; neither agree or disagree; disagree; and strongly disagree. This scale allowed for the quantification of subjective opinions, enabling the analysis of respondents' levels of agreement or disagreement with specific statements [33]. The remaining five questions were open-ended to obtain qualitative feedback on student experiences. These questions allowed students to provide detailed and descriptive responses, offering insight into their personal experiences of the SPLE weeks, any challenges they experienced, and any suggestions on how the SPLE weeks could be improved in future iterations. The qualitative data gathered through these open-ended questions provided the project team with an understanding of the students' overall perspectives and allowed for a more nuanced analysis.

Utilising Canvas analytics, the team were able to efficiently export the student evaluation responses and download it into a Microsoft Excel file. By pulling descriptive statistics from the excel file, the team were able to showcase the analysis of respondents' levels of agreement or disagreement with specific statements, offering valuable insights into the students' perceptions and potential areas for improvement in future iterations. Drawing on Braun and Clark [34,35] as a foundation, thematic analysis of the data from the open-ended questions was conducted, adhering to the distinct stages of analysis. Thematic analysis was chosen due to its theoretical freedom, providing a flexible and useful research tool, enabling one of the researchers (SF) to present a rich and detailed account of the data. Initially the student responses were read multiple times to foster familiarity with the data while simultaneously noting down early themes and ideas. Subsequently, the dataset was coded to identify noteworthy characteristics within the data. Finally, a comprehensive interpretation of the data were synthesised through the generation of themes. The ability to easily access, export, and analyse these data ensured that the analytical process was both thorough and efficient, leading to a summary of the key patterns and themes from the student responses.

2.3. Ethical Implications

The SPLE project was not designed as a primary research study; hence, no formal ethics was sought or approved from the institutions ethical committee. At the time the project was developed, the primary focus was on reducing the impact of COVID-19 on year one students' clinical practice hours, and data were collected via the questionnaire evaluation to establish if the SPLE was effective and to explore student satisfaction. Although ethical approval was not sought and written informed consent was not obtained from all students, they were informed verbally by the project lead (AT) on numerous occasions that an analysis of the evaluation data would be generated to produce a project report that would be discussed and presented to faculty and disseminated to our clinical partners.

The final evaluation questionnaire was set up as a quiz and the data were downloaded in an excel format. This ensured that all students responses were fully anonymised, and the excel sheet contained no identifying data safeguarding the student's privacy and individual responses could not be traced, ensuring the protection of students' rights, dignity, and overall well-being. Additionally, the students were free to choose how many questions they answered and the level of detail they wished to provide as not all questions needed to be answered. The students were not coerced into completing the full evaluation and had freedom to choose which questions they wished to answer. An announcement was sent to the cohort of students informing them of future publications and if any student had any queries/questions on the use of their data to contact the project lead. No students contacted the project lead.

3. Results

3.1. Quantitative

A total of 216 students participated in the simulated practice learning weeks across the spring semester in 2023 with a response rate of 98–100% across all four SPLE weeks. Student numbers attending each week ranged from 198 to 216 (see Table 1) with the variation in the sample size per week accounting for sickness, non-engagement, and students taking a break from their programme of study.

Table 1. Numbers of students who completed SPLE evaluation questionnaires per week.

SPLE Week	Completed Questionnaire
Maternity Care	216
Leaning Disability	205
Child Health	198
Community Care	199

The overall satisfaction from the four-week SPLE evaluation yielded positive results. When combining the responses of "agree" (35%) and "strongly agree" (53%), the total satisfaction score by the students reached 88% (see Figure 2) with Figure 3 illustrating the satisfaction in response rates for each individual SPLE week. Students appeared to be most satisfied with the maternity week and less satisfied with the child health week.

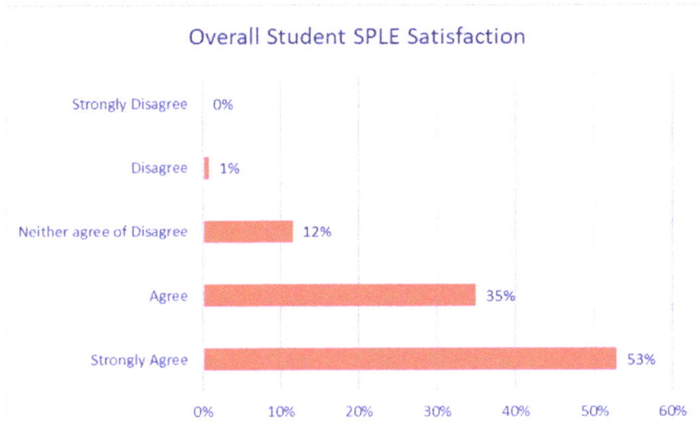

Figure 2. Overall student SPLE satisfaction graph.

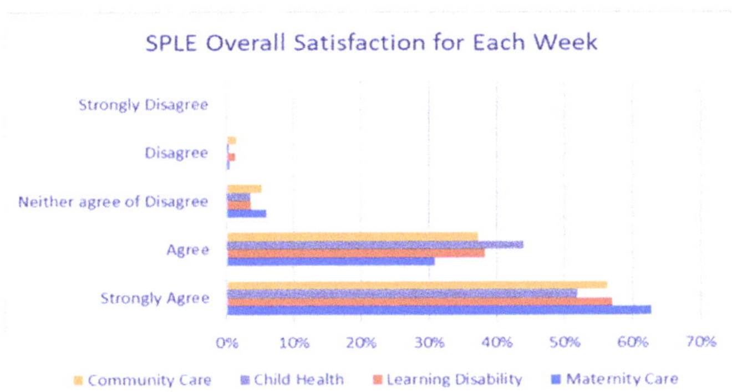

Figure 3. Overall student satisfaction for each individual SPLE week graph.

On average, across all SPLE weeks, 92% of students either agreed or strongly agreed that the virtual space was easy to access and navigate, reflecting the platform's user-friendliness and effectiveness in facilitating their practice learning experience—see Figure 4.

Additionally, 95% of students either agreed or strongly agreed that participating in the SPLE weeks significantly enhanced their knowledge of that specialist field of nursing, with learning disability being a popular choice with the students—see Figure 5.

The high response rate indicates that students fully engaged in the simulated practice learning experience weeks. Student responses suggest that overall, they were satisfied with the SPLE as a replacement for practice learning. The positive results suggest the content and organisation of the week highlights the success of both the virtual platform and the SPLE content in advancing students' practice learning development and practical understanding. Furthermore, the results suggest that the content of the SPLE was appropriately aligned with the practice learning outcomes and the material was relevant and accessible for the students. The maternity week appeared to be more popular with the students, which could be explained with the first use of Thinglink in this week. The immersive environment provided by this platform offering a fresh and interactive perspective on the various stages of maternity care could be a factor in this result. The positive results on the overall organisation and delivery of the SPLE suggest that each week was structured and executed in a manner that appears to have met students' practice learning needs and expectations.

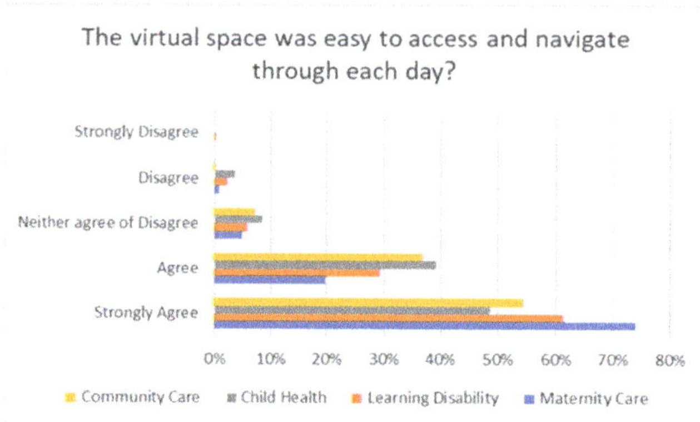

Figure 4. Ease of navigating the virtual space graph.

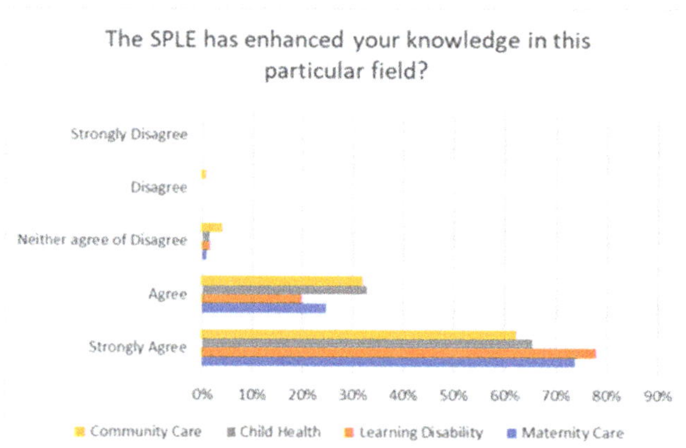

Figure 5. Impact of SPLE on knowledge enhancement in each field graph.

3.2. *Qualitative*

The qualitative responses from the questionnaire showed several key themes that reflected student experiences and perceptions of the SPLE. The themes were categorised into four main headings: transferable skills and personal growth; the value of peer learning; the benefits of learning within the virtual environment; appreciation of service user; and healthcare professional's input. The findings demonstrate the fundamental value and impact students experienced in fostering essential skills and facilitating collaborative learning experiences from the SPLE.

3.2.1. Transferable Skills and Personal Growth

Many students reported how the SPLE was pivotal to their personal growth and preparation for upcoming direct practice learning placements, attributing their sense of readiness and confidence to the comprehensive nature of the SPLE:

> *"I enjoyed this week very much. My knowledge of maternity care has been developed to a satisfactory level. Thus, I feel more confident to apply these skills as a future nurse caring for new mothers and their partners and supporting them with their questions".*

> *"I feel it was very beneficial to learn about maternity care, as made me aware of so much more than just the role of the midwife in maternity care, but how pregnancy can impact on the other branches of nursing too".*

> *"I felt that I gained so much knowledge which I will be able to take forward into practice and help me in my personal life with my family".*

> *"I enjoyed how interactive it was, allowing us to take the information and apply it to the referral forms and care plans".*

3.2.2. Peer Learning

Many of the student responses showcased the benefits of peer learning through small group discussion and activities plus the debrief sessions during the day with clinical staff and service users:

> *"The drop in's and end of day discussions each day were extremely helpful hearing other students' opinions and questions on the material we were learning that day".*

> *"I enjoyed having the opportunity to interact with the other students and lecturers. The days were easy to follow and had very interesting chats".*

> *"The end of the day discussion was valuable as it rounded off the learning and gave opportunities to ask questions".*

> *"I enjoyed being able to see things from a different perspective. This allowed me to challenge my knowledge and help me think on the spot/problem solve".*

3.2.3. Benefits of Learning Within the Virtual Environment

Considering virtual placements are a relatively novel concept in the field of nursing education, it was reassuring to receive student feedback reporting their perceived benefits of virtual learning. The students' reported their experience was notably enhanced by the diverse range of learning methods employed, including videos, live sessions, and interactive tasks. They highly praised the interactive nature of the sessions and the inclusive learning environment, which encouraged engagement through group work, lively discussions, and a supportive learning community. The students also valued the opportunity to collaborate and share perspectives and found engaging with both lecturers and healthcare professionals from various disciplines particularly enriching. This multifaceted interaction not only provided real-world insights but also made their learning process dynamic and engaging:

> *"I really enjoyed all parts of it. At first, I was unsure how well virtual placement would be with it being online but by the end of the first day I thought it was amazing and worthwhile. The lecturers definitely made you want to go research further as you can tell they are so passionate about it".*

> *"I enjoyed working in groups as it allowed us to communicate in different ways and build confidence".*

> *"I truly enjoyed SPLE weeks. The content was good, with excellent explanations, and the materials were accessible and informative".*

> *"I liked the layout of having a lot of live calls with the lecturers and staff, it made it feel very inclusive and you felt a part of everything".*

3.2.4. Appreciation of Service User and Healthcare Professional Input

The students highly valued the opportunity to hear personal stories and real-life experiences from guest speakers, families, and professionals, particularly in the learning disability sector. These narratives provided deep insights and encouraged emotional connections, significantly enhancing their understanding and empathy. The real-world perspectives shared by these individuals offered practical knowledge and contextual understanding, which was deemed invaluable in preparing the students for real-life applications in their future training. By engaging in these activities, students developed a deeper understanding of how theoretical knowledge underpins practical skills and decisions, thereby enhancing their overall competence and confidence in their field

"The participation of the families, speech therapist, learning disability nurses, and their information helped to improve my skills".

"I particularly enjoyed listening to the CALMS meeting as we got to see a real-life scenario".

"The guest speaker was great, her shared experience was more than a book I could ever have read".

"I really appreciated the real-life experiences we had from parents, learning disability nurses, and speech and language therapists".

3.2.5. Areas for Improvement

While students recognised the value of the SPLE's organisation, delivery, and content, they also provided feedback highlighting areas for improvement. It was acknowledged that differing student learning approaches made it challenging to allocate a set timeframe for tasks that suited everyone. A small number of students commented on the pacing, with remarks such as:

"If anything, a little more content would have been good, however I do understand it was like this purposefully not to overwhelm students".

"Lots of information within a short period".

Some students felt that the actual practice experience would have been more beneficial. As one student noted:

"As much as I enjoyed the information, I personally think being on a maternity ward or being on an actual placement would have been more beneficial".

Additionally, a few students found navigating the virtual space stressful, as one student shared:

"It was only the first day and was so overwhelming with information overload and instructions coming from lectures over team meetings. The attempt to navigate my way through the computer and learn was stressful and tense for that day...".

With another student suggesting more flexibility in the timing of activities:

"Have opportunity to complete quizzes earlier, but understand it for timing of days".

This feedback reflects the varying educational support needs of students and emphasises the importance of considering diverse learning preferences when designing future iterations of the SPLE.

4. Discussion

As discussed in the background, there is limited research specifically focusing on simulated practice learning in a virtual environment in nursing, with insights from other healthcare practitioners providing valuable perspectives on the benefits and challenges associated with virtual clinical placements. The COVID-19 pandemic and its impact on the healthcare system led to disruptions in practice learning, prompting the NMC [2] to modify their standards to incorporate virtual approaches. This pushed nurse educators to be innovative and creative to maintain practice learning placements for student nurses, with many United Kingdom HEIs adopting virtual or simulated practice learning experiences [2]. This was a point in time where nurse educators needed to adopt a mindset that encouraged creativity, problem-solving, and the implementation of new ideas, as highlighted by Leary et al. [1]. The aim of this evaluation was to explore if simulated practice learning experience could offer an effective viable alternative to conventional student nurse practice learning placements and what impact it would have on student satisfaction.

The quantitative findings suggests that students overall had a positive experience and were satisfied with their simulated practice learning placements, with 92% agreeing that the virtual platform was easy to access and navigate, highlighting its user-friendliness. Additionally, 95% reported significant knowledge enhancement in their specialist nursing fields, showing that SPLE could be a viable alternative to conventional practice placements. Students reported their satisfaction with the content and organisation, which aligned with practice learning outcomes and provided relevant and accessible practice material. The maternity week was popular possibly due to the immersive nature of Thinglink, offering an interactive perspective on maternity care. Overall, the results indicate that the SPLE weeks were effectively structured to meet students' learning needs, reflecting the success of the platform and content in advancing their practice learning development. It is encouraging to note that these results reflect recent findings by Holt [4] who found that students were satisfied with their simulated practice learning experiences if the SPLE material and environment was organised, included people who use services and their carers, and had students work with authentic and "real life" clinical scenarios. Student satisfaction was rated high due to the equitable nature of the SPLE, allowing all students the opportunity to access practice learning from a diverse range of experiences not available in conventional practice placements which is evident SPLE project.

The qualitative findings are also consistent with similar results documented in the literature, where students identified the following themes that helped them feel prepared for future practice placements.

4.1. Transferable Skills and Personal Growth

Billett [36] highlights the importance of transferable skills in the integration of learning experiences across educational and practical settings, emphasising their necessity for student nurses to effectively transition into professional practice. Despite being in year one of the programme, the students were able to acknowledge the significance of transferable skills in nursing. They recognised the importance of these skills due to the diverse nature of nursing and the array of challenges that nurses face in practice. The SPLE played a pivotal role in their personal growth, significantly improving their communication abilities and deepening their grasp of holistic care approaches, thereby enhancing their readiness to tackle the complex demands of nursing practice. The virtual placement was particularly valued for its practical application of theoretical knowledge. Students found activities such as completing referral forms and conducting assessments highly beneficial. These hands-on experiences not only reinforced their learning but also enabled students to consolidate their knowledge and develop crucial skills for their future roles in clinical practice. Practice placements offer students "hands on" practical skill development, exposure to real healthcare settings, interprofessional collaboration, and, furthermore, patient interaction. The SPLE's were instrumental in preparing them for their future nursing placements, equipping them with the necessary knowledge, skills, and attributes to deliver safe and effective patient care [37] while simultaneously facilitating their personal growth as emerging professionals.

4.2. Peer Learning

The value of peer learning through group work was found to be a benefit of the SPLE. The students discussed how this allowed them to consider aspects of care and hear varying perspectives which encouraged them to consider their own values, create a supportive learning environment that inspires collaboration, enhances skill acquisition, and, furthermore, prepare for the collaborative nature of healthcare work [38]. It adopts a supportive learning community, encourages diverse perspectives, and prepares individuals for teamwork in nursing practice [39]. By leveraging the power of peers, nursing students and professionals can enhance their learning experiences, develop essential skills, and contribute to their professional growth and development. Amankwaa et al. [20] emphasise that learner engagement approaches, such as blended learning and small group discussions, are vital for establishing knowledge acquisition in the online learning environment. These methods facilitate interaction and collaboration among students, which are essential for effective learning. However, they also note that many papers in the review merely described the transition of face-to-face teaching content to an online format without detailing the necessary modifications to ensure student engagement. This suggests that simply replicating in-person teaching online may not be sufficient for effective learning. This was closely linked to the importance students placed on the daily debrief sessions during the SPLE weeks, which provided a safe space for them to consolidate their learning in the safe presence of their peers, maximising educational benefits [20].

4.3. Benefits of Learning Within the Virtual Environment

Students expressed a growing interest in healthcare technology and recognised its relevance to their future careers [10]. Triemstra et al. [16] and Twogood et al. [14] report that virtual placements offer student flexibility, eliminate geographical restrictions, provide exposure to diverse clinicians, and enhance critical thinking skills. These insights from the literature align with the findings from this project evaluation where students positively expressed the flexibility and control they had over their own learning process, particularly with the ability to work at their own pace and, furthermore, expressed how they enjoyed the possibility of independent learning within a comfortable environment. It is, therefore, evident that the students appreciate the immersive SPLE learning environment and the ability to apply theoretical knowledge to virtual scenarios.

4.4. Appreciation of Service User and Healthcare Professional Input

Service user involvement in nursing education not only enriches the learning experience but also prepares the students to become more effective and compassionate healthcare providers [40]. The students' appreciation for the input of service users and healthcare professionals stands out as a critical component of their simulated practice learning experience. Engaging with personal stories and real-life scenarios, particularly in the learning disability SPLE, offered students a profound emotional connection and a deeper understanding of the complexities involved in patient care [41]. The firsthand accounts from families, speech therapists, and learning disability nurses were highly valued as they provided practical, real-world insights that textbooks alone could not offer. These interactions helped bridge the gap between theory and practice, enriching students' empathy, which is essential in healthcare. As students reflected on these experiences, they highlighted how this exposure enhanced their understanding of how theoretical knowledge is applied in clinical decision-making and skill development. This opportunity not only boosted their confidence but will prepare them for future professional challenges. Student feedback emphasised that the participation of guest speakers and professionals added significant value to the simulated practice learning environment, making the content both relevant and impactful.

4.5. Areas for Improvement

While students recognised the value of the SPLE's organisation, delivery, and content, their feedback also highlighted areas for improvement, reflecting some challenges discussed in the literature. Virtual practice learning has been associated with anxiety, motivation concerns, social isolation, and mental health issues [42,43]. Similarly, a small number of students in this project evaluation reported difficulties, such as navigating the virtual space and adjusting to the pacing and structure of activities. For instance, some students found the first day overwhelming, citing "information overload" and "stressful" attempts to adapt to the virtual format. This aligns with Poon et al. [44] who noted that adapting to new learning formats can increase stress levels.

Additionally, some students expressed a preference for in-person practice learning, echoing findings from other studies that emphasise the benefits of meaningful patient contact [16,18]. As one student commented, *"Being on an actual placement would have been more beneficial"*. This reflects ongoing concerns about the limitations of virtual placements in promoting hands-on clinical experience.

However, while these concerns are valid, the SPLE evaluation suggests that many initial uncertainties about the online format were mitigated by its clear organisation, diverse resources, and innovative tools like Thinglink. Students praised the use of interactive elements, particularly during the maternity care week, which provided a realistic authentic clinical experience.

These findings highlight the importance of student feedback in future iterations to address both common and context-specific challenges of SPLE, ensuring that virtual placements are inclusive, adaptable, and responsive to varying student needs.

4.6. Strengths

The project evaluation has effectively identified numerous advantages of SPLE. One of the key strengths lies in the collection of data from a large cohort of students, which adds significant credibility to the findings and reinforces the reliability of the conclusions drawn. The use of novel and unique methods and tools to enhance practice learning has been particularly noteworthy, demonstrating a commitment to innovative educational approaches.

Furthermore, the SPLE ensured equity across all students as each participant was exposed to the same level of learning and practice opportunities, promoting an inclusive practice education environment supported by Holt [4]. As recommended in the scoping review by Amankawaa et al. [20], the incorporation of debriefing sessions at the end of each day provided a safe space for students to reflect on their experiences, guided by experienced clinicians, which enhanced their learning and professional development. Additionally, the emphasis on group work and communication encouraged collaboration among students, helping them to develop essential teamwork skills that are critical in healthcare settings.

The sustainability of the SPLE is further demonstrated by its successful validation by the NMC in 2024, leading to its integration into the Adult and Mental Health BSc Nursing programmes. This achievement reinforces its effectiveness as a long-term practice learning platform, providing a comprehensive and supportive learning experience for students. Together, these strengths underscore the SPLE's value as a recognised component of nursing education, ensuring its ongoing contribution to student practice learning. Each iteration of the SPLE will require the team to review and refine each category of feedback questions to maintain effectiveness and ensure student satisfaction.

4.7. Limitations

The findings are based solely from the feedback provided by first-year students. Therefore, the conclusions drawn cannot be generalised to represent the opinions of student nurses from all years across nursing programmes. The evaluation questionnaire was designed and developed for this project and was only piloted with two year four students.

4.8. Future Considerations and Recommendations

The positive outcomes from this evaluation reinforce the importance of influencing emerging technologies to sustain the effective design and structure of future simulated practice learning experiences. Through simulation, augmented reality immersive technologies, and the virtual shadowing of clinicians and service users, students can engage in more dynamic and interactive learning experiences. These innovations not only enhance critical thinking and bridge the theory–practice gap but also create flexible, scalable solutions for training nurses to meet the evolving demands of healthcare. By harnessing these tools collectively, we can further ensure students are well equipped to provide safe, compassionate care in real-world settings [45].

Nevertheless, the long-term impact of SPLEs remains underexplored due to the varying placement areas assigned to students. Future research should focus on how simulated practice learning influences students' clinical experiences over time. By examining future cohorts through longitudinal studies, we can assess the sustained effectiveness of SPLEs and adapt these innovations to continuously improve nursing education. This iterative approach not only strengthens practice education but also ensures it remains at the forefront of technological advancements in healthcare training.

5. Conclusions

In summary, this project evaluation has proven that simulated practice learning experiences can be effective and students are satisfied with their practice learning experience. The findings underscore both the benefits and challenges of simulated practice learning placements with the positive outcomes of the acquisition of transferable skills, the value of peer learning, and the appreciation of input from service users and healthcare professionals demonstrating the effectiveness of virtual environments for enhancing practice learning.

As the landscape of nursing evolves, simulated placements offer unique opportunities for flexibility and access to diverse practice experiences. This forward-thinking approach not only prepares students for the immediate demands of their roles but also cultivates critical thinking and adaptability for their future careers in healthcare. Moving forward, it is essential to maintain this momentum of innovation, ensuring that the practice education strategies employed not only address current needs but also anticipate future developments in the field of nursing education. By integrating both technological advancements and key elements of traditional practice, we can better prepare future healthcare professionals to meet the growing demands of the profession and deliver safe, compassionate care in a rapidly changing healthcare setting.

The second iteration of the SPLE (2024) will further refine and build on these strengths, focusing on sustainability and continuous improvement.

Author Contributions: S.F. and A.T. contributed to this project evaluation and the writing of this paper. All authors have read and agreed to the published version of the manuscript.

Funding: This project evaluation received no external funding.

Institutional Review Board Statement: Ethical review and approval were not required for this project evaluation as the students completed the evaluation during the scheduled SPLE sessions as part of their regular timetabled programme.

Informed Consent Statement: Students were informed that the data collected would be used to evaluate the project, with a view to inclusion in future publications. Verbal consent was considered appropriate due to the evaluative nature of the project, and all students agreed to participate, fully understanding the purpose of their involvement. The evaluation was regarded as a routine part of the SPLE project.

Data Availability Statement: Students provided consent for their data to be used for evaluative purposes with a view to inclusion of future publication only.

Public Involvement Statement: No public involvement in any aspect of this project evaluation.

Guidelines and Standards Statement: The project evaluation did not adhere directly to specific reporting guidelines; however, it broadly followed improvement methodology to inform the evaluation process.

Use of Artificial Intelligence: AI or AI-assisted tools were not used in drafting any aspect of this manuscript.

Acknowledgments: The authors would like to extend their gratitude to the student nurses who contributed valuable feedback for the evaluation of this simulated practice learning experience (SPLE) project. Their insights were instrumental in shaping the study's outcomes, and their participation is deeply appreciated. The authors would also like to thank the clinical and wider university staff who assisted in the design, development, and delivery of the SPLE weeks. Their support and collaboration were essential to the success of the project.

Conflicts of Interest: The authors declare no conflicts of interest.

References

1. Leary, M.; Demiris, G.; Brooks Carthon, J.M.; Cacchione, P.Z.; Aryal, S.; Bauermeister, J.A. Determining the innovativeness of nurses who engage in activities that encourage innovative behaviors. *Nurs. Rep.* **2024**, *14*, 849–870. [CrossRef]
2. Nursing and Midwifery Council. *Current Recovery Programme Standards*; NMC: London, UK, 2022.
3. Nursing and Midwifery Council. *Standards Framework for Nursing and Midwifery Education*; NMC: London, UK, 2023.
4. Holt, P.J. *Simulated Practice Learning in Pre-Registration Nursing Programmes: An Evaluation of the Experiences of Universities Approved to Deliver Up to 600 Hours Practice Learning Hours Through Simulation*; NMC: London, UK, 2024.
5. Hegland, P.A.; Aarlie, H.; Strømme, H.; Jamtvedt, G. Simulation-based training for nurses: Systematic review and meta-analysis. *Nurse Educ. Today* **2017**, *54*, 6–20. [CrossRef] [PubMed]
6. Bland, A.J.; Topping, A.; Tobbell, J. Time to unravel the conceptual confusion of authenticity and fidelity and their contribution to learning within simulation-based nurse education: A discussion paper. *Nurse Educ. Today* **2014**, *34*, 1112–1118. [CrossRef] [PubMed]
7. Lavoie, P.; Deschênes, M.-F.; Nolin, R.; Bélisle, M.; Blanchet Garneau, A.; Boyer, L.; Lapierre, A.; Fernandez, N. Beyond technology: A scoping review of features that promote fidelity and authenticity in simulation-based health professional education. *Clin. Simul. Nurs.* **2020**, *42*, 22–41. [CrossRef]
8. Salje, J.; Moyo, M. Implementation of a virtual student placement to improve the application of theory to practice. *Br. J. Nurs.* **2023**, *32*, 434–441. [CrossRef]
9. Roberts, E.; Kaak, V.; Rolley, J. Simulation to replace clinical hours in nursing: A meta-narrative review. *Clin. Simul. Nurs.* **2019**, *37*, 5–13. [CrossRef]
10. Pit, S.W.; Velovski, S.; Cockrell, K.; Bailey, J. A qualitative exploration of medical students' placement experiences with telehealth during COVID-19 and recommendations to prepare our future medical workforce. *BMC Med. Educ.* **2021**, *21*, 431. [CrossRef] [PubMed]
11. West, R. Adapting to online placements. *Br. J. Nurs.* **2021**, *30*, 694. [CrossRef]
12. Mian, A.; Khan, S. Medical education during a pandemic: A UK perspective. *BMC Med.* **2020**, *18*, 100–102. [CrossRef] [PubMed]
13. Inman, A.G.; Soheilian, S.S.; Luu, L.P. Telesupervision: Building bridges in a digital era. *J. Clin. Psychol.* **2019**, *75*, 292–301. [CrossRef] [PubMed]
14. Twogood, R.; Hares, E.; Wyatt, M.; Cuff, A. Rapid implementation and improvement of a virtual student placement model in response to the COVID-19 pandemic. *BMJ Open Qual.* **2020**, *9*, e001107. [CrossRef] [PubMed]

15. Peart, A.; Wells, N.; Yu, M.; Brown, T. 'It became quite a complex dynamic': The experiences of occupational therapy practice educators' move to digital platforms during the COVID-19 pandemic. *Aust. Occup. Ther. J.* **2022**, *69*, 38–49. [CrossRef]
16. Triemstra, J.D.; Haas, M.R.C.; Bhavsar-Burke, I.; Gottlieb-Smith, R.; Wolff, M.; Shelgikar, A.V.; Samala, R.V.; Ruff, A.L.; Kuo, K.; Tam, M.; et al. Impact of the COVID-19 Pandemic on the clinical learning environment: Addressing identified gaps and seizing opportunities. *Acad. Med.* **2021**, *96*, 1276–1281. [CrossRef] [PubMed]
17. Hammond, D.; Louca, C.; Leeves, L.; Rampes, S. Undergraduate medical education and COVID-19: Engaged but abstract. *Med. Educ. Online* **2020**, *25*, 1781379. [CrossRef] [PubMed]
18. Walker, M.; Stapleton, E. Undergraduate experience of ENT teaching during the coronavirus disease 2019 pandemic: A qualitative study. *J. Laryngol. Otol.* **2021**, *138*, 741–745. [CrossRef]
19. Franklin, G.; Martin, C.; Ruszaj, M.; Matin, M.; Kataria, A.; Hu, J.; Brickman, A.; Elkin, P.L. How the COVID-19 pandemic impacted medical education during the last year of medical school: A class survey. *Life* **2021**, *11*, 294. [CrossRef] [PubMed]
20. Amankwaa, I.; Boateng, D.; Quansah, D.Y.; Akuoko, C.P.; Desu, A.P.B.; Hales, C. Innovations in nursing education in response to the COVID-19 pandemic: A scoping review. *Nurs. Prax. Aotearoa N. Z.* **2022**, *38*, 1–16. [CrossRef]
21. Barrett, D.; Twycross, A. Impact of COVID-19 on nursing students' mental health: A systematic review and meta-analysis. *Evid. Based Nurs.* **2022**, *25*, 8–9. [CrossRef]
22. Jowsey, T.; Foster, G.; Cooper-Ioelu, P.; Jacob, S. Blended learning via distance in preregistration education: A scoping review. *Nurse Educ. Pract.* **2020**, *44*, 102775. [CrossRef] [PubMed]
23. Divya, K.Y.; Binil, V. E-learning challenges in nursing education during COVID-19 pandemic: A narrative review. *Indian J. Forensic Med. Toxicol.* **2021**, *15*, 2317–2322. [CrossRef]
24. Nursing and Midwifery Council. *Standards of Proficiency for Registered Nurses*; NMC: London, UK, 2024.
25. Wiskow, K.M.; Subramaniam, S.; Montenegro-Montenegro, E. A comparison of individual and group equivalence-based instruction delivered via Canvas. *J. Appl. Behav. Anal.* **2024**, *57*, 262–274. [CrossRef] [PubMed]
26. Burton, C.W.; Rodrigues, S.M.; Jones-Patten, A.E.; Ju, E.; Abrahim, H.L.; Saatchi, B.; Wilcox, S.P.; Bender, M. Novel pedagogical training for nursing doctoral students in support of remote learning: A win-win situation. *Nurse Educ.* **2021**, *46*, E79–E83. [CrossRef] [PubMed]
27. Batista, J.A.F.A.; Souza, M.M.P.; Barros, T.D.; Nishu, G.; Reis, M.J.C.S. Using the ThingLink computer tool to create a meaningful environmental learning scenario. *EAI Endorsed Trans. Smart Cities* **2022**, *6*, e3. [CrossRef]
28. Jeffery, A.J.; Rogers, S.L.; Jeffery, K.L.A.; Hobson, L. A flexible, open, and interactive digital platform to support online and blended experiential learning environments: Thinglink and thin sections. *Geosci. Commun.* **2021**, *4*, 95–110. [CrossRef]
29. Nursing and Midwifery Council. *Standards for Student Supervision and Assessment*; NMC: London, UK, 2023.
30. Creswell, J.W.; Plano Clark, V.L. *Designing and Conducting Mixed Methods Research*, 3rd ed.; Sage Publications: Los Angeles, CA, USA, 2017; pp. 154–196.
31. Fitzpatrick, J.L.; Sanders, J.R.; Worthen, B.R. *Program Evaluation: Alternative Approaches and Practical Guidelines*, 4th ed.; Pearson: London, UK, 2011.
32. NHS Education for Scotland. *Indicators for the Quality Standards for Practice Learning*; NES: Edinburgh, UK, 2020.
33. Joshi, A.; Kale, S.; Chandel, S.; Pal, D.K. Likert scale: Explored and explained. *Br. J. Appl. Sci. Technol.* **2015**, *7*, 396–403. [CrossRef]
34. Braun, V.; Clarke, V. Using thematic analysis in psychology. *Qual. Res. Psychol.* **2006**, *3*, 77–101. [CrossRef]
35. Braun, V.; Clarke, V. *Thematic Analysis: A Practical Guide*; Sage: London, UK, 2021.
36. Billet, S. Integrating learning experiences across tertiary education and practice settings: A socio-personal account. *Educ. Res. Rev.* **2014**, *12*, 1–13. [CrossRef]
37. Henderson, A.; Briggs, J.; Schoonbeek, S.; Paterson, K. A framework to develop a clinical learning culture in health facilities: Ideas from the literature. *Int. Nurs. Rev.* **2011**, *58*, 196–202. [CrossRef]
38. Christiansen, A.; Bell, A. Peer learning partnerships: Exploring the experience of pre-registration nursing students. *J. Clin. Nurs.* **2010**, *19*, 803–810. [CrossRef]
39. Stone, R.; Cooper, S.; Cant, R. The value of peer learning in undergraduate nursing education: A systematic review. *Int. Sch. Res. Not.* **2013**, *2013*, 930901–930911. [CrossRef]
40. Kuti, B.; Houghton, T. Service user involvement in teaching and learning: Student nurse perspectives. *J. Res. Nurs.* **2019**, *24*, 183–194. [CrossRef] [PubMed]
41. Smith, P.; Ooms, A.; Maran-Marks, D. Active involvement of learning disabilities service users in the development and delivery of a teaching session to pre-registration nurses: Students' perspectives. *Nurse Educ. Pract.* **2016**, *16*, 111–118. [CrossRef] [PubMed]
42. Perone, A.K. Surviving the semester during COVID-19: Evolving concerns, innovations, and recommendations. *J. Soc. Work* **2021**, *57*, 194–208. [CrossRef]
43. Aldridge, M.D.; McQuagge, E. "Finding my own way": The lived experience of undergraduate nursing students learning psychomotor skills during COVID-19. *Teach. Learn. Nurs.* **2021**, *16*, 347–351. [CrossRef]

44. Poon, S.H.J.; Chow, M.S.C.; Lam, W.W.T. Medical education and mental wellbeing during COVID-19: A student's perspective. *Med. Sci. Educ.* **2021**, *31*, 1183–1185. [CrossRef] [PubMed]
45. Odro, A.; Clancy, C.; Foster, J. Bridging the theory-practice gap in student nurse training: An evaluation of a personal and professional development programme. *J. Ment. Health Train. Educ. Pract.* **2010**, *5*, 4–12. [CrossRef]

nursing reports

MDPI

Article

Pre-Implementation Strategies to Support Adaptation of Thrive: A Care Transitions Model for Economically Disadvantaged Patients with Serious Mental Illness

J. Margo Brooks Carthon [1,*], Celsea Tibbitt [1], Kelvin Eyram Amenyedor [2], Amanda P. Bettencourt [3], Erin Babe [4], Pamela Z. Cacchione [5] and Heather Brom [1]

[1] Center for Health Outcomes & Policy Research, Leonard Davis Institute of Health Economics, University of Pennsylvania School of Nursing, 418 Curie Blvd., Philadelphia, PA 19104, USA; ctibbitt@nursing.upenn.edu (C.T.); hmbrom@upenn.edu (H.B.)

[2] Yale School of Medicine, Yale University, 333 Cedar St., New Haven, CT 06510, USA; kelvin.amenyedor@yale.edu

[3] Center for Health Outcomes & Policy Research, Penn Implementation Science Center, Leonard Davis Institute of Health Economics, University of Pennsylvania School of Nursing, 418 Curie Blvd., Philadelphia, PA 19104, USA; paamanda@nursing.upenn.edu

[4] Center for Health Outcomes & Policy Research, University of Pennsylvania School of Nursing, 418 Curie Blvd., Philadelphia, PA 19104, USA; erinbabe@upenn.edu

[5] Penn Presbyterian Medical Center, Leonard Davis Institute of Health Economics, University of Pennsylvania School of Nursing, Philadelphia, PA 19104, USA; pamelaca@nursing.upenn.edu

* Correspondence: jmbrooks@nursing.upenn.edu

Abstract: Background: Economically disadvantaged patients diagnosed with serious mental illness (SMI) experience post-hospitalizations disparities due to fragmented care transitions. Purpose: To describe the pre-implementation strategies used to adapt and implement a nurse-led transitional care intervention (Thrive) to meet the needs of economically disadvantaged patients diagnosed with an SMI. Methods: Two pre-implementation strategies, Evidence Based Quality Improvement (EBQI) meetings and Formative Evaluation (FE) research, were used to adapt intervention components. FE data included semi-structured interviews analyzed using Rapid Qualitative Analysis. Findings: Adaptations were made to core components of Thrive and strategies to support implementation were identified. Conclusions: Participatory strategies help to adapt interventions that are person-centered and tailored to the organizational context. Trial: NCT06203509.

Keywords: serious mental illness; Medicaid; transitional support; pre-implementation research; health services research

1. Introduction

Over 14 million Medicaid-insured adults live with a mental illness, such as major depressive disorder, bipolar disorder, and schizophrenia [1,2]. Medicaid is the largest payer of mental healthcare services, providing coverage for 21% of adults living with a mental illness, and 26% of adults living with a serious mental illness (SMI) [2]. When hospitalized with co-occurring mental and physical health conditions, Medicaid-insured individuals with SMI experience higher rates of readmissions and emergency department (ED) utilization compared with non-Medicaid insured individuals with SMI [3–9]. These disparities may be related in part to socioeconomic inequities, such as unstable housing, concerns over copays, or barriers in accessing medications [5,7,10–12]. Deficits in transitional care support, including limited access to community resources may also contribute to higher rates of readmission and ED utilization [5].

To address the post-discharge needs of people insured by Medicaid our team leveraged principles of human-centered design leading to the development of a clinical innovation

Nurs. Rep. **2024**, *14*, 3803–3818. https://doi.org/10.3390/nursrep14040278 https://www.mdpi.com/journal/nursrep

called Thrive [13]. Thrive provides intensive wrap-around services including connections to medical and community-based social services to people insured through Medicaid who are transitioning from hospital to home. Now in its fifth year, Thrive has been recognized by the American Academy of Nursing as an Edge Runner for nurse-led innovations. The Thrive model involves an academic clinical partnership between Penn School of Nursing, Penn Medicine Homecare and Hospice services and three large urban hospitals.

A core feature of Thrive is our focus on addressing health-related social needs such as challenges with transportation and food insecurity as a central facet of transitional care support. Services provided through Thrive were designed with the understanding that many disparities experienced by people insured through Medicaid are driven by social and economic factors and the distribution of healthcare resources in such a way that disadvantages some groups over others [14]. Thrive optimizes the post discharge management process by intensifying resources and interdisciplinary collaborations across settings for patients at risk for experiencing health disparities. The published results of Thrive have demonstrated sizable improvements in post-discharge utilization outcomes for Thrive enrollees including higher rates of primary care connections and fewer readmissions and ED visits compared with patients receiving usual care [15].

A notable finding of our early work was the recognition that at least a third of Medicaid-insured participants receiving Thrive services, were also diagnosed with a co-occurring serious mental illness (SMI) [16]. While Thrive services are designed to support non-psychiatric admissions, we frequently witnessed the effects of unstable mental health needs following hospitalization, including a lack of connection to therapy and medication services. Patients with SMI experience a higher burden of medical comorbidities, and frequently follow intricate drug schedules prescribed by multiple healthcare professionals to treat their mental and physical comorbidities. These factors are often complicated by communication difficulties, cognitive impairment, and a lack of social support rendering them more at risk for readmission and ED utilization. Ref. [17] To better understand the experiences of Thrive participants with co-occurring SMI, we undertook a mixed methods pilot study to examine the extent to which Thrive services met the needs of Medicaid-insured patients with co-morbid SMI diagnoses. Findings from the quantitative arm of the pilot study found no significant differences in 30-day ED and readmission rates between Thrive participants with ($n = 62$) or without SMI ($n = 190$). Despite the literature supporting a much higher 30-day (15.9% vs. 11.7%) and 90-day (16.1% vs. 13.2%) readmission rates for those with SMI compared with those without SMI [18,19]. Interviews, however, revealed that while Thrive participants diagnosed with SMI ($n = 5$) expressed satisfaction with services, they reported that their mental health needs were never fully assessed. One participant revealed "*it would have been helpful*" if someone had asked about their mental health needs, but they did not [16].

Like many transitional care programs, Thrive was not developed to meet the specific needs of people diagnosed with SMI. The current literature suggests that many transitional care programs designed for people with SMI focus primarily on support following psychiatric hospitalizations [20]. Components of these programs frequently include transitions of care coach, medication management, and connections to psychiatric providers, though lack attention to health-related social needs such as transportation, food resources, and stable housing. This raises concerns that the transitional care needs of people diagnosed with SMI and hospitalized for non-psychiatric conditions are largely going unmet. For people insured with Medicaid, who experience the additional burdens of economic concerns, the period after hospitalization can be perilous.

Using evidence from our prior findings, we designed a study entitled. "SMI-Thrives: An equity-focused intervention to Improve care transitions for Medicaid insured individuals with co-occurring serious mental health" (hereafter, SMI-Thrives). Using a Hybrid Type I implementation and effectiveness design, and a stepped wedge approach, SMI-Thrives extends and adapts the current Thrive model to address the transitional care needs of patients who are Medicaid-insured, diagnosed with a co-morbid SMI, and hospitalized for a non-psychiatric illness. This article has two aims: First, to describe the pre-implementation evaluation to identify needed components for the adapted Thrive model. Second, we sought to systematically identify barriers and facilitators to the implementation of SMI-Thrive and link them to specific strategies to influence initial adoption.

The SMI-Thrives study is a Type 1 Hybrid Effectiveness-Implementation Stepped Wedge Cluster Randomized Controlled Trial that compares intensive transitional care support to usual care [21]. In the current Thrive model, Medicaid-insured individuals are (1) identified while hospitalized by nurse case managers and referred to home care services using an electronic medical record (EMR) flag. Following discharge, Thrive participants go on to receive (2) home care services where nurses perform medication reconciliation, intensive teaching and chronic disease management. Next, Thrive participants (3) receive continued clinical oversight by our interdisciplinary team including the discharging hospital-based physician or Advanced Practice Provider (APP) who facilitate care continuity if there is an absence of available primary care support. Finally, the nurse led Thrive Care Management Team (4) facilitates weekly interdisciplinary case management meetings for a full month where connections are made to community, primary, and specialty services [22]. The goal of this paper is to describe the pre-implementation processes used by our team to adapt the Thrive care model to meet the transitional care needs of people with co-occurring serious mental health diagnoses hospitalized for a non-psychiatric admission. For our purposes our adaptation followed a thoughtful and deliberate alteration of the design or delivery of Thrive with an aim of improving its fit or effectiveness in a given context [23,24].

We began our pre-implementation process by engaging staff, mental health experts, and community advisors using a participatory process which included a series of "meet and greets" with institutional partners. Next, we launched an Evidence-Based Quality Improvement (EBQI) workgroup to prioritize additional components to the current Thrive care model. To evaluate the context required for the adaptation of the intervention, we used a Formative Evaluation (FE) approach through interviews of clinicians and leadership who would have direct engagement with referrals to Thrive. The University of Pennsylvania Institutional Review Board approved this study.

Figure 1 outlines the pre-implementation research process. In the following, we provide an overview of the EBQI and FE approaches.

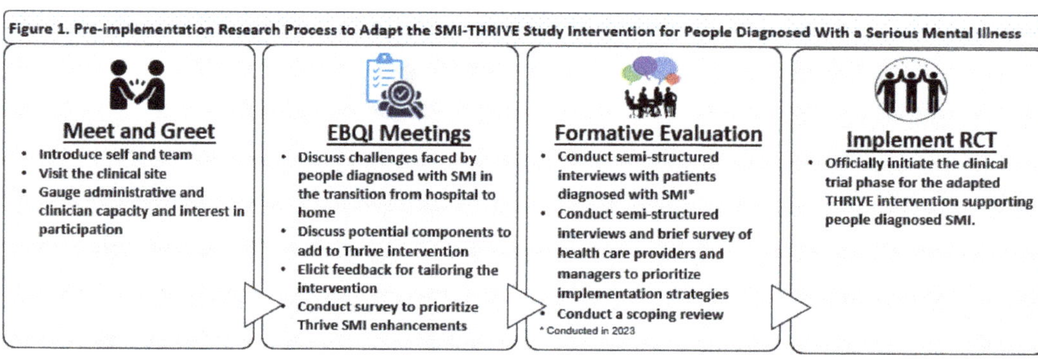

Figure 1. Author's work. Legend: EBQI—Evidence Based Quality Improvement; RCT—Randomized Controlled Trial, SMI—Serious Mental Illness.

2. Methods

2.1. Evidence-Based Quality Improvement Workgroup

We conducted pre-implementation research using Formative Evaluation (FE) and Evidence-Based Quality Improvement (EBQI) methods to identify additional SMI-sensitive adaptations for the Thrive model and implementation into the trial protocol. The combined strengths of these approaches ensured that the perceptions of diverse stakeholders, including clinicians, administrators, and those diagnosed with SMI, were considered during the adaptation and implementation phases.

2.2. EBQI Recruitment and Procedures

The EBQI approach was used to ensure that the added Thrive adaptations were acceptable to stakeholders and consistent with the evidence [25]. For our purposes, the EBQI workgroup members offered perspectives on the challenges faced by patients diagnosed with SMI following hospitalization, and offered suggestions on essential components to consider as adaptations to the Thrive model. Given our goal, we sought workgroup participants such as clinicians with expertise in the care of people diagnosed with SMI, managers from the study site, community representatives, and caregivers of patients with SMI [26]. To ensure we were including perspectives of people with SMI and to protect their privacy, we consulted with two external people diagnosed with SMI who provided feedback throughout the Workgroup process but who preferred not to be identified by their diagnoses. Workgroup members were recruited using both criterion and snowballing techniques which resulted in wide representation.

Our EBQI workgroup first received endorsement from the Hospital Executive team, which helped engender support during workgroup recruitment. The Hospital Executive team was composed of the Nurse Senior Executive and a Clinical Quality Improvement Officer who provided the team with the names of clinicians and managers who could add valuable contributions to the workgroup discussion. In addition, the study team sought the participation of clinicians and content experts (e.g., individuals with experience caring for people diagnosed with SMI) as well as individuals or caregivers of individuals with SMI. The study PI sent personal emails requesting participation in three one-hour work group meetings in early November 2023, with one follow up reminder sent a week after the first. A total of 20 invitations were emailed, with a total of 10 responses. An additional 3 members of the research team were included on the EBQI workgroup bringing the total members to 13. Non-research affiliated workgroup members were provided with a USD 100 honorarium for each one-hour meeting attended.

We hosted three one-hour EBQI workgroup meetings. During meetings, workgroup members offered perspectives on the challenges faced by patients diagnosed with SMI following hospitalization, described current mental health screening practices for non-psychiatric admissions, and prioritized essential components that should be considered as adaptations to the Thrive model. One critical aspect of our work was a review of practices currently operating within the hospital to assess and address the needs of patients diagnosed with co-occurring SMI. Examining existing clinical practices and support systems within the hospital and home care setting helped to set the stage for potential adaptations to the Thrive care model. We aimed to identify gaps and areas for improvement. During each meeting the facilitator stressed the importance of engaging a wide range of perspectives while emphasizing flexible aspects that should be considered. During our final meeting, the workgroup discussed the strengths and merits of 13 possible adaptations to Thrive. Using a consensus approach, participants were asked to rank order their preferences of proposed adaptations. The research team facilitated the consensus process, summarized the results, and then adopted those components that achieved majority support of the 10 non-research workgroup participants.

2.3. Formative Evaluation Research

Formative evaluation (FE) is defined as a "rigorous assessment process designed to identify potential and actual influences on the progress and effectiveness of implementation efforts" [26]. For our purposes, FE was used to assess whether Thrive was believed to address the significant needs for patients diagnosed with SMI. In addition, we sought to understand the community and organizational contexts, elicit potential barriers and facilitators, and prioritize implementation strategies to ensure a smooth launch of Thrive at a new site. Our FE processes were informed by the Health Equity Implementation Framework (HEIF), an adaptation of the Integrated Promoting Action on Research in Implementation in Health Services [i-PHARIS] framework [27]. The FE included semi-structured interviews of clinicians and administrators who would be directly involved in the referrals and clinical care management of patients enrolled to Thrive. The HEIF framework proposes determinants that are believed to predict successful and equitable implementation of an intervention. The three health equity domains of HEIF are cultural factors, clinical encounter factors, and societal contexts. Engaging in this participatory process allowed us to increase buy-in from stakeholders and overcome barriers prior to the launch of the study.

2.4. Semi-Structured Interview Recruitment

We used a criterion sampling framework to select interview participants. Criterion sampling involves choosing a setting, group, and/or individuals because they represent one or more criteria [28]. For our purposes, we were most interested in gaining the perspectives of individuals who would have direct interface in referring to Thrive, providing clinical oversight or managerial support. Hence, participants deemed eligible for semi-structured FE interviews included case managers, social workers, and healthcare providers affiliated with the study hospital or home care setting. Eligible participants included those who had been employed with the healthcare system for at least 3 months.

2.5. Semi-Structured Qualitative Interviews

The formative evaluation (FE) qualitative data were derived from interviews conducted virtually via Teams. Interviews were collected between February and March 2024, after the piloting of the interview guide by two study team members and authors (MBC, HB). Interview questions, informed by the Health Equity Implementation Framework, asked participants to reflect on perceived appropriateness of Thrive, challenges faced by patients following hospitalization, anticipated barriers to intervention acceptance, and organizational and workflow challenges, if any (Table 1). Interviewers obtained verbal consent to record the interviews and memos were taken throughout the duration of the encounter. Twelve eligible participants were contacted by email for interviews and a total of eight agreed to be interviewed, which is sufficient to elicit rich and in-depth perspectives from study participants [16,29].

Table 1. Health Equity Implementation Framework-informed interview guide.

Domain	Example Interview Questions
Clinical Encounter	• What types of difficulties do patients with significant social needs and/or SMI encounter after hospitalization?
Cultural Factors	• Considering the challenges in accepting services that carry stigma, like behavioral health resources, what tactics or communication techniques do you find most effective in motivating patients to agree to post-discharge support upon discharge?
Societal Context	• We understand that your hospital has a unique organizational structure with the health system. Are there any unique community collaborations that would support (or hinder) your ability to implement the clinical intervention?

Procedures. All eligible participants were contacted by email. The recruitment email included a link where potential participants could access information about the study and a consent document and select dates for interviews. Once the interview time was selected, the participant received confirmation by email and a unique Teams link. Recruitment emails were sent in three waves at the beginning of the study and in two-week increments as a reminder. A reminder email was sent 24 h prior to each interview. Each interview lasted approximately 40 min and was followed by a brief 5 min survey that asked for demographics, and 36 questions related to preferred implementation strategies and feasibility of the Thrive intervention. Detailed memos were taken throughout the interviews by the research program manager (KA). Twelve of these items included Proctor's implementation outcomes that assess the acceptability (how fair or reasonable Thrive is deemed), appropriateness (to what extent Thrive seems suitable), and feasibility (the practicality and ease of delivering Thrive). Each construct is four-items assessed on a five-point Likert scale asking participants to rate how much they agree or disagree with each item. The items are averaged with higher scores indicating greater acceptability, appropriateness, or feasibility [30]. The survey also asked participants to rank the usefulness of 12 implementation strategies drawn from the ERIC taxonomy. Participants were asked to select either "most useful" or "least useful" for each potential implementation strategy. Finally, readiness for change was assessed using the 12-item Organizational Readiness for Implementing Change instrument. Participants rated their level of agreement or disagreement with statements about their organization on a five-point Likert scale. The items are averaged with higher scores indicating more agreement that the organization is ready for change [30].

Reflexivity Statement. Our interview team purposely included individuals with expertise in equity and implementation science. One interviewer is Black, and the other is White. Both interviewers have background clinical experience working across hospital and community settings and with patients with chronic illnesses including SMI. Half of the authorship team identify as persons of color and all have substantial research experience in the fields of equity, mental health, implementation science, and nursing. Weekly meetings held throughout the interview process included discussion on how our social and clinical identities or closely held assumptions may influence our interpretation of participant's responses.

2.6. Semi-Structured Interview Data Analysis

Structured template and matrix display. A multistep process was used to summarize interview recordings using rapid qualitative analysis (RQA) procedures [25,31]. The RQA process is a well-established process ideal for use during the pre-implementation process when a deductive approach is in use and when evaluating the feasibility or appropriateness of an intervention. Using Hamilton's and Finley's, 2019, method, we began by identifying interview responses corresponding to each interview question [31–33]. Our interview guide was developed based on the domains of HEIF. Interview questions explored participant's views on the appropriateness of Thrive, aspects of the clinical encounter that might influence acceptance of Thrive, workflow facilitators and barriers, as well as community and organizational context.

Qualitative team members read the transcripts and noted particularly rich responses that were detailed and meaningful. We then developed a structured template to standardize the way to capture the interview content. The domains of HEIF were listed on the template for each study team member (HB and MBC) to summarize interview key ideas. To ensure inner rater reliability and applicability to the interview, two study team members used the template to separately code the same transcripts. The summaries of the two team members were used to confirm the relevancy of the template by comparing and modifying the template as needed. The two team members then divided the remaining interviews and summarized them using the template and HEIF domains. Responses that entailed representative quotes were timestamped for future exploration [34].

The researchers mapped each template onto a visual matrix after summarizing each transcript. The visual matrix consists of a single column per interview transcript, with each HEIF domain represented by a row. Once the findings were entered onto the visual matrix, each row was interpreted, and key ideas were synthesized to assess convergence and divergence across participants.

Rigor was established by adhering to the four dimensions for qualitative research outlined by Guba and Lincoln [35] (1981) which include the following: credibility (e.g., training interviewer with relevant expertise), confirmability (e.g., leveraging methodological triangulation using a brief follow up survey), dependability (e.g., maintaining a detailed audit trail), and transferability (developing an operations definition to achieve saturation).

3. Results

3.1. Evidence-Based Quality Improvement (EBQI) Workgroup Demographics

The EBQI workgroup included thirteen participants, six of whom were female. Four participants were Black, two identified as White, and two identified as other. The educational level of the workgroup members ranged from a baccalaureate degree to doctoral degree. The workgroup consisted of one SMI caregiver, two SMI healthcare professionals, one home care nurse manager, two case managers, two physicians, one advanced practice provider, one quality improvement officer, and three researchers.

3.2. FE Interview Participant Demographics

There were eight interview participants, each with an average of 2 years of experience in their current positions. All participants were female, four participants were Black, three participants were White, and one participant identified as "other". The highest level of education attained was a doctoral degree. Other characteristics of the formative evaluation (FE) participants are detailed in Table 2.

Table 2. Interview Participant Demographics (n = 8).

Variable	
Age, mean (SD)	38.9 (11.3)
Years at current job setting, mean (SD)	2.0 (1.4)
Female, *n* (%)	8 (100%)
Race *n* (%)	
Black or African American	4 (50%)
White	3 (37.5%)
Other	1 (12.5%)
Ethnicity, *n* (%)	
Hispanic	0
Highest level of education, *n* (%)	
Baccalaureate degree	1 (12.5%)
Master's degree	5 (62.5%)
Doctoral degree	1 (12.5%)
MD	1 (12.5%)
Primary job, *n* (%)	
Case manager	2 (25.0%)
Social worker	2 (25.0%)
Physician	1 (12.5%)
RN clinical practice lead	1 (12.5%)
Hospital nurse manager	1 (12.5%)
Home care nurse	1 (12.5%)

3.3. Evidence-Based Quality Improvement (EBQI) Workgroup Discussion Results

The EBQI workgroup held a total of three meetings. In the first meeting, the current Thrive model was introduced, and participants shared their current transitional care challenges for people diagnosed with SMI. Chief concerns raised during the discussion included the following: a lack of care integration/coordination, limited access to outpatient mental health services, need for medication management and reconciliation of psychiatric meds, mistrust and stigma, training healthcare professionals, need for formal mental health screening. The focus of the second meeting included proposed adaptations to the existing Thrive model. Examples of proposed adaptations included the following: addition of mental health screening during discharge process and integrated behavioral health assessments during Thrive case management meetings. The third and final EBQI workgroup meeting used a consensus process to decide on the proposed elements of the final adapted Thrive model. Table 3 displays the workgroup priorities and level of agreement with proposed elements of the Thrive model.

Table 3. Workgroup Priorities for Seven Identified SMI-focused Enhancements to the Thrive Intervention.

Intervention Enhancements, %	Very Important	Important	Somewhat Important	Not Important
Comprehensive integration of mental health into weekly Thrive virtual management calls (e.g., create a formal checklist that reviews mental health diagnosis and current treatment).	71.4%	28.6%	-	-
Integration of mental health in discharge planning (e.g., discussing Thrive during afternoon team huddles)	71.4%	28.6%	-	-
In-person discussions for patients who initially refuse services	71.4%	14.3%	14.3%	-
Presentation of Thrive information to Thrive-eligible individuals with a focus on physical, SDOH, and mental health: elevator pitch by case managers and social workers	57.1%	42.9%	-	-
Trauma-informed care as part of Thrive training	42.9%	42.9%	14.2%	-
Care package that focuses on self-care and mental health concept	28.6%	71.4%	-	-
Thrive training of staff nurses	14.3%	85.7%	-	-

3.4. Evidence-Based Quality Improvement (EBQI) Workgroup Members Endorsed the Following Elements to the Adapted Thrive Model

The team discussed a wide range of potential adaptations to the Thrive intervention to support the needs of patients diagnosed with SMI. Of the seven potential adaptations, the three that received at least 2/3 endorsements by EBQI members included ensuring the comprehensive integration of a mental health assessment during the Thrive weekly interdisciplinary team meetings. This involved creating a standardized inclusive checklist pertaining to all mental health diagnoses, documenting the status (active vs. remission) of mental health diagnoses, and determining current behavioral treatments or levels of engagement with a mental health provider. Participants also endorsed the need to integrate mental health screening into discharge planning during afternoon team huddles. Finally, recognizing that some participants would be hesitant to receive Thrive or home care services, it was proposed that a member of the Thrive team conduct bedside visits to share further information about Thrive.

3.5. Formative Evaluation (FE) Results

Table 4 provides an overview of the FE results analyzed using rapid qualitative analysis and based on the domains of the HEIF. These domains include perceptions of the Thrive innovation, the needs of eligible intervention recipients, community resources, and organizational, healthcare system, and provider factors.

Table 4. Results of rapid qualitative analysis based on the domains of the Health Equity Implementation Framework.

HEIF Domain	Summary	Exemplar Quote
Characteristics of the Innovation: The extent to which the innovation is simple (ease of use), intuitive, and considered to be beneficial or useful (effectiveness). How the proposed integration of the Thrive referral or follow up by APPs or Hospitalists would increase (time) or change workflow	• Overwhelming support from all participants to institute Thrive • Low-burden addition to the inpatient workflow • Aligned with organizational priorities including reduced readmissions and ED utilization • Enthusiastic about improving continuity of care through the intervention • Intervention viewed as necessary since many patients have co-occurring serious mental illness (SMI)	"I really think that having something like this [Thrive], even if you can't save all, you'll be able to save a lot more than what we're able to do now" (Participant 3)
Clinical Encounter: Clinical workflows leading to interactions between patient and provider or between recipients. Includes consideration of unique characteristics and preferences affecting engagement with populations of interest and techniques used by providers to gain trust/improve communication	• Very important to build patient–provider trust so that patients will be open to accepting a home care/Thrive referral • Shorter lengths of stay can be a barrier to fully understanding all the patient's health-related social needs once discharged • Clinicians found it helpful to use communication techniques that met the patient where they were—e.g., good eye contact, normalizing their health or mental health condition	"'you know what's best for you', so encouraging and reminding patients that they have the autonomy and decision" (Participant 2) "there's a care team that's responsible for you but there's a person on this team and that person is you, like you're a part of it and so you have to do that part. You need people who aren't afraid to have those conversations" (Participant 3)
Patient Factors: Specific to a patient or member of the healthcare team and can refer to believes, acceptance, training and knowledge communication, or engagement preferences. Also includes attitudes towards relevant stakeholders of institutions	• Many complex social needs that remain unaddressed • Lack connections to community resources (e.g., primary care providers, mental health service providers) • High levels of co-occurring serious mental illness and substance use disorder • May be resistant to services/providers they do not already know • Many barriers post discharge (e.g., lack of housing, transportation, caregiver, financial concerns) • High burden placed	"we've assisted with like keeping their electricity on but they don't necessarily do their part to kind of make sure that they stay up to date with things;" (Participant 3) "We know you can offer people referrals to community resources, community health workers, substance abuse and they're like 'no'" (Participant 2) "Don't want people in their homes. Fear that people are going to judge them" (Participant 2) "Need support for caregivers—they are burdened with family member's complexity" (Participant 8)

Table 4. *Cont.*

HEIF Domain	Summary	Exemplar Quote
Provider Factors: Specific to a member of the healthcare team and can refer to believes, acceptance, training and knowledge communication or engagement preferences. Also includes atttudes towards relevant stakeholders of institutions	• Providers unable to attend to all of the needs patients have • Needing to meet patients where they are in understanding their life circumstances • Risk of burnout and compassion fatigue when caring for patients who can't follow discharge recommendations related to a lack of community services/supports • Frustration that despite efforts to connect patients to resources that patients are still returning repeatedly to the hospital • Limited expertise to meet the needs of people diagnosed with co-occurring SMI and SUD	"Sometimes all we can do is give a list of resources" (Participant 1) "I think as healthcare workers we have this perception that patients come to use for a service and they should follow our rules and do what we say but that's not life and most of our providers and clinicians and nurses, we can't relate to how they live outside of the hospital so it's no way you can say abide by their rules when we don't know what their life is like" (Participant 3) "mix of like some patients have tremendous support and other don't, so, it can feel, it can certainly contribute to burn out. It can certainly contribute to ambivalence about how effective we are . . . when we suspect or worry that many of the recommendations won't be able to be done for the various barriers that the patients are facing" (Participant 5)
Context: Inner/outer (community/health system/organization factors) Outer: Formal policies, previous experiences specific to the hospital Inner: What factors related to the hospital may have influenced the success of prior interventions Organizational level: community hospital, merger with a larger health system, safety net Community and Local: metro/urban area in the northeast, availability of behavioral health resources Healthcare system—neighborhood clinics, relationship with HUP—Spruce	Fractured community resources Long-wait times for mental health connections once discharged to the community Co-located FQCH seen as a strength Great external resources (PMHC) Disconnection between the front line and senior leadership related to the necessary resources to meet patient needs Unequal distribution of resources between hospitals in the same system Overlapping programs and lack of coordination among programs that have similar aims	"I still don't think as a health system we understand how people in this community really live and what they don't have" (Participant 3) "I think the elephant in the room really is how the communication between home health and the hospitals. How can me make that a little bit more fluid" [Participant 8]
Societal factors: Structural and economic factors that may significantly affect healthcare disparities and implementation drivers, including federal or state, or local policies	New CMS policies requiring SDOH screen has increased the focus on health-related social needs and making connections	

Interview participants provided perspectives about the challenges faced by potential Thrive recipients, including unaddressed complex social needs such as high levels of co-occurring SMI and substance-use disorder. Post-discharge barriers were frequently assessed (e.g., lack of housing, transportation, financial concerns, food insecurity), yet connections to community resources, primary care providers, and mental health services were often lacking. Of note, interview participants voiced that eligible patients may be resistant to Thrive services due to fear or mistrust. One case manager noted,

"... you can offer people referrals to community resources, community health workers, substance abuse and they're like 'no'".

"[They] don't want people in their homes. Fear that people are going to judge them".

When speaking to the context of the health system and community connections, participants reported fractured coordination to community resources and a disconnect between the front-line staff and senior leadership. Participants noted the unequal distribution of resources between hospitals within the same system. While simultaneously noting there are overlapping programs and a lack of coordination among those that have similar aims.

"I think the elephant in the room really is how the communication between home health and the hospitals. How can we make that a little bit more fluid" (Case Manager)

Participants also described a disconnect between the context of the community in which patients diagnosed with SMI currently live and the resources they need post-discharge. Another case manager noted,

"I still don't think as a health system we understand how people in this community really live and what they don't have".

FE interview participants also revealed their perceptions of provider-specific factors contributing to transitional care challenges for patients with SMI. Some participants disclosed limited understanding of the social barriers faced by many patients which may influence the way they are able to connect with patients faced with SMI or economic challenges. One case manager noted,

"I think as healthcare workers we have this perception that patients come to us for a service and they should follow our rules and do what we say but that's not life and most of our providers and clinicians and nurses, we can't relate to how they live outside of the hospital so it's no way you can say abide by their rules when we don't know what their life is like".

When considering any barriers or facilitators to implementing Thrive, participants conveyed overwhelming support. They noted that Thrive appeared to be a low-burden addition to their inpatient workflow. Participants noted that Thrive was well-aligned with organizational priorities already in place including reducing readmissions and ED use. Participants were enthusiastic about improving continuity of care through the intervention.

"I really think that having something like this [Thrive], even if you can't save all, you'll be able to save a lot more than what we're able to do now". (Social Worker)

Interview participants were asked to provide their preferences for up to 13 implementation strategies. Proposed strategies and level of endorsement are detailed in Table 5. Of the thirteen potential strategies, six were unanimously endorsed including identifying champions, audit and feedback, quarterly updates with leadership, educational meetings and training, train-the-trainer strategies, and the inclusion of a reminder flag in the EHR. Strategies that received unanimous support from interview participants were discussed during EBQI workgroup meetings and integrated into the launch of the Thrive intervention.

Table 5. Usefulness Ratings of Implementation Strategies.

Proposed Implementation Strategies	Hypothesized Mechanism of Action	Most Useful	Least Useful
Identify and Prepare Champions	People who will dedicate themselves to supporting, marketing, and driving the intervention, overcoming resistance in an organization. Those who expressed curiosity at first and immediately saw the benefit to patients of Thrive.	100%	0
Audit and Feeback to Clinicians	Giving periodic feedback at regular intervals helps monitoring, evaluation, and course correction as needed	100%	0
Quarterly Meetings with Leadership	Align project with strategic initiatives	100%	0
Conduct Educational Meetings	Information dissemination and knowledge on process for patient referral	100%	0
Train the Trainer Strategies	Designating clinicians to train peers makes education accessible and credible	100%	0
EHR Flag in Electronic Medical Record	The flag reminds clinicians to refer to Thrive	100%	0
Develop Academic Partnerships	Bidirectional relationship—research, coordination, data analytic and clinical skills, local knowledge, passion, influence	85.7%	14.3%
Provide Professional Incentives	Making clinician more engaged, feeling fulfilled in the work they do	85.7%	14.3%
Email Reminders Sent after Initial Orientation Training	The email helps clinicians recall training information and act on it	85.7%	14.3%
Use Mass Media: Use of Educational Flyers and Buttons, etc.	Items spread the word about the innovation among clinicians	85.7%	14.3%
Place Info. About Thrive into Hospital-wide Townhall Hosted by CEO or Board Meetings	Influential opinion leader promotes program and shares success	85.7%	14.3%

4. Discussion

Our use of an Evidence-Based Quality Improvement (EBQI) workgroup and Formative Evaluation (FE) approaches allowed us to engage a wide range of stakeholders to inform the adaptation and implementation of Thrive in a new clinical setting. Through this process of participatory engagement, we successfully adapted the Thrive model to suit the needs of Medicaid-insured patients diagnosed with a co-occurring SMI and discharged from a non-psychiatric hospitalization.

Our final adaptation of the Thrive model was informed by the QUERI Roadmap for Implementation and Quality Improvement (2020) which outlines the following steps for adaptation, (1) assessing the fit to ensure that the adaptation of Thrive met the needs of our local setting, (2) assessing the importance of the adaptation to end users, (3) including stakeholders in what and how to adapt Thrive, and (4) making final adaptations prior to launching the trial [21]. The workgroup discussion and interview results conveyed the shared sentiments of perceived value and the need for the services offered through Thrive. Our team sought input from end-users and those affected by SMI to support each step of the adaptation and implementation strategy selection process resulting in the revised Thrive care model.

4.1. THRIVE Final Adapted Model

The adapted Thrive model has several new key processes and core components. The first process includes the conduct of a screening for serious mental illness prior to hospital discharge (see Figure 2). The mental health screen is completed by a Nurse Case Manager or Social Worker and incorporated into the readiness assessment that all patients receive as a part of discharge planning. Next, because mistrust was identified as a potential threat to acceptance as well as a lack of time by social workers and case managers to fully explain the benefits of Thrive, a second process adaptation was added to the Thrive model, namely "bed-side visits', conducted by a Thrive team member. During bed-side visits, the Thrive virtual care coordinator or program manager visits eligible patients during hospital admission to provide an in-depth overview of the Thrive program and to answer any questions. This approach was believed to offer the benefits of more time for engagement and question answering and to relay experiences of prior Thrive participants. In addition to bedside visits, case managers and social workers reported other strategies to engage and increase trust among patients with SMI. They incorporate normalizing questions about mental health as routine, like other physical health-related questions. They also encouraged patients to exercise their agency in centering their personal goals in the discharge planning process. Finally, a key core component to the Thrive model includes the inclusion of a comprehensive behavioral health assessment during weekly virtual case conferences. This additional assessment by the Thrive care team includes a careful review of all mental health diagnoses and psychiatric medications, including the last date filled and the prescriber. A note with this information is sent to the social worker and the need for further mental health intervention is reviewed. The level of connection to a current mental health provider is assessed and, if needed, referrals for mental health support are provided.

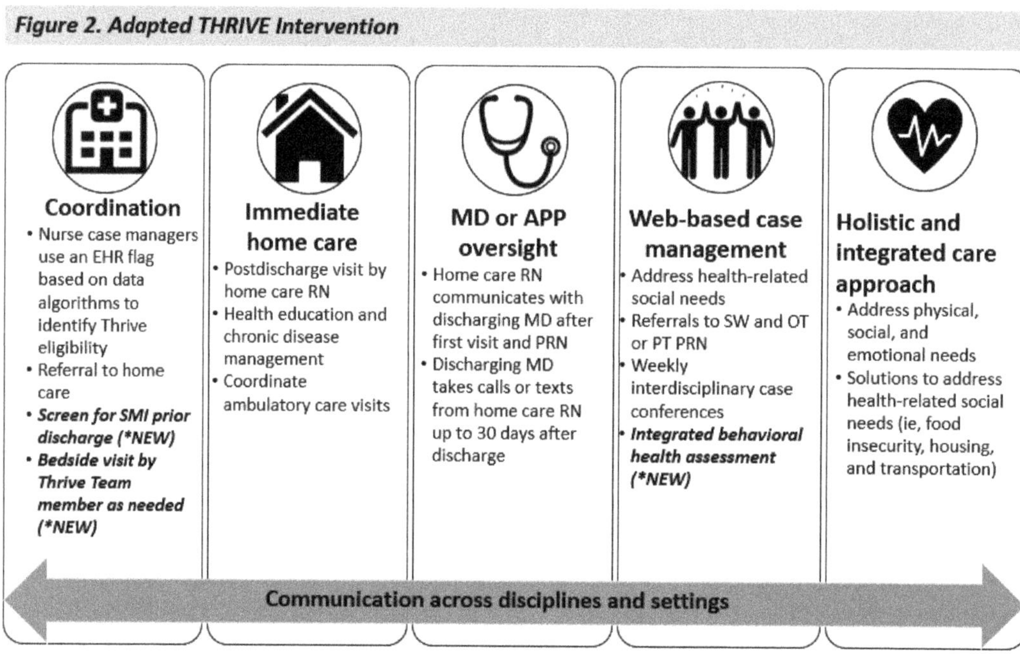

Figure 2. Adapted from Brooks Carthon et al. "Transitional care innovation for Medicaid-insured individuals: early findings" [15].

Finally, consistent with recent calls for integrating implementation science and readiness for change into pre-trial planning [36–38], our FE and EBQI workgroup helped guide the use of implementation strategies to implement and support the successful launch of this study. Of note, selected implementation strategies included the following: identifying and preparing champions who were defined as dedicated clinicians embedded in the health system that could support, market, and drive the Thrive intervention. These individuals were viewed as stakeholders who could help overcome resistance in the organization. For our purposes, a Social Work Manager was selected as a Thrive champion who would bring Thrive up during daily team meetings and help to answer any questions raised by colleagues. A second implementation strategy included providing audit and feedback sessions to clinicians monthly. This feedback was viewed as a useful way to monitor, evaluate, and course correct as needed. Quarterly meetings with health system leadership were also endorsed as a way to ensure that the project remains aligned with strategic initiatives. The addition of interactive and educational meetings with staff involved in implementing Thrive—using train the trainer sessions—to facilitate Thrive peer training were offered to ensure training was accessible and credible. Finally, the inclusion of an EHR Thrive reminder flag was endorsed by all participants as a tool to embed a reminder into usual workflows.

4.2. Limitations

There are several limitations to our use of EBQI and FE approaches. First, we were limited to individuals connected to a single hospital and homecare setting situated in a large northeast setting. Hence, the perspectives of necessary resources, challenges, and necessary Thrive adaptations and implementation strategies may vary by clinical setting and geographical region. However, future research should be multi-site to increase generalizability and could consider adapting the Thrive model for patients experiencing a psychiatric hospitalization. Finally, we conducted a relatively small number of FE interviews. Interviewing a larger number, though not necessary for qualitative research, could have nonetheless yielded deeper insights on implementation processes and perceived barriers.

5. Conclusions

Our use of a rigorous pre-implementation process helped adapt the nurse-led Thrive transitional care model for people who are economically disadvantaged and diagnosed with a serious mental illness. These participatory approaches helped engage individuals with diverse viewpoints and resulted in intervention and implementation strategies, that are person-centered and tailored to the organizational context.

Author Contributions: Conceptualization, J.M.B.C., H.B., P.Z.C. and A.P.B.; Methodology, J.M.B.C., H.B. and A.P.B.; Formal Analysis, J.M.B.C., K.E.A. and H.B.; Data Curation, J.M.B.C., K.E.A. and H.B.; Writing—Original Draft Preparation, J.M.B.C., C.T., P.Z.C., A.P.B., K.E.A., E.B. and H.B.; Writing—Review and Editing, J.M.B.C., C.T., P.Z.C., A.P.B., K.E.A., E.B. and H.B.; Funding Acquisition, J.M.B.C. All authors have read and agreed to the published version of the manuscript.

Funding: This work was supported by the Agency for Healthcare Research and Quality under Grant number 1R18HS029815 (Brooks Carthon PI); and the National Institute of Nursing Research under Grant number T32-NR-007104 (McHugh, PI).

Institutional Review Board Statement: This study was conducted according to the guidelines of the Declaration of Helsinki and approved by the Institutional Review Board of the University of Pennsylvania (IRB #8, Protocol 854422 on 4 October 2023), including a HIPAA waiver of informed consent for clinical data derived from the EHR.

Informed Consent Statement: Informed consent was obtained from all subjects involved in this study.

Data Availability Statement: We will preserve and share de-identified data products with the Inter-university Consortium for Political and Social Research (ICPSR) data repository. We will follow the comprehensive de-identification standards set forth in the ICPSR "Guide to Social Science and Data Preparation and Archiving, 6th Ed" for both quantitative and qualitative data, including the removal of any direct identifiers, date-shifting of indirect identifiers (e.g., dates of service), creating pseudonyms, and collapsing/combining variables that might potentially be identifiable (e.g., clinician roles) in the context of the entire qualitative transcript corpus.

Public Involvement Statement: No public involvement in any aspect of this research.

Guidelines and Standards Statement: This manuscript was drafted against the Standards for Reporting Implementation Studies (StaRI) Statement for reporting implementation science studies (Pinnock, H.; Barwick, M.; Carpenter, C.R.; Eldridge, S.; Grandes, G.; Griffiths, C.J.; Rycroft-Malone, J.; Meissner, P.; Murray, E.; Patel, A.; et al. Standards for Reporting Implementation Studies (StaRI) statement. *BMJ* **2017**, *356*, i6795).

Use of Artificial Intelligence: AI or AI-assisted tools were not used in drafting any aspect of this manuscript.

Conflicts of Interest: The authors declare no conflicts of interest. Research reported in this publication was supported by the National Institute of Nursing Research of the National Institutes of Health under Award Number T32NR007104. The content is solely the responsibility of the authors and does not necessarily represent the official views of the National Institutes of Health. The authors report no competing interests to declare. The authors have no other competing interests to declare.

References

1. National Institute of Mental Health. Mental Illness. 2023. Available online: https://www.nimh.nih.gov/health/statistics/mental-illness#part_2538 (accessed on 6 July 2023).
2. Zur, J.; Musumeci, M.; Garfield, R. *Medicaid's Role in Financing Behavioral Health Services for Low-Income Individuals*; The Henry J. Kaiser Family Foundation: Menlo Park, CA, USA, 2017.
3. McDermott, K.W.; Elixhauser, A.; Sun, R. Trends in hospital inpatient stays in the United States, 2005–2014: Statistical brief # 225. *Healthcare Cost Util. Proj.* **2017**, *24*, 1–18.
4. Ferro, E.G.; Secemsky, E.A.; Wadhera, R.K.; Choi, E.; Strom, J.B.; Wasfy, J.H.; Wang, Y.; Shen, C.; Yeh, R.W. Patient readmission rates for all insurance types after implementation of the hospital readmissions reduction program. *Health Aff.* **2019**, *38*, 585–593. [CrossRef] [PubMed]
5. Boutwell, A.; Maxwell, J.; Bourgoin, A.; Genetti, S.; John Snow Inc.; Collaborative Healthcare Strategies, Inc. (Eds.) *Hospital Guide to Reducing Medicaid Readmissions*; Agency for Healthcare Research and Quality: Rockville, MD, USA, 2014.
6. Singer, A.J.; Thode, H.C.; Pines, J.M. US Emergency Department Visits and Hospital Discharges Among Uninsured Patients Before and After Implementation of the Affordable Care Act. *JAMA Netw. Open* **2019**, *2*, e192662. [CrossRef] [PubMed]
7. Germack, H.D.; Mahmoud, K.; Cooper, M.; Vincent, H.; Koller, K.; Martsolf, G.R. Community Socioeconomic Disadvantage Drives Type of 30-day Medical-Surgical Revisits Among Patients with Serious Mental Illness. *BMC Health Serv. Res.* **2021**, *21*, 1–9. [CrossRef]
8. Shim, R.S.; Druss, B.G.; Zhang, S.; Kim, G.; Oderinde, A.; Shoyinka, S.; Rust, G. Emergency department utilization among Medicaid beneficiaries with schizophrenia and diabetes: The consequences of increasing medical complexity. *Schizophrenia* **2014**, *152*, 490–497. [CrossRef]
9. Baicker, K.; Allen, H.L.; Wright, B.J.; Taubman, S.L.; Finkelstein, A.N. The effect of Medicaid on management of depression: Evidence from the Oregon Health Insurance Experiment. *Milbank Q.* **2018**, *96*, 29–56. [CrossRef]
10. Jiang, H.J.; Boutwell, A.E.; Maxwell, J.; Bourgoin, A.; Regenstein, M.; Andres, E. Understanding patient, provider, and system factors related to Medicaid readmissions. *Jt. Comm. J. Qual. Patient Saf.* **2016**, *42*, 115–121. [CrossRef]
11. Medicare Payment Advisory Commission; Medicaid and CHIP Payment and Access Commission. *Data Book: Beneficiaries Dually Eligible for Medicare and Medicaid*; MACPAC: Washington, DC, USA, 2018.
12. Tepper, M.C.; Cohen, A.M.; Progovac, A.M.; Ault-Brutus, A.; Leff, H.S.; Mullin, B.; Cunningham, C.M.; Cook, B.L. Mind the gap: Developing an integrated behavioral health home to address health disparities in serious mental illness. *Psychiatr. Serv.* **2017**, *68*, 1217–1224. [CrossRef]
13. Brooks Carthon, J.; Brom, H.; Kim, V.; Hedgeland, T.; Ponietowicz, E.; Cacchione, P. How innovation and design thinking can improve care. *Am. Nurse. J.* **2021**, *16*, 30–33.
14. Jones, C.P. Levels of racism: A theoretic framework and a gardener's tale. *Am. J. Public Health* **2000**, *90*, 1212.
15. Brooks Carthon, J.M.; Brom, H.; French, R.; Daus, M.; Grantham-Murillo, M.; Bennett, J.; Ryskina, K.; Ponietowicz, E.; Cacchione, P. Transitional care innovation for Medicaid-insured individuals: Early findings. *BMJ Open Qual.* **2022**, *11*, e001798. [CrossRef] [PubMed]
16. Nikpour, J.; Langston, C.; Brom, H.; Sliwinski, K.; Mason, A.; Garcia, D.; Grantham-Murillo, M.; Bennett, J.; Cacchione, P.Z.; Brooks Carthon, J.M. Determining the Post Discharge Care Needs of Medicaid-Insured Adults with Co-occurring Chronic Medical and Serious Mental Illnesses. *J. Nurs. Care Qual.* **2025**, *40*, 76–83. [CrossRef] [PubMed]
17. Germack, H.D.; Weissinger, G.; Bizhanova, Z.; Martsolf, G.R. Psychiatric medication changes associated with increased rate of medical readmissions in patients with serious mental illness. *J. Nerv. Ment. Dis.* **2021**, *209*, 66–173. [CrossRef]
18. Cook, J.A.; Burke-Miller, J.K.; Razzano, L.A.; Steigman, P.J.; Jonikas, J.A.; Santos, A. Serious mental illness, other mental health disorders, and outpatient health care as predictors of 30-day readmissions following medical hospitalization. *Gen. Hosp. Psychiatry* **2021**, *70*, 10–17. [CrossRef]

19. Browne, J.; Rudolph, J.L.; Jiang, L.; Bayer, T.A.; Kunicki, Z.J.; De Vito, A.N.; Bozzay, M.L.; McGeary, J.E.; Kelso, C.M.; Wu, W.-C. Serious mental illness is associated with elevated risk of hospital readmission in veterans with heart failure. *J. Psychosom. Res.* **2024**, *178*, 111604. [CrossRef]
20. Brom, H.; Sliwinski, K.; Amenyedor, K.; Carthon, J.M.B. Transitional care programs to improve the post-discharge experience of patients with multiple chronic conditions and co-occurring serious mental illness: A scoping review. *Gen. Hosp. Psychiatry* **2024**, *15*, 106–114. [CrossRef]
21. Brooks Carthon, J.; Brom, H.; Amenydor, K.A.; Harhay, M.; Grantham-Murillo, M.; Nikpour, J.; Lasater, K.B.; Golinelli, D.; Cacchione, P.; Bettencourt, A. Transitional Care Support for Medicaid Insured Patients with Serious Mental Illness: A Type 1 Hybrid Effectiveness Implementation Stepped-Wedge Cluster Randomized Trial. *JMIR Res. Protoc.* **2024**, *12*, e64575. [CrossRef]
22. Thrive: Transforming Healthcare Equity. Available online: https://thrive-care.org/ (accessed on 19 November 2024).
23. Goodrich, D.E.; Miake-Lye, I.; Braganza, M.Z.; Wawrin, N.; Kilbourne, A.M. *The QUERI Roadmap for Implementation and Quality Improvement Pre-Implementation—The QUERI Roadmap for Implementation and Quality Improvement—NCBI Bookshelf*; Department of Veterans Affairs (US): Washington DC, USA. Available online: www.nih.gov (accessed on 5 September 2024).
24. Wiltsey Stirman, S.; Gamarra, J.M.; Bartlett, B.A.; Calloway, A.; Gutner, C.A. Empirical examinations of modifications and adaptations to evidence-based psychotherapies: Methodologies, impact, and future directions. *Clin. Psychol. Sci. Pract.* **2017**, *24*, 396.
25. Koenig, C.J.; Abraham, T.; Zamora, K.A.; Hill, C.; Kelly, P.A.; Uddo, M.; Hamilton, M.; Pyne, J.M.; Seal, K.H. Pre-implementation strategies to adapt and implement a veteran peer coaching intervention to improve mental health treatment engagement among rural veterans. *J. Rural. Health* **2016**, *32* (Suppl. S2), S418–S428. [CrossRef]
26. Stetler, C.B.; Legro, M.W.; Wallace, C.M.; Bowman, C.; Guihan, M.; Hagedorn, H.; Kimmel, B.; Sharp, N.D.; Smith, J.L. The role of formative evaluation in implementation research and the QUERI experience. *J. Gen. Intern. Med.* **2006**, *21*, S1–S8. [CrossRef]
27. Woodward, E.N.; Singh, R.S.; Ndebele-Ngwenya, P.; Melgar Castillo, A.; Dickson, K.S.; Kirchner, J.E. A more practical guide to incorporating health equity domains in implementation determinant frameworks. *Implement. Sci. Commun.* **2021**, *2*, 61. [CrossRef] [PubMed]
28. Palinkas, L.A.; Horwitz, S.M.; Green, C.A.; Wisdom, J.P.; Duan, N.; Hoagwood, K. Purposeful sampling for qualitative data collection and analysis in mixed method implementation research. *Adm. Policy Ment. Health Ment. Health Serv. Res.* **2015**, *42*, 533–544. [CrossRef] [PubMed]
29. Malterud, K.; Siersma, V.D.; Guassora, A.D. Sample size in qualitative interview studies: Guided by information power. *Qual. Health Res.* **2016**, *26*, 1753–1760. [CrossRef] [PubMed]
30. Weiner, B.J.; Lewis, C.C.; Stanick, C.; Powell, B.J.; Dorsey, C.N.; Clary, A.S.; Boynton, M.H.; Halko, H. Psychometric assessment of three newly developed implementation outcome measures. *Implement. Sci.* **2017**, *12*, 1–12. [CrossRef] [PubMed]
31. Shea, C.M.; Jacobs, S.R.; Esserman, D.A.; Bruce, K.; Weiner, B.J. Organizational readiness for implementing change: A psychometric assessment of a new measure. *Implement. Sci.* **2014**, *9*, 1–15. [CrossRef] [PubMed]
32. Nevedal, A.L.; Reardon, C.M.; Opra Widerquist, M.A.; Jackson, G.L.; Cutrona, S.L.; White, B.S.; Damschroder, L.J. Rapid versus traditional qualitative analysis using the Consolidated Framework for Implementation Research (CFIR). *Implement. Sci.* **2021**, *16*, 67. [CrossRef]
33. Hamilton, A.B.; Finley, E.P. Qualitative methods in implementation research: An introduction. *Psychiatry Res.* **2019**, *280*, 112516. [CrossRef]
34. Hamilton AB. Qualitative Methods in Rapid Turn-Around Health Services Research. PowerPoint Present 2013 VA HSRD Cyberseminar Spotlight Womens Health. Published Online 2013. Available online: www.hsrd.research.va.gov/for_researchers/cyber_seminars/archives/video_archive.cfm?SessionID=780 (accessed on 16 November 2020).
35. Guba, E.G. Criteria for assessing the trustworthiness of naturalistic inquiries. *ECTJ* **1981**, *29*, 75–91. [CrossRef]
36. Watson, A.K.; Hernandez, B.F.; Kolodny-Goetz, J.; Walker, T.J.; Lamont, A.; Imm, P.; Wandersman, A.; Fernandez, M.E. Using implementation mapping to build organizational readiness. *Front. Public Health* **2022**, *10*, 904652. [CrossRef]
37. Kowalski, C.P.; Kawentel, L.M.; Kyriakides, T.C.; Davis, L.; Bowersox, N.W.; Kilbourne, A.M.; Huang, G.D.; Nevedal, A.L. Facilitating future implementation and translation to clinical practice: The Implementation Planning Assessment Tool for clinical trials. *J. Clin. Transl. Sci.* **2022**, *6*, e131. [CrossRef]
38. Stensland, K.D.; Sales, A.E.; Damschroder, L.J.; Skolarus, T.A. Applying implementation frameworks to the clinical trial context. *Implement. Sci. Commun.* **2022**, *3*, 109. [CrossRef] [PubMed]

nursing reports

MDPI

Article

Knowing, Being and Becoming a Person-Centred Nurse Leader: Findings from a Transformative Professional Development Programme

Clare Cable [1], Tanya McCance [2] and Brendan McCormack [3,*]

1 Queen's Nursing Institute Scotland, Edinburgh EH1 2EL, UK; clare.cable@qnis.org.uk
2 Institute of Nursing and Health Research, Ulster University, Belfast BT15 1AP, Northern Ireland, UK; tv.mccance@ulster.ac.uk
3 Sydney Nursing School, Faculty of Medicine and Health, University of Sydney, Camperdown, NSW 2006, Australia
* Correspondence: brendan.mccormack@sydney.edu.au

Abstract: *Background/Objectives* Leadership is central to the development of effective workplace cultures and as such should be viewed as a practice that is relational, exercised through a process of mutual and reciprocal influence. Person-centred leadership is an approach to leadership that supports a way of being that is authentic, prioritising values lived out in action. However, there is an increasing recognition that leadership development has not been impactful in relation to workplace culture. This paper reports on the ongoing evaluation of an innovative development programme (Queen's Nurse Development Programme), the overall aim of which was to illuminate the participants' experiences of engaging in transformative learning and development and identify the technical and transformative outcomes arising. The programme focused on developing leadership capacity for societal change and maximising the health impact of community nursing leaders. *Methods* The methodological framework for evaluation was underpinned by a Collaborative Critical Creative Inquiry. Twenty community nurses were selected to undertake the programme during 2020. The collection and analysis of data was consistent with the Collaborative Critical Creative Inquiry and was conducted as a one-day workshop, with participants engaged in a cycle of creative hermeneutic analysis. *Results* A total of seven themes were identified, including: sense of belonging; personal growth; developing new skills; finding voice; importance of self-care; and creating a safe place. This illuminated how the transformative learning and development processes within this programme were experienced and how these enabled participants to explore how they influence their practice and workplace. It is the journey with self that generates a sense of belonging and enables personal growth and the ability to care for self and others. *Conclusions* The key learning from this innovative development programme is the importance of focusing on the attributes of practitioners and the key building blocks for knowing, being, and becoming a person-centred practitioner.

Keywords: community nursing; leadership; transformative practices; person-centred practice; collaborative inquiry

1. Introduction

Person-centredness is a global movement in healthcare because it reflects the importance of keeping people at the centre of healthcare systems. It prioritises the human experience and places compassion, dignity and humanistic caring principles at the centre of planning and decision making and is translated through relationships that are built on effective interpersonal processes. A unique perspective of person-centredness can be viewed through the lens of the person-centred practice framework developed by McCance and McCormack [1], which is a theoretical model developed from practice, for use in practice.

Nurs. Rep. **2024**, *14*, 3165–3177. https://doi.org/10.3390/nursrep14040230 https://www.mdpi.com/journal/nursrep

This framework enables the articulation of the dynamic nature of person-centredness, recognising complexity at different levels within healthcare systems, and identifies healthfulness as THE outcome arising from the development of person-centred workplace cultures. Healthfulness means ensuring that the environment in which healthcare is experienced places individual health and the wellbeing of all persons as the core concern.

Leadership is central to the development of effective workplace cultures, and as such, should be viewed as a practice that is relational, exercised through a process of mutual and reciprocal influence [2]. Person-centred leadership is described as a "complex, dynamic, relational and contextually embedded practice that fosters healthful relationships and growth" [3]. This is an approach to leadership that supports a way of being that is authentic, prioritising values lived out in action. Enghiad et al. [4], in a recent integrative literature review exploring clinical leadership in long term care, confirmed the influence of a leader's beliefs and values on the motivation for providing high-quality care. Therefore, it is not surprising that leadership development is complex and context dependent, particularly so for nurses who are directly involved in providing care. In a recent systematic review focusing on nurses' clinical leadership in a hospital setting, Guibert-Lacasa and Vazquez-Calatayud [5] concluded that interventions for leadership skill development required cognitive, interpersonal and intrinsic competences. They proposed the development of multicomponent programmes to address these aspects, including psychological empowerment skills, emotional intelligence and critical reflexivity.

There is an increasing recognition that leadership development has not been impactful in relation to workplace cultures. Some of the reasons for this were presented in a discussion paper by Edmonstone [6] and included assumptions that leadership is context free and there is over-emphasis on competence rather than capacity. Furthermore, Edmonstone suggests there is a focus on the development of individual leaders as opposed to leadership and highlights the importance of leadership development for social capital and the need to view leadership as a practice-based activity. The programme described in this paper was established with this challenge in mind and deliberately set out with a focus on developing leadership capacity for societal change and maximising the health impact of community nursing leaders. So, the emphasis shifted from leadership development to a transformative development programme with a focus on individual transformation for social change in communities with a focus on health and wellbeing.

The Queen's Nursing Institute Scotland (QNIS) is a charitable organisation that is founded on a commitment to enable nurses to make a positive difference in communities, with a focus on maximising the potential of nursing for social justice. In recognition of the need to develop enhanced 'change-making' skills in community nurses, the organisation designed a programme underpinned by the QNIS Excellence Profile, which focuses on helping participants to develop excellence qualities relating to: inspiring others by making a difference; inspiring others with tenacity and resilience; inspiring others by bringing people with them; and inspiring others with humility and reflection. Two complementary theoretical frameworks were chosen to inform the programme design: theory U [7] and the person-centred practice framework [1]. In a previous paper, McCormack et al. [8], described the programme in more detail and the links between theory U and the person-centred practice framework:

"Like Theory U, person-centred practice requires us to connect with our inner selves as human beings with feelings, emotions, thoughts and desires that guide us as persons. It is the sum of these that guide us towards 'that which really matters' and a connection with our unique humanness as persons—our embodied knowing" (p. 4).

To co-create healthful cultures, the Queen's Nurse Development Programme invites participants on a journey of awareness-based systems change, which is transformational. This is beautifully captured in theory U, which sets out the journey that we are to make, individually and collectively, to sense the emerging future. It requires learning new ways of sensing, using all five senses, and a deepening awareness. Theory U sets out a set of principles that can be presented as five movements that follow the path of the U, including:

co-initiating, co-sensing, co-presencing, co-creating, and co-evolving. The programme is structured as a nine-month journey of discovery, weaving together residential workshops, individual co-active coaching (through an individually assigned coach) [9], with an issue for development, which the participants explore as they become their best selves as skilled facilitators of change.

This programme began in March 2020, the year when COVID-19 redefined ways of working. It has been recognised that during the pandemic, community nurses went above and beyond, continuing to care for the most vulnerable and frail citizens wherever they lived. Some nurses were working in full PPE for over a year, sweating through long shifts encased in plastic, donning and doffing dozens of times a day, struggling with flimsy aprons outside in the wind and rain, working behind visors and steamed up spectacles. Others spent hours on the phone on videoconferencing systems trying to connect with people who were isolated and anxious and on MS Teams negotiating to ensure the needs of their teams and communities were met. This made relationships more complex and brought significant stresses and challenges that impacted on leadership practices.

This paper reports on the ongoing evaluation of this innovative development programme and builds on the outcomes reported in an initial evaluation [8]. This paper provides insights into the impact of the programme, on individuals, their practice, and more widely within their teams and the communities where they work.

2. Methods

The overall aim for the programme evaluation was stated as follows:

To illuminate the participants' experiences of engaging in transformative learning and development, and to identify the technical and transformative outcomes arising.

The methodological framework for evaluation was underpinned by a collaborative critical creative inquiry (CCCI) methodology. A CCCI methodology combines collaborative inquiry [10] with critical creativity [11]. Critical creativity combines being critical with being creative, i.e., integrating cognitive critique with creative practices. This framework is based on key theoretical and methodological assumptions that have a primary focus on human flourishing as both a process and outcome. The aim that guided this component of the evaluation was as follows:

To understand if and how the transformative learning and development processes experienced have enabled participants to create the conditions required for their continued flourishing as community nurses.

The focus was primarily on the impact of the programme on individuals, their practice, and their wider communities. More specifically, it focused on the following evaluation objectives as outlined in the evaluation framework:

1. Understand the influence of the programme in shaping and informing individual and collective development.
2. Determine the technical and transformative outcomes arising from participation in the programme.
3. Build an ongoing body of knowledge about transformative learning and development, its impact on individual and collective action, and the contexts that sustain it.

2.1. Selection of Participants

Twenty community nurses were selected to undertake this transformational development programme during 2020. Following nomination by the executive lead in their organisation, which ensures employer support from the outset, each nominee submitted a written application. A selection panel shortlisted the candidates to be invited for the second stage. Shortlisted candidates attended a selection day that included focus groups and multiple mini-interviews. The focus was on in-depth exploration of the quality of the match between each candidate and the Excellence Profile developed by QNIS.

2.2. Data Collection and Analysis

The data collected in this project consisted of three types of data, constituting the everyday inquiry records maintained by participants—creative expressions, reflective diaries and journals, and project notes of specific discussions. These methods are described in detail elsewhere [8]. Throughout the programme, the participants retained their own data in an 'evidence folio' provided by the programme leaders and were asked to bring their folio of evidence to the data analysis workshop. They were also asked to anonymise any data they wished to and redact any data they did not feel comfortable sharing with others. In this way, participants retained control of their data and its analysis. The analysis of data was consistent with CCCI and was conducted as a one-day workshop. The participants engaged in a cycle of creative hermeneutic analysis focusing on the key questions below:

(i) What impact has the programme had on your practice and workplace?
(ii) How did the programme content enable you to deal with uncertainty, anxiety and trauma through the pandemic?

The critical creative hermeneutic process followed the steps outlined in Figure 1, which was adapted from the data analysis described in the Evaluation Framework [8]. Participants worked as a whole group (all 20 participants), in small groups of 6–7 people, in dyads and as individuals as they moved through the steps of data analysis. All of the data sources were revisited to provide a robust audit trail for the common themes identified through the critical creative hermeneutic process. A detailed data extraction process was developed and following review of the outcomes from this process, further refinement was undertaken by the authors of this paper and a final set of themes was generated as described in the results section of this paper.

2.3. Ethical Considerations

This collaborative enquiry was underpinned by a robust ethical framework that reflected the principles of person-centred research and was embedded throughout the delivery and evaluation of the programme, which, consistent with the underpinning values of collaborative inquiry and the shared values of the development programme, participants hold one another accountable for working with and adhering to these shared values. The key ethical considerations in undertaking this component of the evaluation focused on: ensuring voluntary participation; assuring anonymity and confidentiality for participants where appropriate; and ensuring the psychological safety of participants throughout the process. Participants were informed of the purpose of the evaluation workshop in advance, enabling individuals to decide if they wished to participate. Ways of working had already been established for the group and were also used as the basis for conducting the workshop. This addressed issues of negotiating anonymity and confidentiality and ensuring participants engaged in self-care if the workshop revealed issues that were potentially distressing or upsetting. For these reasons, formal ethics approval was not sought for this evaluation, as was the case for the initial evaluation [8], the rationale being that evaluation is integral to the programme.

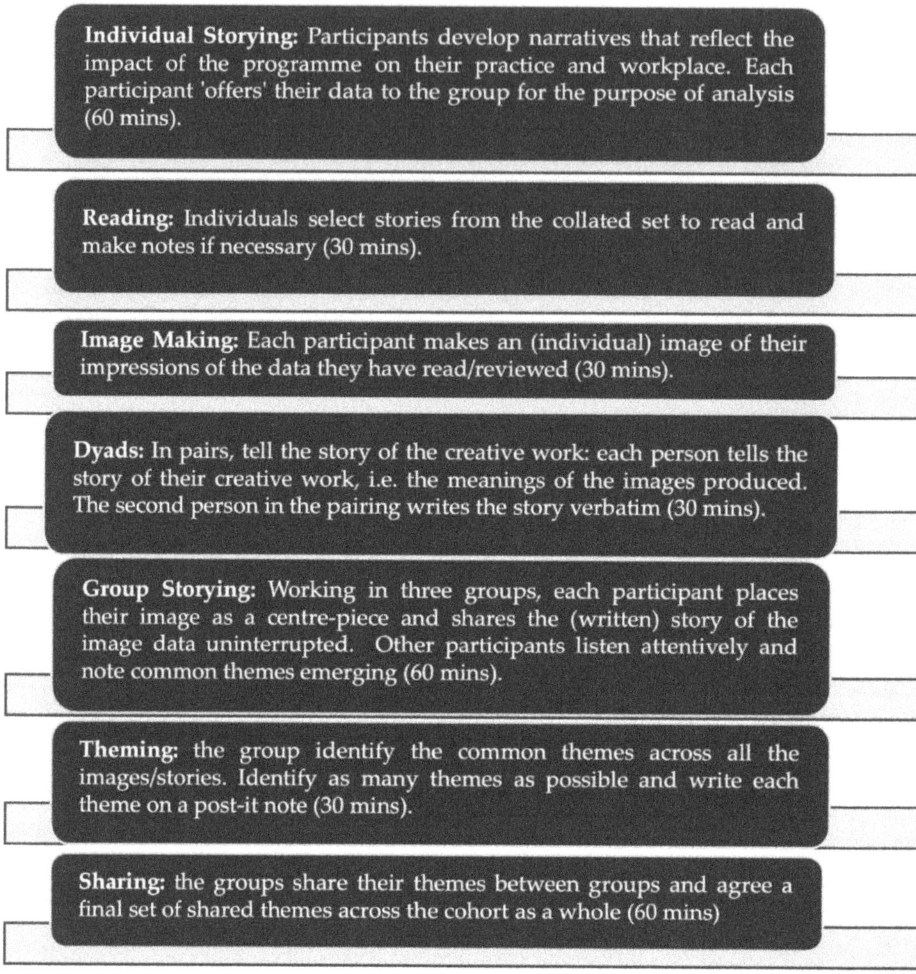

Figure 1. Overview of Collaborative Critical Creative Inquiry (CCCI) Methodology.

3. Results

A total of seven themes were identified, which illuminated how the transformative learning and development processes within the Queen's Nurse Programme were experienced and how these enabled participants to explore how they influenced their practice and workplace. The findings also provide insights into how the participants' journeys were experienced in the context of the ongoing pandemic. The themes are presented in Figure 2, and each is discussed in turn below. The audit trail supporting the themes is drawn from the different stages of the CCCI methodology presented in Figure 1.

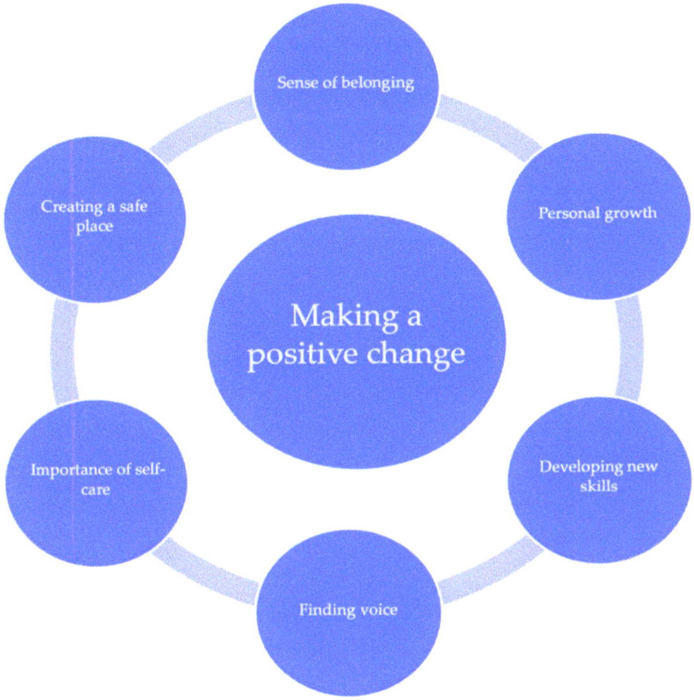

Figure 2. Overview of themes.

3.1. Sense of Belonging

The Queen's Nurse Development Programme offered a space for participants to link with like-minded practitioners who understood the role of a community nurse. Being seen by others was central to this theme: "Others see us as different, we see each other" (Participant 4). Linked to this was the freedom to be their authentic self back in the workplace.

> "It also allowed us as Queens Nurses not to wear a different mask. With all these tools allows a sense of togetherness and (other) staff a sense of involvement" (Participant 7)

For some, they felt isolated and had lost their identity as a nurse, but the programme provided an opportunity to reaffirm their passion for nursing and develop an appreciation of the breadth of skills and expertise held by community nurses, and the types of environments in which they work.

> "But realising being part of a team of QNIS nurses, who always have your back, helped me become the leader I am today and the passion to continue to be the best I can be and to take others with me along the way". (Story 1)

3.2. Personal Growth

The opportunity for participants to explore self in the context of their own professional development was central to the experience within the Queen's Nurse Development Programme. The gift of being able to take time out, to slow down and to reflect enabled exploration of what was important and how this related to self-knowing. Participants talked about the different roles they undertook, personally and professionally, but self knowledge offered clarity on what was important and the ability to be authentic.

> "The program starts a deep reflection within who am I how can I make a difference. Speakers who inspire, strong people who know who they are and are "compassionate" A question to develop and probe into my core. What is important to me, how can I influence, support, develop, be true to myself, but open to opportunity as they arise". (Story 9)

> "Prior to becoming a Queens nurse, I had real struggles with my own identity and professional direction. Honestly not really knowing who "the real me" was, and feeling like I wore different "masks" for my different roles as: mum, wife, nurse, friend, colleague, daughter . . . I am now a confident practitioner who has greater understanding of the impact I have in others. Importantly, I no longer feel like I need to wear masks, I have an understanding of who I am and realise I now quite like who that person is". (Story 5)

Having a personal coach to facilitate this process was a further enabler in the process, and supported exploration of self, in the context of being a community nurse.

> "Time out for me to stand back and reflect. I have been 10 years in this post and hit the ground running and now it's like my treadmill emergency button has been pulled with stillness and calmness. Leisurely walks picking flowers. This was not easy to begin with trying to restart the treadmill at times. Wow! Permission to focus on me! Coaching? My own coach!" (Story 4)

3.3. Developing New Skills

The development of new skills was frequently referenced by participants. Elements core to the programme included reflection and deep listening. The development of these skills was directly connected to the ability to approach issues differently in the workplace. One participant described how she worked differently to support her team during the pandemic, drawing on the skill of deep listening. Creating a safe space to engage in meaningful dialogue, focusing on issues that were important to the team, led to a more bonded team dynamic.

> *"I very quickly recognised, what I had to do, it was my responsibility as deputy manager at the time to use what skill I had learned the week before with QNIS to support my staff team. The first thing I done was set up twice weekly huddle meetings. This allowed me a platform to create a safe space for staff to attend. The staff initially thought this was a space to receive updates about the pandemic and while it did do that, I also had another agenda—to use one of the practises I had learned at the beginning of my QNIS journey. I began by truly and deeply listening to the staff each week learning what they were feeling and using the time to enable them to fully express themselves where they had my full attention. This enabled me to support them to find their own coping strategies. We spent time talking at length. I showed my own fears and worries in a professional manner, this helped us all bond as a team". (Story 13)*

Using skills from the programme, however, was not always easy for participants. One of them describes a sense of distrust from colleagues when she tried a different approach, which was fuelled by lack of motivation and low morale. The importance of using processes that enabled collaboration with all members of the team was an enabler in achieving a positive outcome.

> "On reflection, there are a lot of things I would have done differently, quicker, in a more meaningful way . . . Using the skills, I had learned at the QNIS programme was difficult at first. Because of staff's experiences, they were fearful, did not want to put trust in me and lacked motivation and enthusiasm for their work. It took a year to build the team back up and "bring them with me". With support from our new manager, I used deep listening, reflection, collaboration and sharing my vulnerabilities with them to allow them to start to trust again and open up". (Story 16)

3.4. Finding Voice

Many participants felt that they had found their voice as a result of engaging with the Queen's Nurse Development Programme. This was particularly important in the context of the pandemic and its impact on staff morale and the need to create a supportive working environment.

This was linked to having the confidence to speak up and to be heard, and to challenge when decisions were being made that did not prioritise people.

> "But it also gave me my voice to go back and challenge decisions that were being made. At this time staff were being deployed into areas where they were not required, our service was struggling as a result". (Story 6)

Those who found their voice described the positive impact on the workplace.

> "I have found my voice and no longer struggle to tell the people how I am feeling. I prioritise myself in order to get the best out of myself and my staff and this directly affects patient care, staff well-being and a safe workplace culture". (Story 7)

Linked to the theme of finding voice was the sense of being brave and taking risks. Examples of being brave provided by participants often related to delivery of the service and in response to the needs of patients, families and of staff. In these situations, the context was often challenging, exacerbated by the pandemic, requiring courage to voice concerns and take positive action.

> "I carried on with my journaling and coaching and self-care practices. Through my reflection it hit me how fortunate I had been to have just been immersed in QNIS in Balbirnie pre-lockdown. I had been trying to raise an issue with regards waiting times and a review of service for the last 4 years. I now had time to prepare and present this again. Lots of questions. Is this wrong at a time when people are immersed in managing COVID. So, I did it, resubmitted it again! To my amazement it was approved and at last those that need to have this awareness were activated in reviewing the service and making it fit for purpose and robust". (Story 4)

3.5. Importance of Self-Care

Fundamental to the Queen's Nurse Development Programme is the necessity to care for self. The development of this awareness and tools to support the ability to engage in self-care were highly valued by participants. It underlined the importance of being able to look after self in order to show care towards others.

> "Commencing the QN programme in March 2020, I felt guilty at being away from the workplace. I didn't feel worthy of my nomination. Participating in all aspects of the programme has allowed me to recognise the importance of self care in order to achieve effective outcomes. And it wasn't until December 2020 when I really understood and experienced the consequences of not looking after myself ... My coach supported me to recognise that I am an emotionally connected leader that is able to tune into others. I have my values at the fore throughout my work/practice and I no longer let work/workload/stress define me". (Story 7)

The importance of self-care became even more prominent in the midst of the pandemic. Participants offered examples of not only engaging in their own self care practices, but also supporting others to do the same. One participant describes how they implemented several practices with staff that were drawn for the programme and the positive impact experienced as a result.

> "We looked at ways to focus on our own self care—putting our oxygen mask on so that we could then be there for our residents, bringing the best versions of ourselves every time we stepped into support with any resident care. We

> explored all kinds of ways as a team to practice self care. I even got them to do the leadership dance—some of the staff really enjoyed this while others thought I was a bit bonkers. Anyway, through doing this every week staff began to fell truly valued and appreciated, it enabled everyone to be heard and processes to be implemented to help everyone. I even implemented a wobble room for staff to go to if they needed this. The feedback from this was that staff felt this was a very safe space and were comfortable to use it because of the bonding we had through our weekly huddle meetings". (Story 13)

3.6. Creating a Safe Place

Participants recognised that creating a safe space was an enabler to how they could engage with staff using the new skills they had developed in the Queen's Nurse Development Programme. There was an appreciation of how the facilitators of the programme had created a safe space for them and how instrumental this was to their personal growth. This, in turn, equipped them to create a safe space for their team. One participant described how, in the midst of the pandemic, they were able to use the practice experiences in the programme to support their staff.

> "The work environment had changed from a calm safe environment to what seemed like utter chaos with no rational decisions being made. Before the Queens Nurse programme I may have joined in on the panic but I had learned to breathe. I knew I had to create a space with my teams that we could all think logically about what support we could offer the acute sector whilst managing the public health nursing service in a way that could continue to support the children, young people and families and provide a safety net for our most vulnerable communities. I created a time to pause, gather my thoughts and use my voice to protect the health visiting service ... The Queens Nurse programme not only taught me to stop and pause in the space but it gave me the tools to create that space in the workplace, in meetings to give time to people to ground themselves so that collectively we could all think clearly about the services, about the children and families and what we needed to prioritise". (Story 6)

A sense of safety and the impact of a calm environment were identified as key elements of creating a safe space.

> "Strength to ensure safety is paramount for my patients, advocating. But, also the new found confidence to lead in a different way supporting, nurturing staff to be the best they can be, be a visible leader, supporting, encouraging those around you, calming the situations". (Story 9)

3.7. Making a Positive Change

Being able to make a positive change is evidenced throughout the previous six themes. Positive outcomes identified by participants focused on the enhanced wellbeing of staff, improved teamworking across both nursing and multiprofessional teams, and improvements in practice and service provision. The data supporting the other themes also supports this. The following offers feedback from participants on the specific outcomes they were able to achieve.

> "As time went on staff and anxieties became less concerning, people started to learn this new way of life in care homes. We all worked together in a way that had never been done before and through time our weekly huddles came to a natural end. I am certain we would not have achieved this positive outcome if it had not been for the experiences and strategies, I had been taught by QNIS, these truly helped me lead my team during one of the most difficult times in my life". (Story 13)

> By giving me the combination of self-belief, bravery and the skills, I have been able to effect change—increasing community nursing establishment. More com-

munity nurse undoubtably is the biggest impact on my workplace. But also, the value those nurses feel. Someone cares—so we are safe to care. Someone listens so we are safe to listen. Someone held that space for us safely. So we can hold that space for someone". (Story 11)

"The most valuable approach to achieving success was my determination to create a more collaborative multi-disciplinary team approach, by calling on the huge wealth of expertise of other community nurses and allied health professionals. Initial contact with Queen's nurse colleagues led to immediate and enthusiastic offers of help and guidance—signposting me to learning resources and key services. As a result, I feel I now have a team of fantastic specialist nurses who I can work with to meet each patient's needs most effectively, as well as gradually improving mutual trust and positive relationships with the care home staff". (Story 12)

4. Discussion

With the person-centred practice framework [1] being the theoretical underpinning for the Queen's Nurse Development Programme, the findings will be placed in the context of the contemporary literature on person-centredness. Figure 3 illustrates how the themes map to the components of the person-centred practice framework. This shows how the transformational processes, brought about by engagement in the Queen's Nurses Development Programme, has the potential to enable nurses to contribute to the development of person-centred practice. Five of the seven themes are positioned within the attributes domain of the framework, with one theme connected to the practice environment and the final theme connected to the creation of healthful workplace cultures.

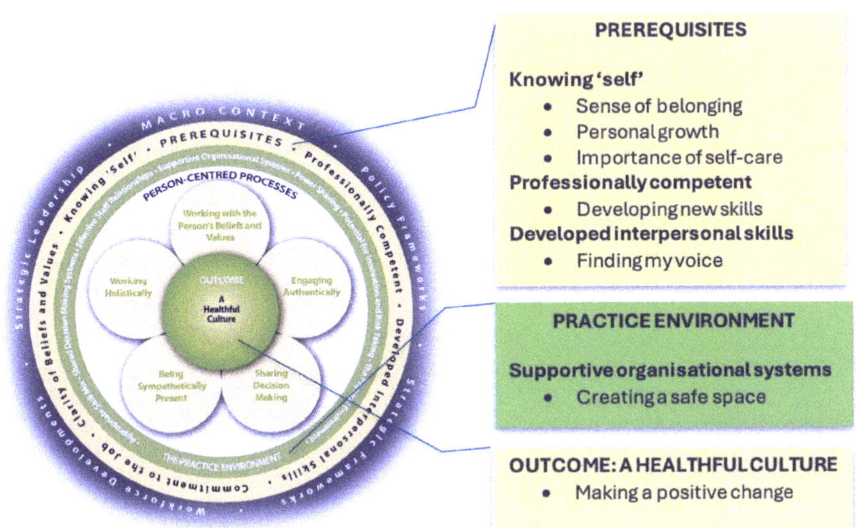

Figure 3. Themes mapped to the person-centred practice framework (McCance & McCormack 2021).

The biggest impact from the Queen's Nurse Development Programme aligns with the attributes domain and in particular 'knowing self'. These findings reflect a way of being in the world, and as emphasised by McCance and McCormack [1], person-centredness requires attention to be paid to our being as persons. They define knowing self as "the way a person makes sense of his/her knowing, being and becoming through reflection, self-awareness and engagement with others" (p. 28). The themes identified under knowing self reinforce the importance of the four modes of being identified by McCance and

McCormack [1]—being in relation, being in a social context, being in place and being with self. Being in relation emphasises the importance of relationships and the interpersonal processes that support the development of positive relationships and it is this that brings about a sense of belonging. Furthermore, personal growth reflects the fundamental need of being with self and gaining clarity about 'that which really matters' and being able to reveal this to others. Interestingly, Nolan et al. [12], in the senses framework that was developed in the context of relationship centred care, identified a sense of belonging as one element that was important in enhancing care environments. This included: enhancing relationships in the team through valuing and showing an interest in one another; being able to confide in people you trust; and feeling part of a valued group who share similar values and beliefs that connect you. This aligns to the sense of belonging described by the participants in this study.

Central to the Queen's Nurse Development Programme are practices that support self-care and personal well-being. Practices learnt in the programme included: being in the body; activating a mindful awareness; embracing stillness through meditation; and the discipline of journalling, through, for example, creating a gratitude list or wellbeing list or recounting the experience of going for a reflective walk (QNIS 2021). These practices added a diversity to the skill set of participants and their use enabled them to function differently in the practice environment. The importance of self-care has been explored in the literature [13,14] but has become more prominent as a consequence of the pandemic [15]. Furthermore, in a systematic literature review, Lee et al. [16] illustrated the nurses' capacity for compassion and the development of skills focusing on self-compassion, self-reflection and self-awareness. The findings from this study are similarly reflected in a review of the literature undertaken by Raab [17] who concluded that using mindfulness interventions for health care workers can reduce perceived stress and increase the effectiveness of clinical care.

The opportunity for participants to develop competence and confidence in their interpersonal ability by finding their voice and speaking out when it was important for patient care is directly related to developed interpersonal skills. McCance and McCormack [1] describe this attribute as "the ability of the person to communicate at a variety of levels with others, using effective verbal and non-verbal interactions that show personal concern for their situation and a commitment to finding mutual solutions" (p. 28). This also links to knowing self, and the importance of knowing and accepting who we are and the personal motivations that drive us, which can help improve interpersonal effectiveness.

The ability to create a safe space reflects the evidence base on psychological safety within healthcare environments. A psychologically safe environment is one where people feel able to focus on the underlying issues without threat of loss of self-identity or integrity [18]. Brown and McCormack [19] conducted an action research study to explore holistic facilitation as an approach to enable healthcare teams to critically analyse practice and enhance patient care. They highlighted the need to create psychologically safe spaces in environments where insufficient support, weak leadership and oppressed behaviours are apparent. Psychological safety enables individuals to feel safe to engage in difficult conversations and consider changes to practice. Supportive organisational systems as described in the person-centred practice framework [1] provide the conditions to create psychologically safe spaces for staff that enable people to flourish. Such systems "support initiative, creativity, freedom and safety of persons" (p. 28). Furthermore, psychological safety connects workplace culture to the health, resilience and well-being of individuals and teams [20], highlighting the relationship with the findings on knowing self.

One of the key findings in this study was the ability of the participants to bring about positive changes in the workplace as a direct result of engaging in the Queen's Nurse Development Programme. This is an impactful finding and is a marker of an effective professional development programme that enables nurses to influence their workplace cultures. The centrality of leadership practices in the development of person-centred workplace cultures is well represented in the literature [21,22]. The positive outcomes presented from the findings of this study, such as enhanced wellbeing of staff and improved teamworking, reflect the development of healthful cultures, the core outcome arising from the development of person-centred practices in teams and organisations as identified in the person-centred practice framework. McCance and McCormack [1] define a healthful culture as one in which "decision making is shared, relationships are collaborative, leadership is transformational and innovative practices are supported" (p. 29). Use of the term healthful reflects a broader notion of health that embraces all dimensions of our being, and once again reflects the themes that were identified in relation to knowing self.

5. Conclusions

The relationship between a systematic approach to transformative professional development and the development of person-centred practices is at the core of this paper. However, what is most striking is the way in which participating in this programme enabled participants to embody the attributes that are a prerequisite for being person-centred. It is the journey with self that generates a sense of belonging, enables personal growth and the ability to care for self and others. This was complemented by the acquisition of new skills that focused on practices such as mindfulness, stillness, deep listening and finding voice. These practices added a diversity to the skill set of participants and their use enabled them to function differently in the practice environment by creating psychologically safe spaces for themselves and their teams. This in turn enabled them to make positive changes in practice, contributing to the development of healthful cultures. The key learning from this innovative development programme is the importance of focusing on the attributes of practitioners and the key building blocks for knowing, being and becoming a person-centred practitioner. This research adds to a growing body of evidence that highlights the importance of healthful workplace cultures for effective person-centred practices and staff wellbeing. However, we are conscious that the work articulated in this paper is intense and requires a high level of commitment from participants and supporting organisations. A key question in moving forward is how we can replicate such programmes at scale and enable these transformative processes to be normalized in all leadership development programmes that have the intent of developing person-centred practitioners and cultures.

Author Contributions: Conceptualization, C.C. and B.M.; methodology, C.C. and B.M.; formal analysis, T.M., B.M. and C.C.; investigation, T.M.; resources, C.C.; data curation, T.M.; writing—original draft preparation, T.M.; writing—review and editing, T.M., B.M. and C.C.; project administration, C.C.; funding acquisition, C.C. All authors have read and agreed to the published version of the manuscript.

Funding: This work was supported by the Queen's Nursing Institute Scotland with generous contributions from The Charles Grant Gordon Charitable Foundation, The Dunhill Medical Trust, and The NHS Lothian Charity.

Institutional Review Board Statement: Ethical review and approval were waived for this study due to the evaluation methods used being considered to be 'routine practice' in the programme.

Informed Consent Statement: All participants agreed to be a part of the evaluation and to share their (anonymised) data with other participants as a part of the analysis processes.

Data Availability Statement: The datasets presented in this article are not readily available because they constitute the everyday inquiry records maintained by participants – creative expressions, reflective diaries and journals, and project notes of specific discussions. Accessing these data would breach confidentiality and anonymity of participants.

Public Involvement Statement: There was no public involvement in any aspect of this research.

Guidelines and Standards Statement: This manuscript was drafted against the guidelines for reporting participatory action research [23].

Use of Artificial Intelligence: AI or AI-assisted tools were not used in drafting any aspect of this manuscript.

Acknowledgments: This work would not have been possible without the participants, facilitators and coaches, who enthusiastically engaged throughout the programme.

Conflicts of Interest: There are no conflicts of interest to declare pertaining to this publication.

References

1. McCance, T.; McCormack, B. The Person-centred Practice Framework. In *Fundamentals of Person-Centred Healthcare Practice*; McCormack, B., McCance, T., Bulley, C., Brown, D., McMillan, A., Martin, S., Eds.; Wiley-Blackwell: Oxford, UK, 2021; pp. 23–32.
2. Middleton, R.; Cardiff, S.; Manley, K.; Dewar, B. Leadership Relationships. In *International Practice Development in Health and Social Care*; Manley, K., Wilson, V., Oye, C., Eds.; Wiley Blackwell: Oxford, UK, 2021; pp. 159–172.
3. Cardiff, S. Person-Centred Leadership: A Critical Participatory Action Research Study Exploring and Developing a New Style of (Clinical) Nurse Leadership. Ph.D Thesis, University of Ulster, Coleraine, UK, 2014.
4. Enghiad, P.; Venturato, L.; Ewashen, C. Exploring clinical leadership in long-term care: An integrative literature review. *J. Nurs. Manag.* **2022**, *30*, 90–103. [CrossRef] [PubMed]
5. Guibert-Lacasa, C.; Vázquez-Calatayud, M. Nurses' clinical leadership in the hospital setting: A systematic review. *J. Nurs. Manag.* **2022**, *30*, 913–925. [CrossRef] [PubMed]
6. Edmonstone, J. What is wrong with NHS leadership development. *Br. J. Healthc. Manag.* **2013**, *19*, 531–538. [CrossRef]
7. Scharmer, C. *The Essentials of Theory U: Core Principles and Applications*; Berrett-Koehler: Oakland, CA, USA, 2018.
8. McCormack, B.; Cable, C.; Cantrell, J.; Bunce, A.; Douglas, J.; Fitzpatrick, J.; Forsyth, N.; Gallacher, J.; Grant, J.; Griffin, L.; et al. The Queen's Nurses collaborative inquiry—Understanding individual and collective experiences of transformative learning. *Int. Pract. Dev. J.* **2021**, *11*, 2. [CrossRef]
9. Kimsey-House, H.; Kimsey-House, K.; Sandahl, P. *Co-Active Coaching: Changing Business, Transforming Lives*; Nicholas Brealey Pub.: Boston, MA, USA, 2011.
10. Bridges, D.; McGee, S. Collaborative Inquiry: Reciprocity and Authenticity. In *Creative Spaces for Qualitative Researching*; Higgs, J., Titchen, A., Horsfall, D., Bridges, D., Eds.; Sense Publishers: Rotterdam, The Netherlands, 2011; pp. 213–222.
11. Titchen, A.; McCormack, B. Dancing with stones: Critical creativity as methodology for human flourishing. *Educ. Action Res.* **2010**, *18*, 531–554. [CrossRef]
12. Nolan, M.; Brown, J.; Davies, S.; Nolan, J.; Keady, J. *The SENSES Framework: Improving Care for Older People through a Relationship-Centred Approach*; University of Sheffield: Sheffield, UK, 2006; ISBN 1-902411-44-7.
13. Rose, J.; Glass, N. Enhancing emotional well-being through self-care: The experiences of community health nurses in Australia. *Holist. Nurs. Pract.* **2008**, *22*, 336–347. [PubMed]
14. Richards, K. Self-care is a lifelong journey. *Nurs. Econ.* **2013**, *31*, 198–202. [PubMed]
15. Hossain, F.; Clatty, A. Self-care strategies in response to nurses' moral injury during COVIS-19 pandemic. *Nurs. Ethics* **2021**, *28*, 23–32. [CrossRef] [PubMed]
16. Lee, M.; Laurenson, M.; Whitfield, C. Can compassion be taught to lessen the effects of compassion fatigue? *J. Care Serv. Manage.* **2012**, *6*, 121–130. [CrossRef]
17. Raab, K. Mindfulness, self-compassion, and empathy among health care professionals: A review of the literature. *J. Health Care Chaplain.* **2014**, *20*, 95–108. [CrossRef] [PubMed]
18. Schein, E.H. *Organizational Culture and Leadership*, 5th ed.; Wiley: Hoboken, NJ, USA, 2016.
19. Brown, D.; McCormack, B. Exploring psychological safety as a component of facilitation within the Promoting Action on Research Implementation in Health Services framework. *J. Clin. Nurs.* **2016**, *25*, 2921–2932. [CrossRef] [PubMed]
20. Shian, M.; Arnold, I.; Germ, A.K. The road to psychological safety: Legal, scientific and social functions for a Canadian National Standard on psychological safety part of facilitation psychological safety in the workplace. *Bull. Sci. Technol. Soc.* **2012**, *32*, 142–162. [CrossRef]
21. Manley, K. Organisational culture and consultant nurse outcomes. Part 1: Organisational culture. *Nurs. Crit. Care* **2000**, *5*, 179–184. [CrossRef] [PubMed]
22. Manley, K.; Sanders, K.; Cardiff, S.; Webster, J. Effective workplace culture: The attributes, enabling factors and consequences of a new concept. *Int. Pract. Dev. J.* **2011**, *1*, 1.
23. Smith, L.; Rosenzweig, L.; Schmidt, M. Best practices in the reporting of participatory action research: Embracing both the forest and the trees. *Couns. Psychol.* **2010**, *38*, 1115–1138. [CrossRef]

nursing reports

MDPI

Article

Functional Capacity of Institutionalized Older People and Their Quality of Life, Depressive Symptoms and Feelings of Loneliness: A Cross-Sectional Study

Fátima Cano [1,2], Elisabete Alves [2,3,*], Lara Guedes de Pinho [2,3,†] and César Fonseca [2,3,†]

1 Local Health Unit of Baixo Alentejo, 7801-849 Beja, Portugal; d52899@alunos.uevora.pt
2 Saão João de Deus School of Nursing, University of Évora, 7000-811 Évora, Portugal; lmgp@uevora.pt (L.G.d.P.); cfonseca@uevora.pt (C.F.)
3 Comprehensive Health Research Centre (CHRC), 7000-811 Évora, Portugal
* Correspondence: elisabete.alves@uevora.pt; Tel.: +351-266-730-300
† These authors contributed equally to this work.

Abstract: Background: The increasing number of institutionalized older individuals worldwide stresses the need to evaluate the association between the functional profile of institutionalized older adults and their quality of life (QoL), depressive symptoms and feelings of loneliness. Methods: A cross-sectional study was conducted in 19 residential facilities in Alentejo, Portugal. Between March and September 2023, all individuals aged ≥65 years were invited to complete a structured questionnaire (n = 1303). Sociodemographic and clinical data were collected, and validated scales for the Portuguese older population were used. Linear regression and unconditional binary logistic models were computed. Results: The highest level of dependence was observed in the self-care dimension (mean (SD) = 2.93 (1.21)), with 40% of participants exhibiting levels of dependence requiring daily care or total replacement. QoL was inversely associated with functionality in all dimensions, as well as with severe or complete dependence, even after adjusting for sex, age and education. Participants with depressive symptoms and feelings of loneliness were, respectively, three and two times more likely to be dependent on care (adjusted OR = 3.69, 95% CI: 1.80–7.52; adjusted OR = 2.04, 95% CI: 1.07–3.87). Conclusions: Public policies and interventions should include social and emotional support strategies alongside traditional medical interventions.

Keywords: institutionalized older; functionality; loneliness; depression; quality of life

1. Introduction

The progressive increase in the older population poses sociological and healthcare challenges, particularly regarding the health policies aimed at people aged 65 years or older [1,2]. In fact, the increasing aging of the population and the increase in average life expectancy are reflected in the higher concern for the care of the older population, especially because of the need to implement long-term care responses [2–4]. This scenario of epidemiological and demographic changes, marked by a notable decrease in mortality and a greater control of early mortality, is responsible for the growing number of people of advanced age. At the same time, demographic aging results in opportunities and challenges of different dimensions on a global scale in the economic, social and health domains. It is undoubtedly one of the main public health concerns due to the increase in noncommunicable chronic diseases due to a decline in the ability to provide self-care [5–9].

The longevity process is a worldwide phenomenon marked by specific biopsychosocial changes [10–13], namely genetic, physiological, behavioral, psychological and social changes [13,14]. It is a natural process of life during which people continue to aspire to maintain their health and quality of life (QoL). In this context, it is not enough to ensure that each person lives longer; it is also necessary to ensure their autonomy, capacity for self-care, independence and QoL. The functional health of older people has been associated with the perception of well-being, socialization and support networks, intellectual conditions, emotional states and attitudes toward individuals and the world [15]. Functional capacity has attracted increasing attention because the loss of functionality increases the number of chronic diseases and compromises the capacity for self-care, often leading to the search for social solutions, namely institutionalization, which requires adaptations by the health and social sectors [16–18].

The ability to maintain functional capacity is directly related to an older person's QoL and to their ability to care for themselves. It is associated with self-esteem, personal well-being, socioeconomic level, health status, emotional stability, social interaction, activity and self-knowledge [19–22]. According to previous literature, older people living in nursing homes or other residential structures tend to feel lonely and dissatisfied and are removed from their social networks in the monotony of day-to-day life. This feeling is aggravated and explained by the growing increase in cases of depression, compromised self-esteem, the permanent desire to return to the family, aggression and suicide attempts [13,20].

Depression and loneliness are significant concerns among older people, especially among those who are institutionalized. Recent studies have shown that loneliness is strongly associated with increased depressive symptoms in the older population [23], which may compromise the mental health and QoL of these individuals [24,25]. Thus, attention to the emotional and social aspects of older individuals is crucial to promoting their general well-being.

Portugal is facing significant demographic challenges, which are characterized by an aging population and a low birth rate, making it one of the countries with the greatest demographic fragility in the European Union [2,11]. These challenges are especially pronounced in the Alentejo region, an area that exemplifies the country's broader demographic problems. The combination of low birth rates, high youth emigration rates and a growing number of older people puts significant pressure on social and health services in the region [26]. Moreover, low population density and depopulation exacerbate feelings of loneliness and social isolation, which are factors that negatively impact the health and well-being of older people [1,2,13].

In this context, a better understanding of how functional capacity is related to the mental health and well-being of older people will contribute to the development of more effective strategies for health promotion in vulnerable populations. Nursing, as an innovative profession, is crucial in addressing these challenges by introducing new approaches, technologies, and practices to improve the quality of care, the autonomy of older adults and the efficiency of services [27]. Thus, this study aims to evaluate the associations between the functional profile of institutionalized older people and their QoL, depressive symptoms and feelings of loneliness according to their sociodemographic and clinical characteristics.

2. Materials and Methods

This cross-sectional study was approved by the Ethics Committee of the University of Évora (Reference 22064). Each participant signed an informed consent form.

Between March and September 2023, 11 institutions in the district of Beja and 8 in the district of Évora were invited to participate in the study. The institutions were contacted by sending an email with all the information about the study to be performed, and all of them agreed to participate. Each institution selected specific collaborators, all of whom were health professionals (nurses, psychologists, physiotherapists, social workers and occupational therapists) who provided care at the participating institutions, to perform the data collection. To ensure consistent training and the quality of the data collection, all health professionals were invited to participate in face-to-face and online training where the study objectives of the study and all procedures to be implemented were clarified, including the presentation and description of the questionnaires to be applied. The training sessions for the professionals took place between January and March 2023.

Data collection from the participants took place between March and September 2023, encompassing a total of 1522 people residing in Central Alentejo and Baixo Alentejo. The present included only participants aged 65 years or older who were institutionalized in a residential structure for older people and who were able to freely sign the informed consent form or who had a guardian or a legally recognized significant other who could do so. Thus, 1396 participants met the inclusion criteria of this study. All the participants answered a structured questionnaire for the collection of demographic and clinical data and for the evaluation of the functionality profile (Elderly Nursing Core Set) and cognitive function of the participants (Mini Mental State Examination). A total of 93 participants who did not respond to the functionality questionnaire were excluded from our sample, and our final sample consisted of 1303 institutionalized people aged 65 years or older. Data, namely sex, age, marital status and education, were collected for the sociodemographic characterization of the participants. Clinical data on the medical diagnoses of the participants were also collected. On the basis of these data, multimorbidity was defined as the diagnosis of two or more chronic diseases.

The Elderly Nursing Core Set (ENCS) is an instrument for assessing the functionality of older adults and consists of 31 questions based on the International Classification of Functioning, Disability and Health (ICF), categorized on a 5-point Likert scale. It assesses four dimensions: self-care (washing, dressing, taking care of body parts, moving around using some type of equipment, walking, performing daily routines, maintaining body position, changing basic body positions, care related to the processes of excretion, use of the hand and arm and drinking and eating); learning and mental functions (emotional functions, orientation functions, attention functions, memory functions, consciousness functions and higher-level cognitive functions); communication (speaking, conversation, communicating and receiving oral messages and family relationships); and relationships with friends and caregivers (personal care providers and personal assistants, health professionals and friends) [11]. The ENCS has high reliability (Cronbach's alpha = 0.963), and there is a strong correlation between items (KMO = 0.947). A higher score indicates a worse functional profile [28,29], with the scores categorized as follows: no problem: 0–4%; mild problem: 5–24%; moderate problem: 25–49%; severe problem: 50–95%; complete problem: 96–100%.

The Mini Mental State Examination (MMSE) assesses cognitive function in six areas: orientation, temporal and spatial, short-term memory (immediate or attention) and recall, calculation, movement coordination and language and visuospatial skills [30]. It is adapted for Portugal, with a score that varies between 0 and 30 [31]. The criterion for the definition of cognitive impairment varies according to the level of education of the participants: a score ≤ 15 for individuals with no formal education; a score ≤ 22 for individuals with <12 years of education; and a score ≤ 27 for individuals with 12 years of education or more [31].

All participants who did not exhibit cognitive impairment ($n = 447$) also completed questionnaires validated for the Portuguese population and adapted for older people to assess QoL (World Health Organization Quality of Life—BREF (WHOQOL-BREF)), depressive symptoms (Patient Health Questionnaire 9—PHQ-9), and feelings of loneliness (Loneliness Scale for Portuguese Elderly—UCLA).

The World Health Organization Quality of Life–BREF (WHOQOL-BREF) measures the QoL of adults in four domains: physical, psychological, social relationships and the environment [32]. The WHOQOL-BREF scale ranges from 0 to 100, with higher scores representing a better QoL. Usable for various disorders and healthy individuals, it allows the calculation of a global indicator of QoL [33].

The 9-item Patient Health Questionnaire (PHQ-9) assesses depressive symptoms via nine questions, each with four response options that reflect the frequency of symptoms, ranging from 0 (none) to 3 (almost every day). This instrument can be used to systematically identify symptoms of depression, and the scores range from 0 to 27: 0–4 points, no depression; 5–9 points, mild depressive disorder; 10–14 points, moderate depressive disorder; 15–19 points, moderately severe depressive disorder; and 20–27 points, severe depressive disorder. The higher the score is, the more severe the depressive symptoms are [34]. It has been validated for the Portuguese population, with good internal consistency and convergent validity [34,35].

The Loneliness Scale for Portuguese Elderly (UCLA) assesses feelings of loneliness with 16 items, which are divided into social isolation and affinities, with responses at four levels. The score ranges from 16 to 64, with scores above 32 indicating significant loneliness [36]. This scale has temporal stability (α (16 items) = 0.985), internal consistency (0.905) and factorial validity, demonstrating high reliability as a diagnostic tool for geriatric loneliness [37].

Data processing was performed via the statistical program STATA 15.1 (College Station, TX, USA, 2017). The sample characteristics are presented as counts and proportions or means and standard deviations. Linear regression models were used to evaluate the crude and adjusted associations and their respective 95% confidence intervals (95% CIs) between the sociodemographic and clinical characteristics of the participants, QoL, depressive symptoms and loneliness with each of the functioning subscales. Unconditional binary logistic regression models were fitted to calculate crude and adjusted odds ratios (ORs) and their respective 95% CIs to assess the determinants of severe or complete functioning.

3. Results

The participants had a mean age of 86 years; more than 70% were female, and 16.7% were married or in a common-law relationship (Table 1). With respect to education, 43.4% had not attended school, whereas 54.1% had attended school but not higher education. The physical health of the participants was marked by a high prevalence of multimorbidity (84.1%) and cognitive impairment (64.7%). Among the participants without cognitive impairment, the mean value (SD) of QoL in general was 52.3 (19.2). The mean (SD) QoL ranged from 53.3 (11.2) for the physical domain to 63.8 (13.7) for the environmental domain. The mean score (SD) for depressive symptoms was 5.1 (5.0), and that for feelings of loneliness was 29.5 (10.2).

Table 1. Sociodemographic, clinical and psychological characteristics of the participants.

	***n* = 1303**
Sex, *n* (%)	
Male	376 (28.9)
Female	927 (71.1)
Age (years)	
Mean (min–max)	86 (65–104)
Marital status, *n* (%)	
Single	146 (11.2)
Married/In a de facto relationship	218 (16.7)
Widower	898 (68.9)
Divorced/Separated	41 (3.2)
Education, *n* (%)	
Did not attend school and cannot read or write	421 (32.3)
Did not attend school, but can read and write	145 (11.1)
Attended school but not higher education	705 (54.1)
Attended higher education	32 (2.5)
Multimorbidity *, *n* (%)	
No	215 (15.9)
Yes	1085 (84.1)

Table 1. *Cont.*

	n = 1303
Cognitive impairment (MMSE) ¥, n (%)	
No	447 (35.3)
Yes	820 (64.7)
Quality of life (WHOQOL-BREF) §, mean (SD) ¶	
Physical domain	53.3 (11.2)
Psychological domain	55.2 (13.1)
Domain of social relationships	60.6 (13.9)
Environmental domain	63.8 (13.7)
General quality of life	52.3 (19.2)
Depressive symptoms (PHQ9) £, median (SD) ¶	
Overall score	5.1 (5.0)
Loneliness (UCLA-16) µ, median (SD) ¶	
Overall score	29.5 (10.2)

* Diagnosis of two or more chronic diseases; ¥ Mini Mental State Examination, MMSE (range: 0–30). Cognitive impairment: a score ≤ 15 for individuals with no formal education; a score ≤ 22 for individuals with <12 years of education; and a score ≤ 27 for individuals with 12 years of education or more. § World Health Organization Quality of Life–BREF, WHOQOL-BREF (range: 0–100); £ 9-Item Patient Health Questionnaire, PHQ-9 (range: 0–27); µ The Loneliness Scale for Portuguese Elderly, UCLA (range:16–64); ¶ n = 447.

The distribution of the results of the functional profile of the sample are shown in Figure 1. Specifically, the highest levels of dependence were observed in the dimensions of self-care (mean (SD) = 2.93 (1.21)) and learning and mental functions (mean (SD) = 2.88 (1.25)). Conversely, the relationships dimension appeared to have the lowest levels of dependence and, consequently, better functionality (mean (SD) = 1.86 (0.65)).

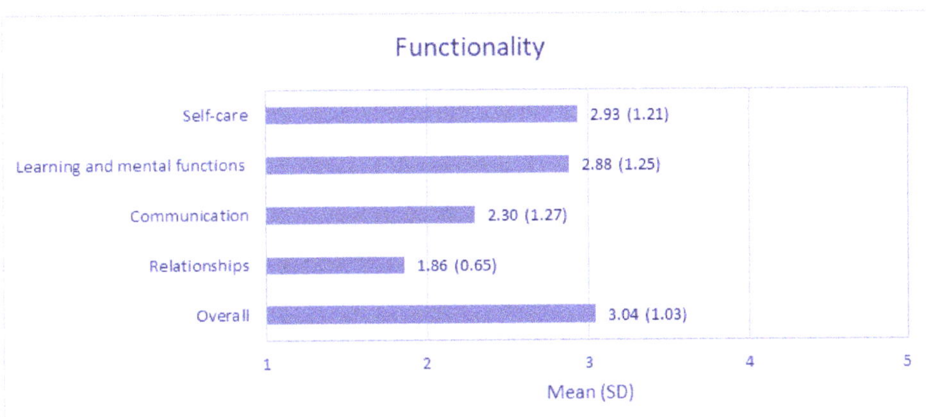

Figure 1. Functional profile of the participants (n = 1303).

The mean (SD) value of the general functional profile (3.04 (1.03)) indicates that more than half of the participants needed help with care. In fact, 27.0% of the participants had moderate levels of dependence, while almost 40% reported high levels of dependence that required daily care (severe problem) or total replacement (complete problem) (Figure 2).

Table 2 shows the associations between the sociodemographic, clinical and cognitive characteristics of the participants and their functionality according to the different dimensions of the ENCS. Women, older participants and those with cognitive deterioration tended to obtain significantly higher scores on the functionality scale, indicating higher levels of dependence in all dimensions. Conversely, participants who had attended school tended to have lower scores than those who did not attend school, indicating a higher level of functionality (general functionality: β = −0.45, 95% CI −0.56 to −0.34; self-care (β = −0.44, 95% CI: −0.57 to −0.31), learning and mental functions (β = −0.57, 95% CI: −0.70 to −0.44), communication (β = −0.48, 95% CI: −0.62 to −0.35) and relationships (β = −0.26, 95% CI: −0.33 to −0.18). Marital status did not seem to be significantly associated with the functionality of the participants.

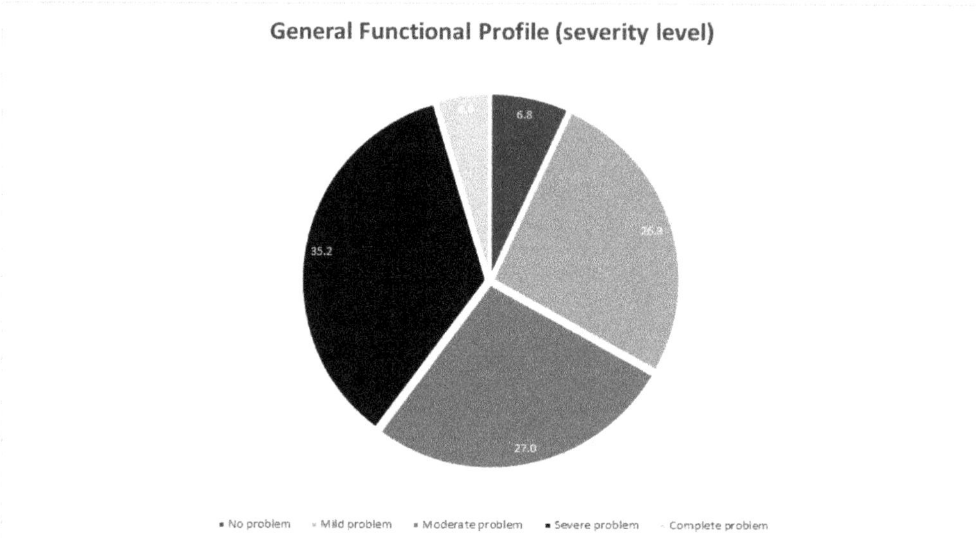

Figure 2. General functional profile of the participants (n = 1303).

Figure 3 depicts the crude and adjusted associations of each of the functionality domains with quality of life, depressive symptomatology and loneliness among institutionalized older adults. Among the participants without cognitive deterioration, QoL was inversely associated with the functionality score in the four dimensions evaluated, whereas depressive symptoms and feelings of loneliness were directly associated with higher levels of functional dependence. The same patterns were described even after adjustment for sex, age and education (Figure 3). Only in the communication and relationship domains of the functionality score, the psychological dimension of QoL (β = −0.00, 95% CI: −0.01 to 0.00; and β = −0.00, 95% CI: −0.01 to 0.00, respectively) and the general dimension of QoL (β = −0.00, 95% CI: −0.01 to 0.00; and β = −0.00, 95% CI: −0.01 to 0.00, respectively) did the associations not reach significance. However, the same association trend was described, despite the lack of statistical significance.

Table 3 shows the sociodemographic, clinical, cognitive and psychological characteristics of the participants that were associated with impaired functionality, taking into account the highest level of dependence (severe and complete disorder). Similar to the results of the analysis of the functionality scale by domain, women (OR = 1.41; 95% CI 1.10–1.81) had a greater prevalence of impaired functionality than did men, whereas education (OR = 0.46; 95% CI 0.37–0.58) was negatively associated with the functional dependence of older individuals. Adults over 65 years of age, institutionalized and with cognitive impairment were 22 times more likely to be dependent on care (OR = 22.07; 95% CI 14.60–33.36) than those without cognitive impairment. Among participants without cognitive impairment, the presence of moderate to severe depressive symptoms and feelings of loneliness were significantly associated with impaired functionality. Quality of life seemed to be inversely associated with severe or complete dependence; however, the results were significant only for the physical domain (adjusted OR = 0.96 (95% CI: 0.93–0.99), social relationship domain (adjusted OR = 0.96 (95% CI: 0.94–0.99)) and environmental domain (adjusted OR = 0.96 (95% CI: 0.93–0.99), both in the raw analysis and after adjustment.

Table 2. Crude association between sociodemographic and clinical characteristics of older adults and functionality.

	Functionality (ENCS) Crude β (95% CI)				
	General	**Self-Care**	**Learning and Mental Functions**	**Communication**	**Relationships**
Sex					
Female vs. male	**0.27 (0.14 to 0.39)**	**0.33 (0.18 to 0.47)**	**0.31 (0.16 to 0.45)**	**0.17 (0.02 to 0.32)**	0.02 (−0.06 to 0.09)
Age (years)	**0.01 (0.01 to 0.02)**	**0.02 (0.01 to 0.03)**	**0.02 (0.01 to 0.03)**	0.01 (−0.00 to 0.02)	0.00 (−0.00 to 0.01)
Marital status					
Married/In a de facto relationship vs. Single, widowed or divorced/separated	−0.01 (−0.16 to 0.14)	−0.02 (−0.20 to 0.15)	0.01 (−0.17 to 0.19)	−0.05 (−0.24 to 0.13)	0.05 (−0.04 to 0.15)
Education					
Attended school vs. Did not attend school	**−0.45 (−0.56 to −0.34)**	**−0.44 (−0.57 to −0.31)**	**−0.57 (−0.70 to −0.44)**	**−0.48 (−0.62 to −0.35)**	**−0.26 (−0.33 to −0.18)**
Multimorbidity *					
Yes vs. No	0.05 (−0.10 to 0.21)	0.06 (−0.12 to 0.24)	0.06 (−0.12 to 0.25)	0.06 (−0.13 to 0.25)	**−0.10 (−0.20 to −0.01)**
Cognitive impairment (MMSE) ¥					
Yes vs. No	**1.24 (1.15 to 1.34)**	**1.28 (1.16 to 1.40)**	**1.53 (1.41 to 1.65)**	**1.38 (1.25 to 1.50)**	**0.36 (0.29 to 0.43)**

Crude β, unstandardized beta; 95% CI, 95% confidence interval. * Diagnosis of two or more chronic diseases; ¥ Mini Mental State Examination, MMSE (range: 0–30). Cognitive impairment: a score ≤ 15 for individuals with no formal education; a score ≤ 22 for individuals with <12 years of education; and a score ≤ 27 for individuals with 12 years of education or more. Bold type indicates statistically significant associations ($p < 0.05$).

Participants with depressive symptoms were three times more likely to be dependent on care (adjusted OR = 3.69 (95% CI: 1.80–7.52)), whereas those who felt lonely were twice as likely to need care (severe problem) or total replacement (complete problem) (adjusted OR = 2.04 (95% CI: 1.07–3.87)) after adjustments for sex, age and education level.

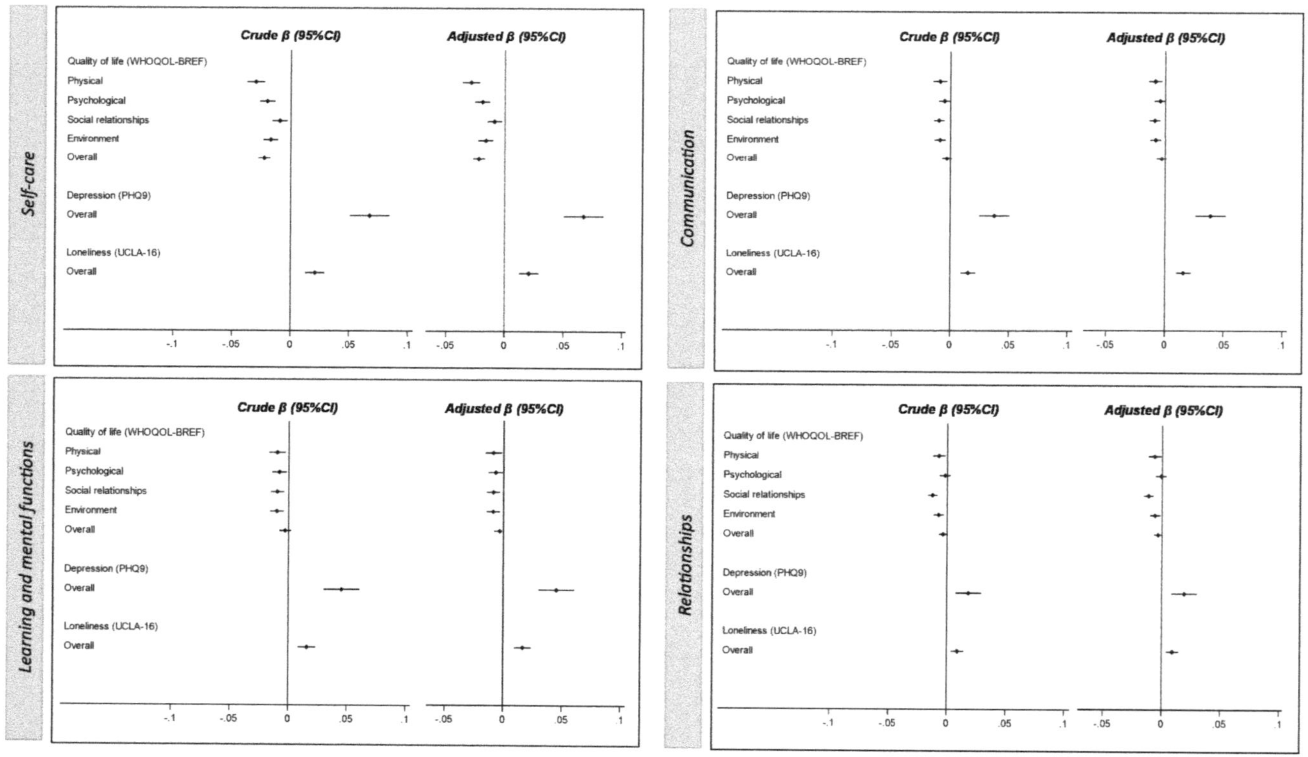

Figure 3. Crude and adjusted associations of the functionality domains with quality of life, depressive symptomatology and loneliness among institutionalized older adults. Crude β, unstandardized beta; 95% CI, 95% confidence interval; adjusted for sex, age and education level.

Table 3. Crude and adjusted associations between participants' sociodemographic, clinical and psychosocial characteristics and severe or complete impaired functioning.

	Functionality (ENCS)	
	Severe or Complete Problem [1]	
	Crude OR (95% CI)	Adjusted OR (95% CI) [2]
Sex		
Male	1	-
Female	**1.41 (1.10–1.81)**	-
Age (years)		
<80	1	-
≥80	0.88 (0.65–1.20)	-
Marital status		
Married/In a de facto relationship	1	-
Single, widowed or divorced/separated	0.91 (0.68–1.22)	-
Education (years)		
Did not attend school	1	-
Attended school	**0.46 (0.37–0.58)**	-
Multimorbidity *		
No	1	-
Yes	1.15 (0.84–1.56)	-
Cognitive impairment (MMSE) ¥		
No	1	-
Yes	**22.07 (14.60–33.36)**	-
Quality of life (WHOQOL-BREF) §		
Physical domain	**0.96 (0.93–0.99)**	**0.96 (0.93–0.99)**
Psychological domain	0.99 (0.96–1.02)	0.99 (0.96–1.02)
Domain of social relationships	**0.96 (0.93–0.98)**	**0.96 (0.94–0.99)**
Environmental domain	**0.96 (0.93–0.98)**	**0.96 (0.93–0.99)**
Overall quality of life	0.99 (0.97–1.01)	0.99 (0.97–1.01)
Depressive symptoms (PHQ9) £		
None, minimal or mild	1	1
Moderate, moderately severe or severe	**3.28 (1.64–6.55)**	**3.69 (1.80–7.52)**
Negative feelings of loneliness (UCLA-16) µ		
No	1	1
Yes	**2.01 (1.07–3.78)**	**2.04 (1.07–3.87)**

* Diagnosis of two or more chronic diseases; ¥ Mini Mental State Examination, MMSE (range: 0–30); Cognitive impairment: a score ≤ 15 for individuals with no formal education; a score ≤ 22 for individuals with <12 years of education; and a score ≤ 27 for individuals with 12 years of education or more. § World Health Organization Quality of Life–BREF, WHOQOL-BREF (range: 0–100); £ 9-Item Patient Health Questionnaire, PHQ-9: none, minimal or mild depressive symptoms, 0–14 points; moderate, moderately severe or severe depressive symptoms, 15–27 points; µ Loneliness Scale for Portuguese Elderly, UCLA: feelings of loneliness, >32 points. [1] Elderly Nursing Core Set, ENCS: no, mild or moderate problem: 0–49%; severe or complete problem: 50–100%. [2] Adjusted for sex, age and education level. Bold type indicates statistically significant associations ($p < 0.05$).

4. Discussion

The results of this study provide a detailed view of the functionality of older people, revealing important associations with the sex, education and cognitive impairment of the participants. These findings provide valuable insights into the variables that influence functional dependence in different populations. Presentation of the data by the dimension of functioning and degree of severity provides a rich and multifaceted analysis of the functioning of the participants, allowing the identification of specific needs, the evaluation of the global impact, the stratification of risks and the customization of interventions. Moreover, the analysis of data on the functionality, QoL, depressive symptoms and loneliness of institutionalized people aged 65 years or older provides a solid basis for the discussion of the challenges faced by this population. Our results revealed very high levels of functional dependence. Although the literature supports a higher prevalence of functional limitations in older people, it is important to note that the severity observed in our sample exceeds some of the previous estimates [5,12], suggesting the need for more targeted and comprehensive interventions to adequately meet the needs of this population.

Women and those with cognitive impairment tend to obtain significantly higher scores on the functionality scale, indicating higher levels of functional dependence in all the dimensions evaluated. This finding is consistent with the literature, which suggests that aging and cognitive impairment are strongly associated with decreased functional capacity [17], imposing a greater burden on both participants and institutions in regard to providing care and requiring more resources and specialized support [5,6,17]. In addition, women often report higher levels of functional dependence, possibly due to greater longevity, a higher prevalence of chronic conditions than that of men, and differences in the social structure and support available to older women [38–40].

The high prevalence of multimorbidity among participants is consistent with recent findings. The literature indicates that multimorbidity is increasingly common among older people, particularly at older ages, affecting approximately 60–80% of the older population [41]. The management of multimorbidity requires a holistic approach that integrates specialized and generalist care to address the multiple needs of patients [42]. The lack of statistical significance in our study between most dimensions of functioning and multimorbidity may be due to the high prevalence of multimorbidity, which makes our population more homogeneous in relation to this variable and makes it difficult to obtain statistically significant results.

Participants who had attended school had significantly lower scores on the functionality scale, indicating greater functional independence. These data suggest that education may be a protective factor against the loss of functionality, possibly due to the constant cognitive stimulation and access to better living conditions that education provides. This result, although in agreement with the literature [43], highlights the existence of social inequalities in health, which affect health throughout the life cycle, stressing the need to intervene early in less-educated populations who are, consequently, more vulnerable to adverse health outcomes.

Among participants without cognitive impairment, better QoL is associated with lower levels of functional dependence, whereas depressive symptoms and feelings of loneliness are directly associated with higher levels of functional dependence. The associations described between quality of life and all domains of the functionality scale are consistent with the literature. This highlights the importance of social interactions and effective communication in maintaining the mental health and well-being of older people [44,45] as well as of their involvement in lifelong learning activities to improve their mental health and QoL [46]. Moreover, depression can decrease motivation and energy, worsening the functional capacity of older individuals [40,47], whereas loneliness can aggravate mental and physical health problems, increasing dependence [47,48]. These findings reinforce the importance of psychological well-being and social support networks in maintaining functionality in individuals without cognitive impairment [17,42,47]. Thus, programs that promote and encourage social interaction and improve communication skills may be beneficial for this population.

This study highlights crucial issues that require interventions and social and emotional support strategies that go beyond traditional medical interventions. The reduced ability of older people to perform daily activities and participate in social activities affects their physical and mental well-being [5,7,20]. Social isolation, a common problem among those whose health conditions limit mobility or cause stigma [17,23], can exacerbate feelings of dependence and loss of autonomy [7,24], leading to an increased psychological and emotional burden [46,47]. Thus, it is essential to implement multidimensional interventions that disseminate programs that promote social engagement, namely through support groups, community groups and recreational activities, to mitigate feelings of loneliness and depression. In addition, access to counseling and therapy services may help older adults cope with depression and the emotional challenges associated with the loss of functionality. In fact, care strategies that combine medical treatment with psychosocial approaches are essential to address the multiple aspects that affect QoL.

One of the main advantages of this study is the deepening of the understanding of the complex interactions among functionality, mental health, loneliness and quality of life in institutionalized older individuals, which should contribute to the design and implementation of integrated approaches that consider both physical and emotional aspects in the well-being of institutionalized older individuals. Also, the use of multiple data collection instruments validated for the Portuguese population and adapted for older people and their ethical and methodological rigor need to be stressed as strengths of the study. Our study presents a relatively large sample size, which was calculated to ensure a power of 80% to demonstrate associations with a magnitude of at least 1.2 (odds ratio) at a 5% significance level. Also, the inclusion of 11 institutions in the district of Beja and 8 in the district of Évora and the small proportion of participants that did not respond to the functionality questionnaire (6.7%) ensures the representativeness of our sample for the Alentejo region.

Some limitations also need to be acknowledged and discussed. The cross-sectional nature of our study prevents the establishment of causal relationships between functionality and quality, depression and loneliness. The data collection by the institution's health professionals, although promoting performance in a safe context where the older people feel comfortable, may have influenced participants to respond in a socially desirable way to the questions about QoL, depression and loneliness [19]. However, in this case, it would be expected that the associations described would be even more pronounced, emphasizing the importance of intervening in mental health as early as possible to optimize the quality of life of people aged 65 years or older. The proportion of women included in our study was higher than that described for the older population (65 years of age or older) in Portugal [49]. In 2021, women accounted for approximately 57% of the older population, reflecting greater female longevity. The Alentejo region, where the study was conducted, has a proportion of older people above the national average, with Central Alentejo and Baixo Alentejo having one of the highest percentages of older people in the country. Thus, the high average age included may also explain the greater participation of women. This phenomenon has been called the "feminization of old age" in scientific literature [50]. However, although women live longer than men, these additional years are generally not accompanied by good health, as they tend to have poorer health throughout their lives and greater economic needs [2]. In the current study, a sensitivity analysis was performed by randomly selecting a similar number of male and female older adults, and the results remained very similar. Finally, the analysis of QoL, depressive symptoms and loneliness was restricted to participants without cognitive impairment, which reduced the sample size and consequently limited the statistical power. However, this procedure is common in most studies in this area because it is commonly accepted that the self-completion of psychosocial assessment scales requires adequate cognitive ability to ensure the attainment of valid and reliable responses [51]. Thus, the restricted application of the QoL, depression and loneliness scales to individuals without cognitive impairment strengthens the internal validity of the study, ensuring that the analyzed data more accurately reflect the perception of each participant, thus ensuring the quality and reliability of the data obtained.

5. Conclusions

The results of this study are in line with the literature and more recent guidelines, which highlight the importance of public policies and interventions focused on education and psychosocial support to improve functionality, QoL and mental health, especially among vulnerable populations [52–55]. The increase in longevity has profound implications for health policies and social responses, requiring strategies that are adapted to the complex needs of older people. In this context, programs that promote healthy aging and preventive and integrated approaches to chronic diseases, including continuing education and social support, may be effective in reducing functional dependence and contribute to improving the QoL and mental health of older people.

The associations described between functionality and QoL, depression and loneliness emphasize the importance of developing and implementing public policies that simultaneously promote mental and physical health through measures aimed at improving the quality of long-term care. Thus, the results of the present study underscore the need to develop multifaceted approaches to promote functionality and independence in aging and cognitively vulnerable populations.

This study is particularly relevant because it focuses on a vulnerable group and offers a robust basis for formulating more effective and personalized health policies that are aligned with the diverse needs of a growing older population. It also contributes to reducing social and health inequalities, with pioneering impacts in health promotion, human rights and health governance through the promotion of an innovative and equitable society that values the physical and mental health of institutionalized older adults simultaneously.

Future investigations should longitudinally explore the impact of specific interventions on the functionality and psychosocial well-being of institutionalized older people. In addition, comparative studies between different regions of Portugal could enrich the understanding of regional variations in geriatric care needs and responses.

Nursing care is fundamental to ensuring that the physical, emotional and psychosocial needs of the older are met holistically, promoting healthy and dignified aging in any care setting. Nurses can play a key role in improving self-care and functionality through the promotion of health education, health literacy, physical exercise and cognitive training [56]. By addressing both the challenges and opportunities associated with population aging, healthy and dignified aging can be promoted for all older citizens in Portugal.

Author Contributions: Conceptualization, F.C., E.A., L.G.d.P. and C.F.; methodology, F.C., E.A. and C.F.; validation, L.G.d.P. and C.F.; formal analysis, F.C., E.A. and L.G.d.P.; investigation, all; resources, all; data curation, E.A. and C.F.; writing—original draft preparation, F.C. and E.A.; writing—review and editing, L.G.d.P. and C.F.; visualization, all; supervision, L.G.d.P. and C.F.; project administration, C.F.; funding acquisition, C.F. All authors have read and agreed to the published version of the manuscript.

Funding: This research was funded by the European Regional Development Fund (ERDF) through the Program Interreg VA España–Portugal (POCTEP) 2014–2020, the International Institute for Research and Innovation in Aging–Capitaliza, "0786_CAP4ie_4_P" and by national funds through the Foundation for Science and Technology, IP national support through CHRC (UIDP/04923/2020).

Institutional Review Board Statement: The study was conducted in accordance with the Declaration of Helsinki and approved by the Ethics Committee of the University of Évora (Reference 22064).

Informed Consent Statement: Informed consent was obtained from all subjects involved in the study.

Data Availability Statement: Data will be available upon request.

Acknowledgments: We thank all participants for their involvement in this study.

Conflicts of Interest: The authors declare no conflicts of interest. The funders had no role in the design of the study; in the collection, analyses, or interpretation of data; in the writing of the manuscript; or in the decision to publish the results.

Public Involvement Statement: No public involvement in any aspect of this research.

Guidelines and Standards Statement: This manuscript was drafted against the STROBE (The Strengthening the Reporting of Observational Studies in Epidemiology Statement) for observational research.

Use of Artificial Intelligence: AI or AI-assisted tools were not used in drafting any aspect of this manuscript.

References

1. Jones, C.H.; Dolsten, M. Healthcare on the brink: Navigating the challenges of an aging society in the United States. *NPJ Aging* **2024**, *10*, 22. [CrossRef] [PubMed]
2. United Nations Department of Economic and Social Affairs (UNDESA). *World Population Aging 2019: Highlights*; ONU: Nova York, NY, USA, 2019. Available online: https://www.un.org/development/desa/pd/news/world-population-ageing-2019 (accessed on 30 May 2024).
3. World Health Organization (WHO). *World Report on Aging and Health*; WHO: Geneva, Switzerland, 2015. Available online: https://www.who.int/publications/i/item/9789241565042 (accessed on 30 May 2024).
4. United Nations Population Fund (UNFPA). 8 Billion Lives, Infinite Possibilities: In Defense of Rights and Choices. *World Population Status Report 2023*. 2023. Available online: https://brazil.unfpa.org/sites/default/files/pub-pdf/swop2023-ptbr-web.pdf (accessed on 30 May 2024).
5. Chen, H.L.; Yu, X.H.; Yin, Y.H.; Shan, E.F.; Xing, Y.; Min, M.; Ding, Y.P.; Fei, Y.; Li, X.W. Multimorbidity patterns and the association with health status of the oldest-old in long-term care facilities in China: A two-step analysis. *BMC Geriatr.* **2023**, *23*, 851. [CrossRef] [PubMed]
6. Maresova, P.; Javanmardi, E.; Barakovic, S.; Barakovic Husic, J.; Tomsone, S.; Krejcar, O.; Kuca, K. Consequences of chronic diseases and other limitations associated with old age: A scoping review. *BMC Public Health* **2019**, *19*, 1431. [CrossRef] [PubMed]
7. Bôas, S.S.V.; de Araújo, C.M.; Prates, R.V.; Novais, M.M.; Pinto, D.S.; dos Reis, L.A. Functional capacity and family support in long-lived elderly people living at home. *Saúde* **2020**, *46*. [CrossRef]
8. Cochar-Soares, N.; Delinocente, M.L.; Dati, L.M. Physiology of aging: From plasticity to cognitive consequences. *Rev. Neurocienc.* **2021**, *29*, 1–28. [CrossRef]
9. Denkinger, M.; Knol, W.; Cherubini, A.; Simonds, A.; Lionis, C.; Lacombe, D.; Petelos, E.; McCarthy, M.; Ouvrard, P.; Van Kerrebroeck, P.; et al. Inclusion of functional measures and frailty in the development and evaluation of medicines for older adults. *Lancet Healthy Longev.* **2023**, *4*, e724–e729. [CrossRef]
10. Menassa, M.; Stronks, K.; Khatmi, F.; Roa Díaz, Z.M.; Espinola, O.P.; Gamba, M.; Itodo, O.A.; Buttia, C.; Wehrli, F.; Minder, B.; et al. Concepts and definitions of healthy ageing: A systematic review and synthesis of theoretical models. *EClinicalMedicine* **2023**, *56*, 101821. [CrossRef]
11. Fonseca, C.; Pinho, L.G.; Lopes, M.J.; Marques, M.C.; Garcia-Alonso, J. The Elderly Nursing Core Set and the cognition of Portuguese older adults: A cross-sectional study. *BMC Nurs.* **2021**, *20*, 108. [CrossRef]
12. Lee, R.Z.Y.; Yang, W.F.Z.; Mahendran, R.; Suárez, L. Psychometric properties of the World Health Organization WHOQOL-AGE Scale in Singapore. *Eur. J. Ageing* **2024**, *21*, 10. [CrossRef]
13. Imaginário, C.; Rocha, M.; Machado, P.; Antunes, C.; Martins, T. Functional capacity and self-care profiles of older people in senior care homes. *Scand. J. Caring Sci.* **2020**, *34*, 69–77. [CrossRef]
14. Lopes, M.; Sakellarides, C. *Os Cuidados de Saúde Face aos Desafios do Nosso Tempo-Contributos para a Gestão da Mudança*; Impresa da Universidade de Évora, Coleção Azulejo: Évora, Portugal, 2021; ISBN 978-972-778-189-8.
15. Schmidt, A.M.; Laurberg, T.B.; Moll, L.T.; Schiøttz-Christensen, B.; Maribo, T. The effect of an integrated multidisciplinary rehabilitation programme for patients with chronic low back pain: Long-term follow up of a randomized controlled trial. *Clin. Rehabil.* **2020**, *35*, 232–241. [CrossRef] [PubMed]
16. Jerez-Roig, J.; de Brito Macedo Ferreira, L.M.; Torres de Araújo, J.R.; Costa Lima, K. Functional decline in nursing home residents: A prognostic study. *PLoS ONE* **2017**, *12*, e0177353. [CrossRef] [PubMed]
17. Birtwell, K.; Planner, C.; Hodkinson, A.; Hall, A.; Giles, S.; Campbell, S.; Tyler, N.; Panagioti, M.; Daker-White, G. Transitional Care Interventions for Older Residents of Long-term Care Facilities A Systematic Review and Meta-analysis. *JAMA Netw. Open* **2022**, *5*, e2210192. [CrossRef]
18. Gomes, G.; Moreira, R.; Maia, T.; dos Santos, M.A.; Silva, V. Factors associated with personal autonomy among the elderly: A systematic review of the literature. *Ciência Saúde Coletiva* **2021**, *26*, 1035–1046. [CrossRef] [PubMed]
19. Geigl, C.; Loss, J.; Leitzmann, M.; Janssen, C. Social factors of health-related quality of life in older adults: A multivariable analysis. *Qual. Life Res.* **2023**, *32*, 3257–3268. [CrossRef]
20. Pinho, L.G.; Lopes, M.J.; Correia, T.; Sampaio, F.; Arco, H.R.; Mendes, A.; Marques, M.C.; Fonseca, C. Patient-Centered Care for Patients with Depression or Anxiety Disorder: An Integrative Review. *J. Pers. Med.* **2021**, *11*, 776. [CrossRef]
21. Tomás, M.T.; Galán-Mercant, A.; Carnero, E.A.; Fernandes, B. Functional Capacity and Levels of Physical Activity in Aging: A 3-Year Follow-up. *Front. Med.* **2018**, *4*, 244. [CrossRef]
22. Nguyen, T.X.; Nguyen, A.H.P.; Nguyen, H.T.T.; Nguyen, T.T.H.; Nguyen, H.L.; Goldberg, R.J.; Thillainadesan, J.; Naganathan, V.; Vu, H.T.T.; Tran, L.V.; et al. Health-Related Quality of Life among Older Adults with Dementia Living in Vietnamese Nursing Homes. *Int. J. Environ. Res. Public Health* **2024**, *21*, 135. [CrossRef]
23. Bäuerle, A.; Steinbach, J.; Schweda, A.; Beckord, J.; Hetkamp, M.; Weismüller, B.; Kohler, H.; Musche, V.; Dörrie, N.; Teufel, M.; et al. Mental health burden of the COVID-19 outbreak in Germany: Predictors of mental health impairment. *J. Prim. Care Community Health* **2020**, *11*, 2150132720953682. [CrossRef]
24. Hwang, T.J.; Rabheru, K.; Peisah, C.; Reichman, W.; Ikeda, M. Loneliness and social isolation during the COVID-19 pandemic. *Int. Psychogeriatr.* **2020**, *32*, 1217–1220. [CrossRef]

25. Ratcliffe, J.; Galdas, P.; Kanaan, M. Older men and loneliness: A cross-sectional study of sex differences in the English Longitudinal Study of Aging. *BMC Public Health* **2024**, *24*, 354. [CrossRef] [PubMed]
26. PORDATA. [Aging Index and Other Aging Indicators]. PORDATA. 2023. Available online: https://www.pordata.pt/portugal/indice+de+envelhecimento+e+outros+indicadores+de+envelhecimento-526 (accessed on 6 June 2024).
27. National Academies of Sciences, Engineering, and Medicine; National Academy of Medicine; Committee on the Future of Nursing 2020–2030. The Role of Nurses in Improving Health Care Access and Quality. In *The Future of Nursing 2020–2030: Charting a Path to Achieve Health Equity*; Flaubert, J.L., Le Menestrel, S., Williams, D.R., Wakefield, M.K., Eds.; National Academies Press (US): Washington, DC, USA, 2021; pp. 99–126. Available online: https://www.ncbi.nlm.nih.gov/books/NBK573910/ (accessed on 8 June 2024).
28. Fonseca, C.; Christian, K. The Dimension of sustainable indicators for rehabilitation nursing care and its implications for people aged 65 and over with self-care deficit: Systematic Review of Literature. *J. Aging Innov.* **2018**, *7*, 33–40.
29. Muszalik, M.; Repka, I.; Puto, G.; Kowal-Skałka, J.; Kędziora-Kornatowska, K. Assessment of Functional Status and Quality of Life of Elderly Patients Undergoing Radiotherapy and Radiotherapy Combined with Chemotherapy—A Cross-Sectional Study. *Clin. Interv. Aging* **2021**, *16*, 9–18. [CrossRef]
30. Folstein, M.F.; Folstein, S.E.; McHugh, P.R. Mini-mental state: A practical method for grading the cognitive state of patients for the clinician. *J. Psychiatr. Res.* **1975**, *12*, 189–198. [CrossRef] [PubMed]
31. Santana, I.; Duro, D.; Lemos, R.; Costa, V.; Pereira, M.; Simões, M.R.; Freitas, S. Mini-mental state examination: Assessment of new normative data in the screening and diagnosis of cognitive impairment. *Acta Med. Port.* **2016**, *29*, 240–248. [CrossRef]
32. Vaz-Serra, A.; Canavarro, M.C.; Simões, M.R.; Pereira, M.; Gameiro, S.; Quartilho, M.; Rijo, D.; Carona, C.; Paredes, T. Psychometric studies of the World Health Organization quality of life assessment instrument (WHOQOL-Bref) for Portuguese from Portugal. *Psiquiatr. Clín.* **2006**, *27*, 41–49.
33. Canavarro, M.C.; Simões, M.R.; Vaz Serra, A.; Pereira, M.; Rijo, D.; Quartilho, M.J.; Carona, C. Instrumento de avaliação da qualidade de vida da Organização Mundial de Saúde: WHOQOL-Bref. In *Avaliação Psicológica: Instrumentos Validados para a População Portuguesa*; Simões, M., Machado, C., Gonçalves, M., Almeida, L., Eds.; Quarteto Editora: Coimbra, Portugal, 2007; Volume III, pp. 77–100.
34. Monteiro, S.; Torres, A.; Pereira, A.; Albuquerque, E.; Morgadinho, R. 2077—Preliminary validation study of a portuguese version of the patient health questionnaire (PHQ-9). *Eur. Psychiatry* **2013**, *28*, 1. [CrossRef]
35. Ferreira, N.; Sousa, I.; Salgado, J. Brief assessment of depression: Psychometric properties of the Portuguese version of the Patient Health Questionnaire (PHQ-9). *Psychol. Pract. Res. J.* **2019**, *1*, 15–23. [CrossRef]
36. Russell, D. UCLA Loneliness Scale (Version 3): Reliability, Validity, and Factor Structure. *J. Pers. Assess.* **1996**, *66*, 20–40. [CrossRef]
37. Pocinho, M.; Farate, C.; Dias, C.A.; Validação Psicométrica da Escala UCLA-Loneliness para Idosos Portugueses. Interações Soc. E Novas Mod. *2010, 10.* Available online: https://www.interacoes-ismt.com/index.php/revista/article/view/304 (accessed on 17 April 2024).
38. Wang, J.; Xiao, L.D.; Wang, K.; Luo, Y.; Li, X. Gender Differences in Cognitive Impairment among Rural Elderly in China. *Int. J. Environ. Res. Public Health* **2020**, *17*, 3724. [CrossRef]
39. Lohman, M.; Dumenci, L.; Mezuk, B. Gender differences in the construct overlap of frailty and depression: Evidence from the Health and Retirement Study. *J. Am. Geriatr. Soc.* **2020**, *68*, 392–398.
40. Lyu, J.; Kim, H.Y.; Han, J.W.; Kim, T.H.; Kim, K.W. Cognitive impairment, depression, comorbidity, and disability as determinants of health-related quality of life in older adults. *Geriatr. Gerontol. Int.* **2021**, *21*, 488–494.
41. Plasencia, G.; Gray, S.C.; Hall, I.J.; Smith, J.L. Multimorbidity clusters in adults 50 years or older with and without a history of cancer: National Health Interview Survey, 2018. *BMC Geriatr.* **2024**, *24*, 50. [CrossRef] [PubMed]
42. Whitty, C.J.M.; MacEwen, C.; Goddard, A.; Alderson, D.; Marshall, M.; Calderwood, C.; Atherton, F.; McBride, M.; Atherton, J.; Stokes-Lampard, H.; et al. Rising to the challenge of multimorbidity. *BMJ* **2020**, *368*, l6964. [CrossRef]
43. Zaninotto, P.; Batty, G.D.; Stenholm, S.; Kawachi, I.; Hyde, M.; Goldberg, M.; Westerlund, H.; Vahtera, J.; Head, J. Socioeconomic Inequalities in Disability-free Life Expectancy in Older People from England and the United States: A Cross-national Population-Based Study. *J. Gerontol. A Biol. Sci. Med. Sci.* **2020**, *75*, 906–913. [CrossRef]
44. Mendes, L.; Oliveira, J.; Barbosa, F.; Castelo-Branco, M. A Conceptual View of Cognitive Intervention in Older Adults with and Without Cognitive Decline-A Systemic Review. *Front. Aging* **2022**, *3*, 844725. [CrossRef]
45. Zhang, X.; Li, J.; Xie, F.; Chen, X.; Xu, W.; Hudson, N.W. The relationship between adult attachment and mental health: A meta-analysis. *J. Pers. Soc. Psychol.* **2022**, *123*, 1089–1137. [CrossRef]
46. Park, S.; Kim, Y.; Yoon, S.; Nam, Y.J.; Hong, S.; Cho, Y.H.; Son, S.J.; Hong, C.H.; Noh, J.S.; Roh, H.W. Association of Geriatric Depressive Symptoms and Government-Initiated Senior Employment Program: A Population-Based Study. *Psychiatry Investig.* **2024**, *21*, 284–293. [CrossRef]
47. Ribeiro, O.; Teixeira, L.; Araújo, L.; Rodríguez-Blázquez, C.; Calderón-Larrañaga, A.; Forjaz, M.J. Anxiety, Depression and Quality of Life in Older Adults: Trajectories of Influence across Age. *Int. J. Environ. Res. Public Health* **2020**, *17*, 9039. [CrossRef]
48. Zhang, D.; Zheng, W.; Li, K. A relação entre o estado civil e o comprometimento cognitivo em idosos chineses: Os múltiplos efeitos mediadores do apoio social e da depressão. *BMC Geriatr.* **2024**, *24*, 367. [CrossRef]
49. Instituto Nacional de Estatística (INE). *Annual Resident Population Estimates*; INE: Lisboa, Portugal, 2023.

50. Davidson, P.M.; DiGiacomo, M.; McGrath, S.J. The Feminization of Aging: How Will This Impact on Health Outcomes and Services? *Health Care Women Int.* **2011**, *32*, 1031–1045. [CrossRef] [PubMed]
51. Smith, S.C. Measuring Health-Related Quality of Life in Dementia. In *Person-Centered Outcome Metrology*; Fisher, W.P., Jr., Cano, S.J., Eds.; Springer Series in Measurement Science and Technology; Springer: Cham, Switzerland, 2023. [CrossRef]
52. Chang, J.; Chen, H.; Wang, Y. Gender differences in disability among older adults in China: Evidence from the China Health and Retirement Longitudinal Study. *J. Aging Health* **2021**, *33*, 82–92.
53. Smith, M.L.; Ory, M.G.; Ahn, S.; Kulinski, K.P.; Jiang, L.; Horel, S. Regional variations in functional disability and health status among older adults with arthritis: Implications for health disparities. *J. Aging Health* **2020**, *32*, 231–244.
54. Verropoulou, G.; Tsimbos, C.; Papadopoulos, A. Gender disparities in health and functional status among older adults in the Mediterranean region: The role of sociodemographic factors. *Eur. J. Aging* **2021**, *18*, 45–58.
55. Bucholc, M.; McClean, S.I.; Cleland, J. Socioeconomic inequalities in health and disability in older adults: Evidence from the UK Biobank study. *J. Epidemiol. Community Health* **2021**, *75*, 485–492.
56. Alves, E.; Gonçalves, C.; Oliveira, H.; Ribeiro, R.; Fonseca, C. Health-related outcomes of structured home-based rehabilitation programs among older adults: A systematic literature review. *Heliyon* **2024**, *10*, e35351. [CrossRef]

nursing reports

MDPI

Article

The Kumagai Method: Feeding Techniques Using the Pigeon Baby Cleft Palate Bottle

Shingo Ueki [1,*], Yukari Kumagai [2], Yumi Hirai [2], Eri Nagatomo [1], Shoko Miyauchi [3], Takuro Inoue [4], Qi An [5], Eri Tashiro [1] and Junko Miyata [1,6]

1 Department of Health Sciences, Faculty of Medical Sciences, Kyushu University, Fukuoka 812-8582, Japan; nagatomo.eri.018@m.kyushu-u.ac.jp (E.N.); tashiro.eri.084@m.kyushu-u.ac.jp (E.T.); miyata.junko.789@m.kyushu-u.ac.jp (J.M.)
2 Department of Nursing, Osaka University Dental Hospital, Osaka 565-0871, Japan; kumagai-y@office.osaka-u.ac.jp (Y.K.); hirai-yu@office.osaka-u.ac.jp (Y.H.)
3 Department of Advanced Information Technology, Faculty of Information Science and Electrical Engineering, Kyushu University, Fukuoka 819-0395, Japan; miyauchi@ait.kyushu-u.ac.jp
4 Department of Informatics, Graduate School of Information Science and Electrical Engineering, Kyushu University, Fukuoka 819-0395, Japan; inoue.takuro.882@s.kyushu-u.ac.jp
5 Department of Human and Engineered Environmental Studies, Graduate School of Frontier Sciences, The University of Tokyo, Chiba 277-8563, Japan; anqi@robot.t.u-tokyo.ac.jp
6 Department of Pediatric Surgery, Graduate School of Medical Sciences, Kyushu University, Fukuoka 812-8582, Japan
* Correspondence: ueki.shingo.388@m.kyushu-u.ac.jp; Tel.: +81-92-642-6748

Abstract: Background/Objectives: This study aimed to identify the P-bottle feeding techniques systematically organized by Ms. Kumagai, an expert in nursing care for children with a cleft lip and/or palate (CLP), which were developed as she gained expertise in feeding affected children. Methods: We recruited three nurses who had mastered the Kumagai method for feeding with a P-bottle. Through analysis of participants' voices and videos during interviews, we focused on aspects such as dealing with a closed mouth, inserting the nipple in cases of unilateral and bilateral CLP, dealing with the child's movements after insertion, and key considerations when squeezing the bottle. Results: The interview analyses revealed numerous techniques used by nurses to manage the difficulties encountered while feeding children, ensuring successful provision of nourishment. Specifically, the nurses employed techniques such as placing the nipple along the midline of the child's tongue and varying the application of force on the nipple depending on the cleft type. The nurses reported that the objectives of these techniques were to prevent ulcer formation and encourage the use of the tongue, simulating original feeding movements. Conclusions: We explored feeding techniques and the management of associated challenges. Our results suggest that the "Kumagai Method" could be valuable in improving feeding practices.

Keywords: cleft lip; cleft palate; child; feeding difficulties; qualitative research

1. Introduction

Cleft lip and/or palate (CLP) is one of the most prevalent congenital facial malformations. A systematic review reported that the global prevalence of CLP was 10.8 cases per 1000 live births [1]. The challenges associated with CLP are multifaceted, encompassing concerns related to feeding, chewing, articulation, and facial esthetics [2]. Among these challenges, feeding difficulties, which are present in 35–67% of children with CLP [3,4], bear considerable significance, and are attributed to factors such as shortened sucking motions, an accelerated sucking pace, an elevated suck–swallow ratio, and an inability to establish negative pressure within the oral cavity [5]. Furthermore, the lack of muscular coordination within the oral region, including inadequate swallowing function and sub-optimal sucking patterns, adds to the complexity of the situation in children affected by

CLP [6]. Regrettably, feeding difficulties arising from these functional irregularities often translate to inadequate weight gain and even malnutrition [7–9]. Notably, the timing of the first surgical intervention for cleft lip repair is based on the often-quoted "rule of tens," which involves "weight of 10 pounds, hemoglobin of 10 g/dL, and age > 10 weeks" [10]. However, the confluence of feeding challenges faced by children with CLP can impede their ability to attain sufficient weight gain within the prescribed timeframe before surgical intervention, potentially causing delays in the surgical schedule [11].

Breastfeeding is known to have various benefits [12,13] and is also recommended for children with CLP [14]. The World Health Organization (WHO) recommends that infants should be fully breastfed for the first six months and has presented a statement entitled "Ten Steps to Successful Breastfeeding" with recommendations for healthcare facilities worldwide [15]. Some tips for breastfeeding were reported, such as "football/twin feeding style with the infant in the semi-upright position," "occluding the cleft with a thumb or finger," "supporting the infant's cheeks to decrease the width of the cleft," "positioning the breast toward the side of the palate that has the most intact bone," "dancer hand position, which supports the infant's chin to stabilize the jaw during sucking," "releasing breast milk into the infant's mouth," "placing the nipple downward onto the tongue," and "taking feeding pauses by removing the breast to allow the infant to breathe" [6,16]. However, most infants with a cleft palate cannot drink enough from the breast directly, necessitating the use a supplementary bottle or cup [16]. Moreover, a recent study has shown that some parents of infants with CLP prefer mixed breastfeeding and bottle-feeding [17]. Therefore, it is necessary to consider the appropriate ways of providing sufficient amounts of milk to infants with CLP other than breastfeeding.

Various special feeding devices are available for children with CLP who cannot create negative oral pressure [14]. The Pigeon Baby Cleft Palate Bottle (P-bottle), characterized by its squeezable design, is a widely adopted option. The P-bottle's nipple features a one-way valve, a Y-cut tip, and an air vent [16]. This bottle was first developed in Japan, and has now gained global usage. A recent Japanese study revealed that approximately 60% of nurses use the P-bottle for feeding children with CLP, applying a variety of feeding techniques [18]. However, contradictory techniques such as "inserting the nipple to not touch the cleft" and "closing the cleft using the nipple to create negative pressure in the oral cavity" were identified. This study concluded that feeding techniques lacked standardization. Notably, most nurses who participated in this study cared for less than five CLP patients annually [18]. Therefore, we consider that these results mostly included inadequate feeding techniques employed by less experienced nurses. Certain studies reported that even with special feeding bottles, children with CLP fed less than healthy children [19], and that simply using special bottles did not provide substantial benefits to the child's growth [20]. These findings indicate the need to elucidate effective strategies for handling specialized bottles, especially the P-bottle.

Although reviews have investigated the techniques used for feeding bottles [16,21–23], the included studies largely focused on the above-mentioned techniques for breastfeeding and were not specific to the P-bottle. Moreover, infants who have difficulty feeding often exhibit a refusal response, turning their face away and pushing the nipple out with their tongues, because they cannot accept feeding. Therefore, it is necessary to know not only how to use the bottle, but also how to respond to the child's movement patterns. A recent scoping review also reported that existing resources, including guidelines for managing the challenges associated with CLP, were inadequate [24], and developing specific feeding techniques is an important issue. Therefore, the purpose of the present study was to identify P-bottle feeding techniques performed by nurses who were experts in feeding children with CLP and feeding difficulties.

2. Materials and Methods

2.1. Study Design

The present study employed a qualitative, descriptive research design in which participants' voices and videos were used as data.

2.2. Participants

The participants were nurses working at a university-affiliated dental hospital in Japan. The hospital, equipped with a CLP center, conducts approximately 400 CLP-related surgeries annually. Consequently, since children with severe CLP from across Japan visit the hospital, this facility frequently deals with cases of feeding difficulties. Additionally, the hospital provides educational support, including on-site feeding guidance, upon request from nearby obstetric hospitals. The head nurse, Ms. Kumagai, who has worked at the hospital for several years, has independently refined feeding techniques, resulting in the name "the Kumagai Method". This method involves two approaches, viz., using a narrow-long nipple and a P-bottle. We have already published the techniques using the narrow-long nipple [25]. The present study was designed to elucidate the P-bottle based techniques.

To acquire proficiency in the Kumagai Method, the hospital conducts specialized training sessions internally. However, only a few participants pass these training sessions. We invited Ms. Kumagai to participate in this study and asked her to provide us with recommendations for nurses who had obtained certification in mastering the Kumagai method with the P-bottle. The researcher (S.U.) provided research explanations to these nurses, and upon obtaining consent, enrolled them as research participants.

2.3. Data Collection

In September 2022, participants were equipped with recording microphones and asked to stand in front of a video camera. A semi-structured, in-depth interview was conducted in Japanese to gather information on the following: dealing with a closed mouth, inserting the nipple in cases of unilateral CLP, inserting the nipple in cases of bilateral CLP, dealing with the child's movements after insertion, and points to note when squeezing the bottle. The "child's movements that should be dealt with" were determined based on the following factors: intense crying, swinging the body widely, pushing out the nipple with the tongue, licking the nipple with the tongue without sucking, pushing up the nipple strongly with the tongue, weak sucking, and spitting out milk (a lot or a little). These movements were confirmed with the participants in advance as undesirable movements that commonly occur in children with feeding difficulties, and were defined before commencing the study.

Participants were requested to demonstrate feeding movements while holding a child doll with an incision in the oral cavity, to simulate CLP, and simultaneously provide verbal explanations. Recordings were made through the microphone and video camera. The collected audio and video files constituted the data for this study.

The interviewer was a researcher (S.U.) with experience as a pediatric nurse in feeding children with CLP, but who was ignorant of the Kumagai method. Therefore, he proceeded with the interview while checking the meaning of each word said by the participant.

2.4. Analysis

We used thematic analysis based on interpretivism [26]. This method is used to identify and report patterns (themes) obtained from interviews. First, the audio data were translated into written text, and the information provided by movements in the video data were added. The text was then mailed to each participant and checked for corrections or additions. After reading to understand the meaning, each technique was intercepted and coded. The codes were grouped by semantic content. The techniques were reviewed among the authors to ensure that the content of the techniques was understandable and that the different techniques were clearly distinguishable. The analysis was conducted by a researcher who specializes in pediatric nursing and has experience in feeding with a P-bottle. After analysis, the results were returned to the participants again for perusal to ensure that there were no discrepancies in each participant's intended meaning, which achieved investigator triangulation and enhanced the validity of the findings. The results were confirmed again by researchers and participants six months after the analysis was completed to ensure reliability.

2.5. Ethical Consideration

The present study was conducted in accordance with the International Committee of Medical Journal Editors guidelines, after obtaining ethical review approval and clinical research registration at Kyushu University. We explained the purpose and methods of the study to the participants and obtained their signatures on a consent form. The participants were informed that participation was voluntary and that they could withdraw at any time. Data collection was conducted in a private room in the hospitals to ensure privacy. In addition, data were managed by serial numbers to ensure that individuals could not be identified.

3. Results

The three nurses who had mastered the Kumagai Method had 19, 28, and 36 years nursing experience, respectively. The interview durations were 17.13, 18.78, and 24.62 min each.

3.1. Dealing with a Closed Mouth

Sometimes children with CLP will not open their mouth even when the nipple is close to their mouth. Three techniques were mentioned for dealing with such a situation: waking the children up with daily care, stimulating the mouth area with fingers or nipples, and lowering the lower jaw with using fingers.

> I encourage the child's sucking reflex and opening the mouth by stimulating their lips with a nipple. It is not a good idea to wait all the time without doing anything or forcing the nipple into the mouth (No.2).

3.2. Inserting the Nipple

The correct and incorrect methods of nipple insertion are listed in Table 1.

Table 1. Methods of inserting a nipple to the mouth.

Correct	Incorrect
• You insert the nipple straight on the middle of the tongue and keep it in that position.	• You insert the nipple in the mouth up to the base of nipple and the child's vomiting reflex is elicited. • The nipple hits the mucosa of the cleft when the child launches the nipple with the tongue.
(In the case of unilateral cleft lip and palate) • You should place the nipple in the middle of mouth and only half against the palate while applying force to the opposite side of the cleft even if the child's tongue tries to insert the nipple into the cleft, so that it is only half compressed by the child's tongue.	• You fit the nipple into the cleft; therefore, the child cannot compress the nipple with the tongue sufficiently and ulcers are formed on the mucous membranes. • You poke with the nipple toward the palate.
(In the case of bilateral cleft lip and palate) • You press the nipple against the raised tongue as the child sucks. • You squeeze the bottle at the same time the child sucks so that the child drinks in as short a time as possible.	• You leave the hard side of the nipple against the mucous membranes. • You do not squeeze the bottle.

It is not enough to simply put the nipple in the mouth. There is a technique to enable children with feeding difficulties to effectively use their tongues to be fed milk. By inserting the nipple straight down the middle against the tongue, the child can wrap the nipple with the tongue. The participant nurses intended to promote learning original feeding movements. The nipple of the P-bottle is shaped like a cylinder, and the depth of insertion is also important.

> Since the nipple is longer than a normal nipple, it is not inserted very deeply. To avoid inducing the gag reflex, do not insert the nipple all the way to the base of the nipple. The nipple is placed in the middle of the tongue so that the child wraps their tongue around the nipple, allowing the tongue to be used as the child could learn to move the tongue for original suckling (No. 2).

In the case of unilateral CLP, the participants called this maneuver "Hikkake-Nomashi" (a Japanese word devised by nurses, which means feeding while hooking the nipple onto the palate), a method that allowed only half of the nipple to be in contact with the palate area, whereas the other half remained untouched, such that the nipple was overhanging the palate (Figure 1). By employing this method, the child can squeeze half of the nipple with the tongue to release milk. The other half of the nipple is not compressed; however, the nipple does not enter the cleft, thus avoiding damage to the mucous membranes and ulcer formation.

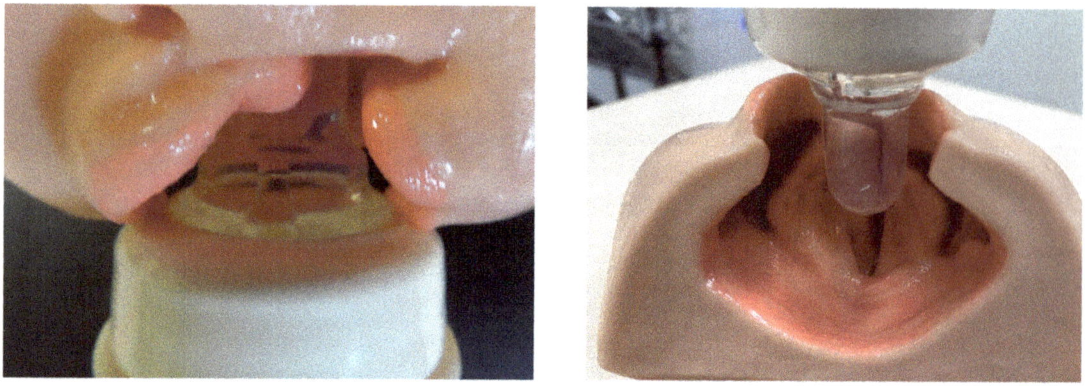

(a) View from above (b) View from the oral cavity

Figure 1. Correct position of the nipple for children with unilateral cleft lip and palate. (**a**) When viewed from above, only half the nipple is visible through the cleft. (**b**) Only half the nipple is in contact with the palate.

> As the child tends to bring the nipple into the cleft with their tongue, I keep the nipple overhanging a little to the palatal side to keep the nipple from getting stuck in the cleft and hold the nipple in the middle of tongue (No.1).

> By placing the nipple slightly against the palate, half of the pressure to the nipple escapes into the cleft. Only half of the nipple gets the pressure to drink. As the situation continues, the child will put the tongue straight up. The child will no longer try to enter the cleft and will not have to apply force in the direction opposite to the cleft. The incorrect way is to leave the nipple as it enters the cleft. Although you feel as if the child drinks well, the nipple is, in fact, not applying any pressure with their tongue at all. In this way, the milk is not released, and the child does not drink as much as they should (No.2).

> If the nipple goes toward the cleft (Figure 2), it will create an ulcer on the mucous membrane, so I do not think it should be done in such a way that the nipple goes in there (No.3).

In the case of bilateral CLP, there is no palate against which the nipple can be applied; hence, the nurses need to feed the child while pushing the face of the nipple in the direction of the tongue. In such cases, the pressure exerted by the child by only pushing up with the tongue is not sufficient to dispense enough milk. Therefore, the nurse has to squeeze the bottle while the child sucks to allow them to drink the milk and to prevent the child from getting tired.

> In the case of bilateral CLP, lightly press the nipple toward the tongue as the nipple cannot be hooked onto the palate, so as to inhibit the child from raising the tongue up too much. Adjust the milk flow by squeezing the bottle; the bottle should be squeezed more forcefully than for children with unilateral CLP. The timing should match the child's sucking. In the case of bilateral CLP, the key is to let the child feel that they are drinking from their own sucking (No.4).

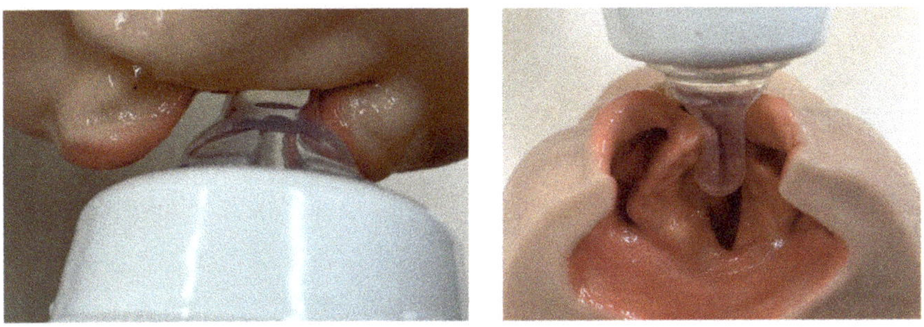

(a) View from above (b) View from the oral cavity

Figure 2. Incorrect positioning of the nipple for children with unilateral cleft lip and palate. (**a**) When viewed from above, the nipple is not visible. (**b**) The nipple is directed toward the cleft.

3.3. Squeezing the Bottle

The P-bottles are soft and can be squeezed to allow milk to flow out. However, the participants appeared to adjust the timing and pressure and not squeeze continuously, ensuring that the child could suck carefully (Table 2).

Table 2. Squeezing the bottle.

Correct	Incorrect
• You squeeze the bottle at the same time the child sucks. • You gradually increase the pressure to squeeze the bottle while making sure the child does not choke.	• You do not squeeze the bottle and let the child just suck. • You squeeze the bottle regardless of the child's breathing. • You continuously squeeze the bottle.

> If I squeeze the bottle too fast, the child may choke; thus, we adjust the amount of milk while looking at whether the child is swallowing properly and not choking (No.3).

> Squeezing in time with the child's breathing and sucking is a very important technique. If I squeeze the bottle at my own pace, without matching the child's breathing and sucking, it may cause choking. Another reason is that the child may learn to drink without sucking, which leads to not sucking (No.2).

3.4. Dealing with Various Child Movements after Insertion

A child with feeding difficulties may exhibit a variety of movements, as shown in Table 3. The first thing that the participants would do in response to the child's movements was to "re-hold" the child. If the child did not stop the movements even after that, the participants would take action, as shown in Table 3.

Table 3. Techniques other than "re-holding" to deal with the child's movement.

Cases	Remedial Steps
• Swinging the body wide • Pushing out the nipple with the tongue • Licking the nipple with the tongue without sucking	• Removing and re-inserting the nipple gently
• Pushing up the nipple strongly with the tongue	• Increasing the flow rate by increasing bottle squeezing
• Intense crying	Squeezing the bottle slightly
• Weak sucking	1st: Stimulating the tongue or lip 2nd: Squeezing the bottle slightly 3rd: Squeezing the bottle depending on how much as the child can swallow, if sucking occurs
• Spitting out milk (a little)	• Continuing the feeding
• Spitting out milk (a lot)	• Removing the nipple and allowing the child's breathing to recover, and then resuming

If the child "swings the body wide," "pushes the nipple out with the tongue," or "licks the nipple with the tongue without sucking," the participants assessed the situation as resistance to feeding and removed the nipple temporarily.

> If the child is quiet and then suddenly arching, I think the nipple might be in a painful place. Thus, I check if I am inserting the nipple correctly and will re-insert again (No.1).

Some children exhibit a tendency to strongly force the tongue to rise and tend to move the nipple into the cleft, even if the participants attempt to perform "Hikkake-Nomashi." In this case, the participants maintain the position of the nipple on the midline of the tongue and squeeze the bottle more to allow the child to focus on swallowing, resulting in the use of appropriate force to raise the tongue.

> If the child's tongue raising is strong, I increase the flow rate of milk. If I am defeated by the child's force of tongue raising and the nipple enters the cleft, an ulcer is formed. Furthermore, when the nipple enters the cleft, the nipple is not compressed sufficiently and the child's force of raising up the tongue becomes even stronger. This strong tongue raising is a response to wanting more milk, so milk flow needs to be increased. By increasing the bottle squeezing, the child will be able to drink the amount they want to drink. As a result, the force of the tongue raising will become moderate (No.2).

When the sucking is weak, it is necessary to apply a stimulus to assess if the sucking power is restored. The way to deal with this situation is to squeeze the bottle slightly and release a little milk to check if the sucking reflex would be initiated.

> Even if I try to stimulate the child's tongue or lips, the sucking reflex still does not occur, I squeeze slightly. I look to check if sucking occurs before swallowing, and if it does, I adjust the force of squeezing bottle to match the force of the child's sucking (No.2).

4. Discussion

The strength of the present study is that it systematically organized the detailed technical patterns that Ms. Kumagai, an expert in nursing care for children with CLP, has achieved over time. After birth, a palatal obturator is fabricated and fitted for children with CLP, and most children are able to drink without special bottle-feeding techniques [27] and achieve breastfeeding. However, it takes about a week to fabricate a palatal obturator. Meanwhile, children with CLP, who cannot create a negative pressure in the oral cavity and cannot be breastfed directly, must become accustomed to the P-bottle. If the child is not helped to drink adequate milk, they will require tube feeding or intravenous infusion, and their natural ability to feed will degenerate [28]. The Kumagai method allows more children to drink milk orally. The other issue in this study is the effectiveness of the techniques of the Kumagai method. Ms. Kumagai recently presented a practical report in Japanese demonstrating the effectiveness of this method in actual children [29]. Implementation of the Kumagai method in children with CLP with ulceration of the nasal septum resulted in reduction of the ulcers in about 80% of children, and they could also drink the target amount of milk within 20 min [29]. Further clinical studies investigating this method with a larger sample of children are warranted to scientifically prove the extent to which the Kumagai method increases feeding volume and contributes to weight gain in children with CLP and feeding difficulties, and that it decreases the frequency of ulcer development compared to other techniques.

The novelty of this study is that we clarified the direction of nipple insertion into the oral cavity (inserting the nipple to rest on the midline of the tongue), depth of insertion (not up to the base of the nipple), and timing (squeezing the bottle at the time of the child's sucking). Furthermore, the direction of the nipple force should be changed depending on the type of CLP (unilateral or bilateral). One of the reasons for this particular direction of pushing force for nipple placement is to prevent ulceration of the nasal septum mucosa. The mucosa of the nasal septum is soft and susceptible to ulceration due to irritation [16]. In addition, children with CLP have a tendency to try to insert the nipple into the cleft with the tongue. If the nurse allows this movement and continues to feed with the nipple inserted into the cleft, the pressure of the nipple causes ulceration. Ueki et al. [18] conducted a survey and found that many nurses use the "fit the nipple into the cleft" method, which may inadvertently cause ulcers. If the Kumagai method becomes the standard for clinical feeding, it may contribute to a reduction in the occurrence of ulcers. Other studies have suggested that the nipple be inserted in a direction without the cleft palate while tilting [30]. This method would also be less likely to result in ulcer development. However, the participants in the present study have insisted that the nipple should be directed along the midline position of tongue. The reason for this is to prevent ulceration and simultaneously promote natural movements of tongue suckling. When a healthy infant feeds, the tongue undulates in a wavy motion as it squeezes the nipple [31]. By placing the nipple on the midline of tongue, the child would be able to catch the nipple firmly with the tongue. Valentim et al. reported that poor tongue habits have a significant impact on the oral environment, with ramifications for the dentition and facial structure [32]. Adherence to the Kumagai method may have a positive impact on the dentition, by averting the characteristic facial features and speech problems that commonly occur in children with CLP.

The P-bottle can be squeezed to release milk, allowing nurses to adjust the amount of milk. However, if this adjustment is not appropriate, it can cause the child to choke. Feeding requires synchronized sucking, swallowing, and breathing [33]. If the child's sucking ability is weak, the amount and timing of releasing the milk should be adjusted so that the three aforementioned elements are in synchronicity. However, if the force of the tongue raising is strong, the nurse should increase the milk flow rate as per the present experience with the Kumagai method. This would allow the child to concentrate on swallowing, and naturally reduce the force of the tongue raising. This flow rate adjustment was one of the techniques used to correct the child's use of their tongue.

One limitation of this study is the small same size, limited to three participants. However, these three nurses have supported many children with feeding difficulties using the "Kumagai method," which is the result of this study. They have demonstrated that this method has enabled children with CLP to feed using the P-bottle. It would be easy to simply increase the number of participants, but it is not easy to find practitioners with exemplary technical skills. Another shortcoming is that the present findings are based only on interviews. Besides the techniques verbally recounted in the interviews, there may be other detailed techniques that these nurses use unconsciously. Moreover, demonstrations with a doll may not have replicated reality. It is necessary to observe the nursing skills of the participants in their daily nursing practice in real children and to investigate whether or not there are other techniques that have not yet been identified.

Thus, although there is still room for further study, this study evinced a pioneering result, being the first research with the potential to expand the application of the Kumagai method as a standard feeding method in the future. Recently, many videos explaining feeding in children with CLP have been disseminated on social networking services (SNS); however, the contents have low validity [34]. To promote the global adoption of the Kumagai method, we released a brief video of the method on social media prior to this study [35,36]. We are now preparing new videos with more detailed explanations based on the results of this study. Additionally, we plan to develop a smartphone application in the future. We also believe that interventional studies utilizing these tools will be necessary to facilitate skill acquisition.

The present study does not explicitly promote bottle-feeding promotion; the WHO's 10 Steps to successful breastfeeding, revised in 2018, have added the following: "9. Counsel mothers on the use and risks of feeding bottles, teats and pacifiers" [15]. Breastfeeding has mutual benefits for the mother and child and should be the first priority. However, when this is not possible, the existence of alternative bottle-feeding techniques, such as the one detailed in this study, would provide support to mothers.

5. Conclusions

The three expert nurses' methods of feeding children with CLP and feeding difficulties using a P-bottle included detailed techniques for dealing with a closed mouth before feeding, inserting the nipple, and squeezing the bottle. In particular, the nipple position was a new perspective, wherein the nipple should be placed on the line in the middle of the tongue, and the nipple should not be inserted to all the way to the base. In addition, it was found that the direction of the nipple force was changed; this means that if the child had unilateral CLP, the nipple was placed against half of the palate, and if the child had bilateral CLP, pressure was applied in the direction of the tongue. These methods had two purposes: to prevent ulcers and to help the child learn the natural tongue movement for suckling. In the future, it is desirable to discover other unconscious practices in these expert nurses' techniques and to scientifically verify the effectiveness of this Kumagai method.

Author Contributions: S.U.: Conceptualization, Methodology, Formal analysis, Investigation, Writing—original draft; Writing—review and editing, Project administration, Funding acquisition. Y.K.: Validation, Writing—review and editing. Y.H.: Validation, Writing—review and editing. E.N.: Investigation, Validation, Writing—review and editing. S.M.: Investigation, Validation, Writing—review and editing. T.I.: Investigation, Validation, Writing—review and editing. Q.A.: Investigation, Supervision, Writing—review and editing. E.T.: Supervision, Writing—review and editing. J.M.: Supervision, Writing—review and editing. All authors have read and agreed to the published version of the manuscript.

Funding: This work was supported by JSPS KAKENHI (Grant No. JP22K17504) from the Japan Society for the Promotion of Science, Ministry of Education, Culture, Sports, Science, and Technology, Tokyo, Japan.

Institutional Review Board Statement: This study was approved by the Institutional Ethics Review Committee of Kyushu University (code, 22136-02; 26 September 2022) and was performed in line with the principles of the Declaration of Helsinki and its later amendments.

Informed Consent Statement: Informed consent was obtained from all individuals involved in the study.

Data Availability Statement: The data and resources utilized in the research can be obtained from the corresponding author upon reasonable request.

Public Involvement Statement: No public involvement in any aspect of this research.

Guidelines and Standards Statement: We report our findings based on the standards for reporting qualitative research (SRQR) guidelines [37].

Use of Artificial Intelligence: AI or AI-assisted tools were not used in drafting any aspect of this manuscript.

Acknowledgments: The authors are deeply grateful to all participants.

Conflicts of Interest: The authors declare no conflicts of interest.

References

1. Salari, N.; Darvishi, N.; Heydari, M.; Bokaee, S.; Darvishi, F.; Mohammadi, M. Global prevalence of cleft palate, cleft lip and cleft palate and lip: A comprehensive systematic review and meta-analysis. *J. Stomatol. Oral Maxillofac. Surg.* **2022**, *123*, 110–120. [CrossRef] [PubMed]
2. Augsornwan, D.; Pattangtanang, P.; Surakunprapha, P. Development of information system for patients with cleft lip and palate undergoing operation. *J. Med. Assoc. Thai* **2015**, *98*, S151–S157.
3. Reid, J.; Kilpatrick, N.; Reilly, S. A prospective, longitudinal study of feeding skills in a cohort of babies with cleft conditions. *Cleft Palate Craniofac. J.* **2006**, *43*, 702–709. [CrossRef]
4. de Vries, I.A.; Breugem, C.C.; van der Heul, A.M.; Eijkemans, M.J.; Kon, M.; Mink van der Molen, A.B. Prevalence of feeding disorders in children with cleft palate only: A retrospective study. *Clin. Oral. Investig.* **2014**, *18*, 1507–1515. [CrossRef]
5. Green, M.A.; Resnick, C.M. Feeding considerations for infants with craniofacial malformations. *Semin. Fetal Neonatal Med.* **2021**, *26*, 101280. [CrossRef]
6. Boyce, J.O.; Reilly, S.; Skeat, J.; Cahir, P.; Academy of Breastfeeding Medicine. ABM Clinical Protocol #17: Guidelines for Breastfeeding Infants with Cleft Lip, Cleft Palate, or Cleft Lip and Palate-Revised 2019. *Breastfeed. Med.* **2019**, *14*, 437–444. [CrossRef]
7. Kaye, A.; Thaete, K.; Snell, A.; Chesser, C.; Goldak, C.; Huff, H. Initial nutritional assessment of infants with cleft lip and/or palate: Interventions and return to birth weight. *Cleft Palate Craniofac. J.* **2017**, *54*, 127–136. [CrossRef] [PubMed]
8. Nyakotey, D.A.; Apprey, C.; Annan, R.A. Malnutrition in children with unrepaired orofacial cleft: A systematic review. *IJPHCS* **2019**, *6*, 67–76. [CrossRef]
9. Tungotyo, M.; Atwine, D.; Nanjebe, D.; Hodges, A.; Situma, M. The prevalence and factors associated with malnutrition among infants with cleft palate and/or lip at a hospital in Uganda: A cross-sectional study. *BMC Pediatr.* **2017**, *17*, 17. [CrossRef] [PubMed]
10. Phalke, N.; Goldman, J.J. *Cleft Palate*; StatPearls Publishing: Treasure Island, FL, USA, 2023.
11. Baylis, A.L.; Pearson, G.D.; Hall, C.; Madhoun, L.L.; Cummings, C.; Neal, N.; Smith, A.; Eastman, K.; Stocker, C.; Kirschner, R.E. A quality improvement initiative to improve feeding and growth of infants with cleft lip and/or palate. *Cleft Palate Craniofac. J.* **2018**, *5*, 1218–1224. [CrossRef] [PubMed]
12. World Health Organization and United Nations Children's Fund. Protecting, Promoting and Supporting Breastfeeding: The Baby-Friendly Hospital Initiative for Small, Sick and Preterm Newborns, Geneva, World Health Organization. 2020. Available online: https://iris.who.int/handle/10665/333686 (accessed on 30 May 2024).
13. Centers for Disease Control and Prevention. Breastfeeding: Recommendations and Benefits. Available online: https://www.cdc.gov/nutrition/infantandtoddlernutrition/breastfeeding/recommendations-benefits.html (accessed on 30 May 2024).
14. Lewis, C.W.; Jacob, L.S.; Lehmann, C.U.; Section on Oral Health. The primary care pediatrician and the care of children with cleft lip and/or cleft palate. *Pediatrics* **2017**, *139*, e20170628. [CrossRef]
15. Aryeetey, R.; Dykes, F. Global implications of the new WHO and UNICEF implementation guidance on the revised Baby-Friendly Hospital Initiative. *Matern. Child. Nutr.* **2018**, *14*, e12637. [CrossRef]
16. Shahzad, F.; Sanati-Mehrizy, P. Feeding protocol in cleft palate patients. In *Surgical Atlas of Cleft Palate and Palatal Fistulae*; Fayyaz, G.Q., Ed.; Springer: Singapore, 2022; pp. 1–14. [CrossRef]
17. Stowe, G.; Schleif, E.P.; Perry, J.L.; Briley, P.M. Impact of insurance status on initiation of breast milk feeding among infants with CL $\pm$ P. *Cleft Palate Craniofac. J.* **2023**, *60*, 858–864. [CrossRef]
18. Ueki, S.; Fujita, A.; Kumagai, Y.; Hirai, Y.; Tashiro, E.; Miyata, J. Bottle-feeding techniques for children with cleft lip and palate experiencing feeding difficulties. *Int. J. Nurs. Sci.* **2023**, *10*, 82–88. [CrossRef]
19. Madhoun, L.L.; O'Brien, M.; Baylis, A.L. Infant-driven feeding systems: Do they "normalize" the feeding experience of infants with cleft palate? *Cleft Palate Craniofac. J.* **2021**, *58*, 1304–1312. [CrossRef] [PubMed]
20. Penny, C.; McGuire, C.; Bezuhly, M. A systematic review of feeding interventions for infants with cleft palate. *Cleft Palate Craniofac. J.* **2022**, *59*, 1527–1536. [CrossRef]
21. Sharma, S. Feeding intervention for cleft lip and palate child. *J. Emerg. Technol. Innov. Res.* **2020**, *7*, 1347–1351.

22. Shetty, M.S.; Khan, M.B. Feeding considerations in infants born with cleft lip and palate. *APOS Trends Orthod.* **2016**, *6*, 49–53. [CrossRef]
23. Gailey, D.G. Feeding infants with cleft and the postoperative cleft management. *Oral. Maxillofac. Surg. Clin. N. Am.* **2016**, *28*, 153–159. [CrossRef]
24. Klein, A.; Uyehara, M.; Cunningham, A.; Olomi, M.; Cashin, K.; Kirk, C.M. Nutritional care for children with feeding difficulties and disabilities: A scoping review. *PLOS Glob. Public Health* **2023**, *3*, e0001130. [CrossRef]
25. Ueki, S.; Kumagai, Y.; Hirai, Y.; Nagatomo, E.; Miyauchi, S.; Inoue, T.; An, Q.; Miyata, J. The Kumagai Method utilizing the Pigeon Bottle feeder with a long nipple: A descriptive study for the development of feeding techniques for children with cleft lip and/or palate. *Children* **2024**, *11*, 365. [CrossRef]
26. Braun, V.; Clarke, V. Using thematic analysis in psychology. *Qual. Res. Psychol.* **2006**, *3*, 77–101. [CrossRef]
27. Buller, M.; Jodeh, D.; Qamar, F.; Wright, J.M.; Halsey, J.N.; Rottgers, S.A. Cleft Palate Fistula: A Review. *Eplasty* **2023**, *23*, e7. [PubMed]
28. Brand, B.M. Cleft Lip and Palate Feeding Intervention: A Scoping Review. Doctoral Dissertation, Stellenbosch University, Stellenbosch, South Africa, 2020.
29. Kumagai, Y.; Hirai, Y.; Ueki, S.; Nagatomo, E.; Kogo, M.; Tanaka, S. Verification of bottle-feeding (Kumagai Method) for children with unilateral cleft lip and palate. *J. Jpn. Cleft Palate Assoc.* **2024**, *49*, 110.
30. Iijima, H. Disease, nutritional guidance and dietary therapy: Feeding disorders in children with cleft lip and palate. *Jpn. J. Pediatr.* **2019**, *72*, 563–566.
31. Ishimaru, A.; Saito, T. Formational change of tongue and nipple during feeding: Smoothness of tongue movements. *Jpn. J. Child. Health* **2002**, *5*, 761–766.
32. Valentim, A.; Furlan, R.; Amaral, M.; Martins, F. Can orofacial structures affect tooth morphology? In *Human Teeth—Key Skills and Clinical Illustrations*; IntechOpen: London, UK, 2020. [CrossRef]
33. Degenaar, H.; Kritzinger, A. Suck, swallow and breathing coordination in infants with infantile colic. *S. Afr. J. Commun. Disord.* **2015**, *62*, e1–e10. [CrossRef] [PubMed]
34. Srivastav, S.; Tewari, N.; Antonarakis, G.S.; Upadhyaya, A.D.; Duggal, R.; Goel, S. How informative is YouTube regarding feeding in infants with cleft lip and palate? *Cleft Palate Craniofac. J.* **2024**, *61*, 774–790. [CrossRef] [PubMed]
35. Osaka University Dental Hospital, Department of Nursing. Kumagai Method #1 Unilateral CLP. 2021. Available online: https://youtu.be/S1nr9E-8JYo (accessed on 18 September 2024).
36. Osaka University Dental Hospital, Department of Nursing. Kumagai Method #2 Bilateral CLP. 2021. Available online: https://youtu.be/RVAoC6fbFAY (accessed on 18 September 2024).
37. O'Brien, B.C.; Harris, I.B.; Beckman, T.J.; Reed, D.A.; Cook, D.A. Standards for reporting qualitative research: A synthesis of recommendations. *Acad. Med.* **2014**, *89*, 1245–1251. [CrossRef]

nursing reports

MDPI

Article

Nurse-Driven Interventions Reduce Central Line-Associated Bloodstream Infection Close to Zero in One Pediatric Oncologic Facility: A Single-Center Retrospective Observational Study

Federico Turoldo [1], Antonella Longo [2], Mariavittoria Sala [3], Denis Valentini [4], Nicole De Vita [2], Sara Toniutti [2], Loredana Zuppel [2] and Natalia Maximova [2,*]

1 Department of Medicine, Surgery and Health Sciences, Hygiene and Preventive Medicine, University of Trieste, Strada di Fiume 447, 34149 Trieste, Italy; federico.turoldo@studenti.units.it
2 Department of Pediatrics, Institute for Maternal and Child Health—IRCCS "Burlo Garofolo", Via dell'Istria 65/1, 34137 Trieste, Italy; antonella.longo@burlo.trieste.it (A.L.); nicole.devita@burlo.trieste.it (N.D.V.); sara.toniutti@burlo.trieste.it (S.T.); loredana.zuppel@burlo.trieste.it (L.Z.)
3 Department of Public Health and Pediatric Sciences, University of Turin, 10136 Turin, Italy; mariavittoria.sala@unito.it
4 Department of Emergency Medicine, Hospital of Cattinara, Azienda Sanitaria Universitaria Giuliano Isontina (ASU GI), Strada di Fiume 447, 34149 Trieste, Italy; denis.valentini@asugi.sanita.fvg.it
* Correspondence: natalia.maximova@burlo.trieste.it; Tel.: +39-040-3785276 (ext. 565); Fax: +39-040-3785494

Abstract: Background: Central line-associated bloodstream infections (CLABSIs) are critical infectious complications among pediatric hematology-oncology patients, and the management of central venous catheters (CVCs) by healthcare personnel can significantly influence the incidence of these infections. This study evaluates the impact of nurse-led changes in CVC management on the incidence of CLABSIs. Methods: This single-center, retrospective observational study was conducted at an urban, tertiary referral, and academic center serving pediatric patients. Results: The study cohort comprised 239 patients and 323 CVCs seen between 2012 and 2022. CLABSI was defined according to the Centers for Disease Control and Prevention definitions. Oncology nurse leaders developed CVC-specific educational modules for CLABSI prevention. All the relevant information during the CVC maintenance period was noted in the patient's CVC logbook. A total of 24 (7%) cases of confirmed CLABSI were identified. The incidence of CVC-related infections was 0.32 cases per 1000 catheter days (95%CI: 0.19–0.45). The incidence decreased by 40% between the first and second three-year study period. Documented exit-site infection was reported in 32 (10%) cases. The correlation between exit-site infection and CLABSI was found in 9 (28%) cases. Our CVC-related infection rates are significantly lower than the incidence reported by the Italian Association of Pediatric Hematology and Oncology, which settles at 3–5 cases per 1000 catheter days. Conclusions: Our data confirm the effectiveness of local CVC management guidelines in preventing CVC-related infectious complications.

Keywords: central venous catheter; pediatric; oncological; central line-associated bloodstream infections; catheter-related bloodstream infections

1. Introduction

Central line-associated bloodstream infections (CLABSIs) and catheter-related bloodstream infections (CRBSIs) are the most critical central line-correlated infectious complications among pediatric hematology oncology patients [1,2]. The incidence of CLABSI among pediatric oncological patients is 1–4.6 per 1000 catheter days for external central venous catheter (CVC) engaging about 25% of this population, with an estimated mortality rate between 12.5% and 25% [3–5]. Patients arc particularly susceptible to infectious complications during episodes of chemotherapy-induced neutropenia, but also non-neutropenic outpatients can suffer from CVC-related infections [6,7].

Nurs. Rep. **2024**, *14*, 2668–2679. https://doi.org/10.3390/nursrep14040197 https://www.mdpi.com/journal/nursrep

The incidence of CLABSI is variable according to modifiable and non-modifiable factors. If patient characteristics such as age, low body weight, disease status, and comorbidities cannot be changed, the "human factor", which determines how a CVC is managed, is improvable. The correct management of the central line, the proper preparation and administration of infusion liquids, the correct dressing techniques, and appropriate drug delivery methods are all modifiable factors that have a certain weight in the incidence of catheter-related infections [8–10]. In our Institute, CVC management is the responsibility of dedicated nursing staff, per standard practice. The decision to conduct this study was dictated by the need to verify whether we can reduce CVC-related infectious complications thanks to the rigorous and collaborative application of local CVC management guidelines.

After introducing the CVC management protocol, designed by highly qualified oncology nurse staff, and its application in all satellite hospitals, we aimed to estimate the incidence of CVC-related infections, placing this question as the study's primary aim.

2. Materials and Methods

2.1. Study Design and Population

This is a single-center retrospective observational study. The study reviewed CVC data routinely collected from January 2012 to July 2022. Three hundred twenty-six consecutive children and adolescents with cancer and hematological disease who initiated care at the Department of Pediatric Hematology Oncology and Bone Marrow Transplantation of the urban, tertiary referral academic medical center Burlo Garofolo Children's Hospital were included in the study group. Inclusion criteria were as follows: CVC inserted in our hospital between January 2012 and July 2022, hematological or oncological diagnosis, age less than 18 at the time of CVC insertion, and informed consent for using clinical data signed by parents at admission. Exclusion criteria were CVC removal within the first 24 h of insertion and personal CVC logbook unavailability.

This was a unit-based quality improvement project designed by nurses with longstanding experience. The study's primary aim was to assess whether the nurses' CVC management recommendations would result in a lower incidence of infectious complications than the rates reported in the literature. The secondary aim was to determine if, among the analyzed variables, it was possible to identify any additional risk factors for CVC-related infectious in a pediatric oncological setting.

Demographic and clinical characteristics data were collected on the patients with an oncologic or hematologic diagnosis who had a CVC placed.

2.2. Ethical Approval and Informed Consent

The study protocol was approved by the Institutional Review Board of the IRCCS Burlo Garofolo (reference No. IRB RC 32/2023), and the study was conducted following the Declaration of Helsinki. The data were collected according to the Authorization to Process Personal Data for Scientific Research Purposes (Authorization No. 9/2014) [11].

According to our Institute regulations, parents or guardians had to give written informed consent on the first visit to use any clinical data in research. The medical records of all the patients were analyzed individually and anonymously.

2.3. Nurse-Led Quality Improvement CVC-Management Protocol

Following a critical evaluation of the best evidence, the oncological nurse team developed changes to the unit's nursing practice on CVC handling guidelines to reduce CLABSI incidence. The differences in the modified guidelines compared to the in-force departmental CVC maintenance protocol were the following:

- The ordinary management of the CVC is exclusively the responsibility of the trained personnel;
- Two-person dressing approach;
- Use an aseptic technique during any CVC manipulation that requires the lumen opening or removal of the CVC exit-site dressing;

- The preparation of injecting drugs or solutions to be infused into the CVC under a laminar flow hood using an aseptic technique;
- A total of 2% chlorhexidine and 70% isopropyl alcohol disinfection of needle-free connectors (NFCs) and cover with a double layer of sterile gauze for biological fluid contamination protection;
- The maintenance of the closed circuit during the use of infusion lines;
- The replacement of infusion lines every 24 h if blood products, total parenteral nutrition (TPN), propofol administration, or closed-circuit interruption; otherwise, replacement is carried out every 72 h;
- The production of the patient CVC logbook, which includes placement information, dressing according to the eventual patient's preferences, any maintenance problems, and any infectious event reported (Figure 1);
- Newly hired and satellite hospital personnel training to prepare them to work independently, maintaining uniform CVC management.

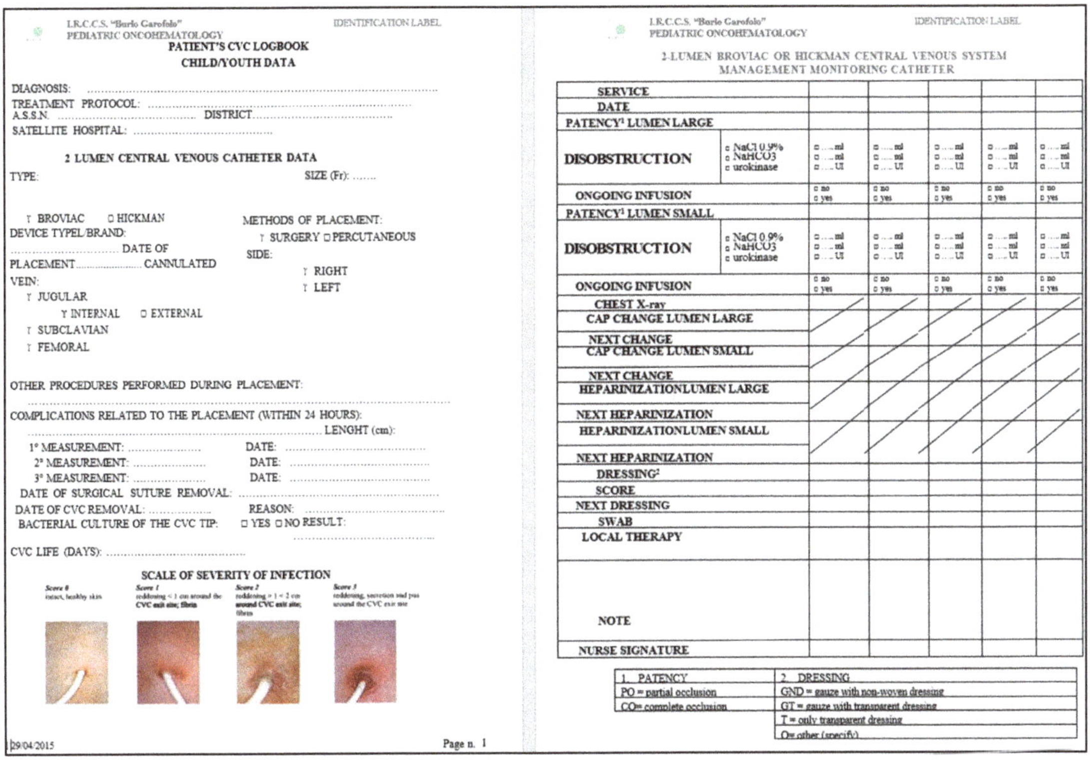

I.R.C.C.S. "Burlo Garofolo"
PEDIATRIC ONCOHEMATOLOGY
IDENTIFICATION LABEL

PATIENT'S CVC LOGBOOK
CHILD/YOUTH DATA

DIAGNOSIS: ....
TREATMENT PROTOCOL: ....
A.S.S.N. .... DISTRICT ....
SATELLITE HOSPITAL: ....

2 LUMEN CENTRAL VENOUS CATHETER DATA

TYPE: SIZE (Fr): ....

□ BROVIAC □ HICKMAN
DEVICE TYPEL/BRAND: .... DATE OF PLACEMENT .... CANNULATED VEIN:
□ JUGULAR
□ INTERNAL □ EXTERNAL
□ SUBCLAVIAN
□ FEMORAL

METHODS OF PLACEMENT:
□ SURGERY □ PERCUTANEOUS
SIDE:
□ RIGHT
□ LEFT

OTHER PROCEDURES PERFORMED DURING PLACEMENT: ....
COMPLICATIONS RELATED TO THE PLACEMENT (WITHIN 24 HOURS): .... LENGHT (cm):
1° MEASUREMENT: .... DATE: ....
2° MEASUREMENT: .... DATE: ....
3° MEASUREMENT: .... DATE: ....
DATE OF SURGICAL SUTURE REMOVAL: ....
DATE OF CVC REMOVAL: .... REASON: ....
BACTERIAL CULTURE OF THE CVC TIP: □ YES □ NO RESULT: ....
CVC LIFE (DAYS): ....

SCALE OF SEVERITY OF INFECTION

Score 0 intact, healthy skin
Score 1 reddening < 1 cm around the CVC exit site; fibrin
Score 2 reddening > 1 < 2 cm around CVC exit site; fibrin
Score 3 reddening, secretion and pus around the CVC exit site

29/04/2015 Page n. 1

I.R.C.C.S. "Burlo Garofolo"
PEDIATRIC ONCOHEMATOLOGY
IDENTIFICATION LABEL

2-LUMEN BROVIAC OR HICKMAN CENTRAL VENOUS SYSTEM MANAGEMENT MONITORING CATHETER

SERVICE						
DATE						
PATENCY[1] LUMEN LARGE						
DISOBSTRUCTION	□ NaCl 0.9% □ NaHCO3 □ urokinase	□ ....ml □ ....ml □ ....UI	□ ....ml □ ....ml □ ....UI	□ ....ml □ ....ml □ ....UI	□ ....ml □ ....ml □ ....UI	□ ....ml □ ....ml □ ....UI
ONGOING INFUSION		□ no □ yes	□ no □ yes	□ no □ yes	□ no □ yes	□ no □ yes
PATENCY[1] LUMEN SMALL						
DISOBSTRUCTION	□ NaCl 0.9% □ NaHCO3 □ urokinase	□ ....ml □ ....ml □ ....UI	□ ....ml □ ....ml □ ....UI	□ ....ml □ ....ml □ ....UI	□ ....ml □ ....ml □ ....UI	□ ....ml □ ....ml □ ....UI
ONGOING INFUSION		□ no □ yes	□ no □ yes	□ no □ yes	□ no □ yes	□ no □ yes
CHEST X-ray						
CAP CHANGE LUMEN LARGE						
NEXT CHANGE						
CAP CHANGE LUMEN SMALL						
NEXT CHANGE						
HEPARINIZATIONLUMEN LARGE						
NEXT HEPARINIZATION						
HEPARINIZATIONLUMEN SMALL						
NEXT HEPARINIZATION						
DRESSING[2]						
SCORE						
NEXT DRESSING						
SWAB						
LOCAL THERAPY						
NOTE						
NURSE SIGNATURE						

1. PATENCY	2. DRESSING
PO = partial occlusion	GND = gauze with non-woven dressing
CO= complete occlusion	GT = gauze with transparent dressing
	T = only transparent dressing
	O= other (specify)

Figure 1. The personal logbook is given to the patient or parent and used by the nursing personnel to add information about placement, dressing, eventual dressing preferences, maintenance problems, and any infectious event reported.

2.4. Central Line Data

We documented all the CVCs, along with the device type, number of lumens, tube size, date of placement, laterality, cannulated vein, duration of CVC, dressing frequency, CVC use (TPN, transfusions, blood sampling, or apheresis), and removal indication. CVCs that had been in place for less than one day were excluded. If a patient underwent multiple CVC placements, it was considered a different entry in the database. CVCs were categorized as tunneled (cuffed and non-cuffed), non-tunneled, and implanted subcutaneously.

2.5. CVC Dressing Protocol

CVC dressings were performed according to the GAVeCeLT protocol (Italian expert group on long-term central venous accesses). They were changed every seven days (planned) or whenever they became damp, detached, or visibly soiled (unplanned). If the dressing and CVC exit site appeared perfect in inpatients, the dressing was postponed to 10 days.

After the adhesive tissue was removed with Remove© wipes (Smith and Nephew, Watford, England, UK), the dressing area's skin was cleaned using a BD ChloraPrepTM applicator (Becton, Dickinson and Company, Franklin Lakes, NJ, USA) that delivers a solution of 2% *w*/*v* chlorhexidine gluconate and 70% *v*/*v* isopropyl alcohol without orange dye. BD Chloraprep™ was applied by rubbing the skin around the exit site back and forth to cover the whole dressing area and let dry for 30 s. When the skin was dry, adhesive transparent dressing IV3000 (Smith&Nephew, Watford, UK) or Tegaderm™ I.V. Advanced (3M, Maplewood, MN, USA) was attached.

2.6. CVC-Associated Infectious Data

CLABSI is defined as a culture of recognized pathogens from one or more blood cultures, with the organism not related to an infection at another site, in patients with a CVC in place within 48 h before detection. If a common skin contaminant is cultured, two or more blood cultures drawn on separate occasions are required, along with specific symptoms [12]. We considered CLABSI in the inpatient setting if the first positive blood culture occurred >48 h after admission or <48 h after hospital discharge. In the outpatients, CLABSIs were considered if the first positive blood culture occurred >48 h after hospital discharge or <48 h after admission [13]. We considered the mucosal barrier injury to reduce the potential overestimation of true CRBSI incidence [14]. The occurrence of skin irritation was defined as the presence of areas of skin loss, erythematous plaques, or vesicles at the site of CVC insertion. We have defined a CVC exit-site infection as hyperemia, induration, and/or tenderness ≤ 2 cm from the catheter exit site with negative blood cultures. The exit site was evaluated using a visual exit-site score [15].

2.7. Statistical Analysis

Data were statistically analyzed using the R software version 4.3.1 (16 June 2023 ucrt) for Windows [16].

Descriptive statistics were used to analyze the demographic data, CVC characteristics, and details on CVC insertion, usage, and complications using the "gtsummary" package [17]. Categorical data were presented as frequency and percentage, while continuous data were presented as the median and interquartile range (IQR). The tests defaulted were the Wilcoxon rank sum test for continuous variables, Pearson's Chi-squared test without Yates' correction for categorical variables with all the expected cell counts ≥ 5, and Fisher's exact test for categorical variables with any expected cell count < 5. Incomplete observations were removed from the analysis.

The incidence of infection was calculated as the number of cases/person-time, and the 95% CI was calculated using the formula CI = rate $\pm$ 1.96 $\times$ sqrt (rate/person-time).

In order to study additional factors associated with infection, the dataset was divided according to CLABSI, and also alternative outcomes were proposed and explored to conduct sensitivity analyses. In this secondary analysis, associations were explored by running a univariate logistic regression on the relative outcome for each variable taken into consideration, and the resulting OR and 95%CI were reported. In the supplements, a survival analysis was conducted to establish the cumulative incidence of infection among different groups of interest with the help of the "survival" package [18].

The statistical significance was arbitrarily set to <0.05.

3. Results

3.1. Patient Population and Device Characteristics

In total, 239 pediatric oncological and hematological patients had a CVC inserted between January 2012 and December 2019, with the last follow-up occurring in December 2022. Some patients had multiple CVC placements, often at different times, with potential variations in patient characteristics or the CVC itself. For this reason, each CVC placement was considered a separate entry. The total number of CVCs inserted during the study period was 323, with 66 (20%) patients requiring one or more CVC replacements. The most common primary diagnoses were acute lymphoblastic leukemia (n = 145, 45%) and solid tumors (n = 100, 31%). In total, 122 (37.8%) patients underwent hematopoietic stem cell transplantation (HSCT), and 245 (75.9%) patients received TPN.

All the CVCs were inserted according to the local standard operating procedures. The median age at placement was 6.7 years (range, 0–18). The most common central device type (n = 210, 6%) was Broviac®—Hickman® (Bard Access Systems). All the central devices were tunneled and cuffed. The median lumen density was 1.46, and the median duration of the central device was 228 days (IQR, 103–320). The following indications for removal were observed: 200 (62%) due to end of therapy, 31 (10%) due to CVC-related infections, 31 (10%) due to malposition and dislodgement, 27 (8.5%) due to death, 19 (6%) due to occlusion and malfunction, and 11 (3.5%) due to breakage. Patient and central device characteristics are shown in Table 1.

Table 1. Main characteristics of the population.

Characteristic	**Frequency [1] (n = 323)**
Sex	
- Female	121 (37.5%)
- Male	202 (62.5%)
Age (years)	6.71 (2.95–11.90)
Duration of CVC (days)	228.0 (103.0–320.5)
Total CVC placements [2]	
- 1 CVC placement	173 (72.4%)
- 2 CVC placements	50 (20.9%)
- 3 CVC placements	14 (5.9%)
- 4 CVC placements	2 (0.8%)
Lumen	
- Monolumen	175 (54.2%)
- Bilumen	148 (45.8%)
Diameter of CVC (French)	8.00 (6.00–9.00)
Diagnosis	
- Acute lymphatic leukemia	145 (44.9%)
- Acute myeloid leukemia	22 (6.8%)
- Myelodysplastic syndromes	26 (8.0%)
- Non-malignant hematological diseases	26 (8.0%)
- Solid Tumors	100 (31.0%)
- Unknown	4

Table 1. *Cont.*

Characteristic	Frequency [1] (*n* = 323)
HSCT	
- Yes	122 (37.8%)
- No	201 (62.2%)
TPN	
- Yes	245 (75.9%)
- No	70 (21.7%)
- Unknown	8
CVC model	
- BARD—BROVIAC/HICKMAN	210 (65.0%)
- LIFECATH/VYGON	47 (14.6%)
- MEDCOMP	52 (16.1%)
- Other	14 (4.3%)
Insertion side	
- Right	237 (73.4%)
- Left	85 (26.3%)
- Unknown	1
Vein	
- Internal jugular	169 (52.3%)
- External jugular	24 (7.4%)
- Subclavian	50 (15.5%)
- Brachiocephalic	64 (19.8%)
- Other	16 (5.0%)
Dressing setting	
- IRCCS Burlo Garofolo	85.1 (52.71–100.0)
- Satellite hospitals	14.91 (0.0–47.29)
Dressing time interval (% of total dressings)	
- 1–6 days	30.43 (22.2–45.7)
- 7 days	50.0 (36.6–60.1)
- 8–10 days	16.1 (8.9–24.2)

[1] categorical variables: frequency and percentage. Continuous variables: median and interquartile range. [2] categorical variables: frequency and percentage (*n* = 239). CVC: central venous catheter; HSCT: hematopoietic stem cell transplantation; TPN: total parenteral nutrition; IRCCS: "Scientific Research and Healthcare Institute".

3.2. Central Line-Associated Infectious Events

During the study period, we identified 24 proven CLABSI events in the hospital's electronic database. The rate of CLABSI was 0.32 infections per 1000 catheter days (95%CI: 0.19–0.45). We analyzed patient and CVC characteristics to find the factors that might increase the risk of infection (Table 2).

Table 2. Proven CLABSI and distribution of main characteristics.

Characteristic	**Not Infection, *n* = 299** [1]	**CLABSI, *n* = 24** [1]	***p*-Value** [2]	**OR (95%CI)** [3]
Patient characteristics				
Age (years)	6.9 (3.1, 12.0)	4.1 (2.7, 10.3)	0.2	0.95 (0.88, 1.04)
Sex			0.4	1.5 (0.6, 3.72)
0—Female	114 (38%)	7 (29%)		
1—Male	185 (62%)	17 (71%)		
Diagnosis			0.12	
1—Acute lymphoblastic leukemia	139 (46%)	6 (25%)	0.042	1
2—Acute myeloid leukemia	20 (6.7%)	2 (8.3%)	0.7	2.32 (0.44, 12.28)
3—Myelodysplastic syndromes	22 (7.4%)	4 (17%)	0.11	4.21 (1.1, 16.13)
4—Non-malignant hematological diseases	22 (7.4%)	4 (17%)	0.11	4.21 (1.1, 16.13)
5—Solid Tumors	92 (31%)	8 (33%)	0.8	2.01 (0.68, 6)
6—Unknown	4 (1.3%)	0 (0%)	>0.9	0 (0, Inf)
HSCT			0.4	1.43 (0.62, 3.31)
0—No	188 (63%)	13 (54%)		
1—Yes	111 (37%)	11 (46%)		
CVC characteristics				
CVC Model			0.3	
1—BARD—BROVIAC/HICKMAN	198 (66%)	12 (50%)	0.11	1
2—LIFECATH/VYGON	43 (14%)	4 (17%)	0.8	1.53 (0.47, 4.99)
3—MEDCOMP	46 (15%)	6 (25%)	0.2	2.15 (0.77, 6.04)
4—COOK	1 (0.3%)	0 (0%)	>0.9	0 (0, Inf)
5—Unknown	11 (3.7%)	2 (8.3%)	0.3	3 (0.6, 15.09)
CVC type			>0.9	
1—CICC	277 (93%)	23 (96%)	>0.9	1
2—PICC	13 (4.3%)	1 (4.2%)	>0.9	0.93 (0.12, 7.4)
3—FICC	1 (0.3%)	0 (0%)	>0.9	0 (0, Inf)
4—PORT	8 (2.7%)	0 (0%)	>0.9	0 (0, Inf)
CVC life and use				
CVC duration (days)	237 (111, 325)	163 (58, 272)	0.1	1.00 (0.995, 1.01)
TPN			0.2	0.48 (0.14, 1.65)
0—No	224 (77%)	21 (88%)		
1—Yes	67 (23%)	3 (13%)		
Unknown	8	0		
At least one occlusion			0.9	0.95 (0.41, 2.18)
0—No	133 (44%)	11 (46%)		
1—Yes	166 (56%)	13 (54%)		

[1] categorical variables: *n* (%); continuous variables: median (IQR). [2] Fisher's exact test; Wilcoxon rank sum test; Pearson's Chi-squared test. [3] univariate logistic regression. CLABSI: central line-associated bloodstream infection; HSCT: hematopoietic stem cell transplantation; TPN: total parenteral nutrition; CICC: Centrally Inserted Central Catheter; PICC: Peripherally Inserted Central Catheter; FICC: Femoral-Inserted Central Catheter; IRCCS: "Scientific Research and Healthcare Institute".

Only ALL diagnosis was associated with a lower incidence of CLABSI ($p = 0.042$). Even if no other statistically significant association with infection was found, older age (>seven years) and insertion in the subclavian vein appear to be protective factors (Figure 1). We found no correlation even between CLABSI and total parenteral nutrition (TPN) or CVC occlusion events in our cohort. The reliability of the results was tested through sensitivity analysis. The sensitivity analysis was also extended to patients with possible CVC-related infection and CVCs removed due to infection (Table 3). Fifty-one cases of possible infection were identified, and in this population, the patients' ages were also lower than the mean cohort age. The incidence of possible infection was 0.67 events per 1000 days of CVC (95%CI: 0.49–0.86). Thirty-one infected CVCs (10%) were removed because of the infection. No other significant association between infection and patient or CVC characteristics was found. Figure 2 shows a survival analysis to investigate the cumulative incidence of CLABSI among the patients, focusing on age and ALL diagnoses.

Table 3. Incidence of infection in groups with different dressing frequency.

Group	N. Subjects	CLABSI	Infection Rate per 1000 CVC Days	(95% CI)
Less frequent dressing	111	8	0.31	(0.09–0.53)
Standard dressing	212	16	0.32	(0.16–0.48)

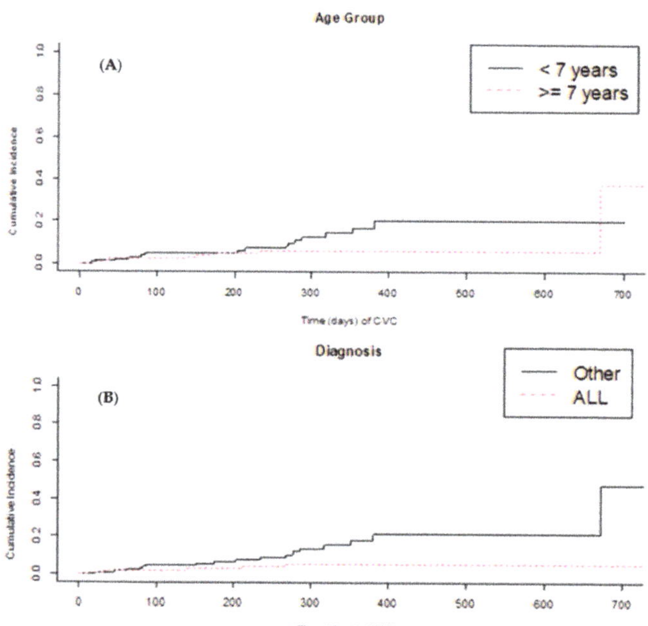

Figure 2. CVC-related infections and patients' variables. (**A**) Age $\geq$ seven years appears to be a protective factor for CLABSI without reaching statistical significance ($p > 0.05$). (**B**) ALL diagnosis was associated with a lower incidence of CLABSI ($p = 0.042$).

The majority of the germs involved in the CLABSI were Staphylococcus aureus (45%), Staphylococcus epidermidis (17%), Pseudomonas aeruginosa (13%), Candida albicans (13%), and Candida parapsilosis (13%). Ten percent (32 events) of all the CVCs analyzed had a positive exit-site culture, with the prevalence of Staphylococcus aureus (50%). The skin site colonization and CLABSI were correlated in nine cases (28%). A strong correlation was found between CVC tip colonization and bloodstream infection: the same pathogen was isolated from blood cultures in 11 out of 18 cases (61%).

3.3. Dressing and CVC Exit-Site Score

We assessed whether the frequency of dressings correlates with CVC-related infections. The median percentage of dressings with 1–6 day intervals was significantly higher in the CLABSI group than in the non-infected group (50% of total dressing, IQR 37–68% vs. 30%, IQR 22–43%; $p < 0.001$). The median percentage of dressings performed once a week was significantly higher in the non-infected group compared to the CLABSI group (50% of the total dressing, IQR 38–61% vs. 31%, IQR 11–45%; $p < 0.001$). No significant differences were found in both groups for dressing performed every ten days (16% of the total dressing, IQR 9–24% vs. 12%, IQR 5–28%, $p = 0.3$). We obtained comparable, statistically significant results by analyzing the correlation between the frequency of dressings and the number of CVCs removed due to infection: 54% vs. 29% for 1–6 day intervals and 31% vs. 50% for once weekly dressing in the CLABSI group and the non-infected group, respectively; $p < 0.001$. To further explore the relationship between dressing frequency and infection, we calculated different infection rates in the subsets of patients whose percentage of dressings falling within the 8–10 days range exceeded a variable threshold. We defined this subgroup of patients with more than 20% of dressing in the 8–10 days range as "less frequent dressing". Table 3 illustrates the infection rate in both groups; there was no statistically significant difference (two-sample test for Poisson rates p-value = 0.075). In the supplements, we tested different threshold values. The infection rate initially reduced even if the patients were subject to less frequent dressing, and then seemed to stabilize around the value of 0.495 cases per 1000 CVC days considering patients who were dressed with an 8–10 days range of more than 30% of the time (Figure S1).

In the event of a suspected or confirmed exit-site infection, it is customary to perform CVC dressings in the pediatric hematology oncology department. Patients with a CVC exit-site score of 0 and without malfunction problems received the medication at home from the appropriately trained staff of the satellite hospitals. For this reason, the relationship between the dressing location and CLABSI was predictable. The median percentage of dressings performed at our department on patients with CLABSI compared to other locations was significantly higher (100%, IQR 69–100% vs. 0%, IQR 0–31%; $p < 0.001$).

We investigated a possible relationship between the visual exit-site score grading and CLABSI. A statistically significant correlation exists between CLABSI and exit-site score ≥ 1. In the patients without CLABSI, the median number of dressings with a score of 0 was 0.93 compared to 0.81 in the CLABSI group ($p = 0.001$).

3.4. CVC Removal Infection-Related Indication

Thirty-one (9.6%) CVCs were removed due to CLABSI. The only variables correlating with CVC removal for infection are ALL and long-time catheterization. ALL diagnosis is a protective factor, with only 26% of the CVCs removed due to infection compared to 47% removed due to other reasons ($p = 0.025$). CVCs that remain in placement longer are frequently removed for reasons other than infection ($p = 0.019$). Other variables, such as CVC model and type, method of insertion, number of lumens, HSCT, TPN, and occlusion events, are not correlated with infection-related removal indication (Table S1).

4. Discussion

The literature data report an incidence of central CLABSI between 1.7 and 11.3 cases for 1000 days catheter. In the oncology and hematology wards, the incidence is 1–4.6 per 1000 catheter days for external CVCs. CLABSI affects about 25% of pediatric patients with oncological and hematological disease, and its estimated mortality rate is between 12.5% and 25% [3]. Infected CVC management differs in pediatric patients compared to adults, particularly in the oncology setting. The necessity of peripheral vein cultures for diagnosing CVC-related infection remains controversial in children because of the poorer venous assets.

Conservative, pharmacologically focused management through CVC remains mandatory, with CVC removal only in selected cases [19]. Therefore, the prevention of CLABSI in this setting of patients becomes a more effective approach.

The nursing initiative was carried out to reduce the incidence of CLABSI through education and bundled intervention implementation in our pediatric oncology hematology department. Their effort and determination achieved significant and sustained decreases in CLABSI over ten years, bringing the incidence consistent with national data to 0.32 proven events for 1000 catheter days only. The protocol's capillary distribution within the satellite hospitals that manage the patients treated in our department and the frequent retraining of the healthcare teams were probably among the most important factors contributing to its effectiveness.

The creation of the CVC logbook is an innovation that allows healthcare workers in any hospital to safely manage every central device inserted in our department. This logbook is compiled for each CVC placed in our department. It reports all the insertion details and specifics of each dressing performed in and outside the department beyond occlusion, dislocation, or exit-site infection episodes. Our study is the first report in the literature of a personal CVC logbook filled out at each notable catheter handling. Another critical point is carefully evaluating the exit site during each CVC dressing. A section where the exit site is classified according to the Visual Exit Site Score has been inserted in the CVC logbook [20]. This tool helps identify the early signs of local infection and prevents microorganism migration and the colonization of the CVC, avoiding CLABSI.

In our cohort, 32 (10%) of the 323 catheters with a positive exit-site swab resulted in a match with a positive blood culture. Of these, only nine (28%) presented with CLABSI, which means that less than one-third of exit-site infections resulted in an extraluminal migration of the pathogen. The sterile technique of handling the infusion lines under a laminar flow hood guarantees a low risk of intraluminal bacterial dissemination.

TPN, multi-lumen devices, chemotherapy treatment, immunosuppression, and the number of days of catheterization were recognized as modifiable risk factors that increased the probability of developing CLABSI [21]. Among the non-modifiable factors is known significant negative surviving correlation with diabetes mellitus, cardiovascular disease, lung disease, chronic kidney disease, the presence of $\geq$3 comorbidities, gut or skin graft versus host disease, patients within 15 days after stem cell transplant, high-risk neuroblastoma, AML, relapsed ALL, and dressing/line concerns or issues within the past 72 h [22,23]. In our study, only a few variables were associated with infection. Presumably, such a low incidence of infections affected the identification of risk factors and discouraged the implementation of further analysis. The association between ALL and a lower infection rate is probably linked to the intensity of chemotherapy protocols. While other malignancies have a strictly programmed time interval for chemotherapy cycles, ALL protocols require a normalized white blood cell count before starting a new cycle, thus exposing patients to a milder infectious risk. In the years ahead, by expanding the data pool, it could be possible to investigate the risk factors and patterns of infection in our setting to be included in new surveillance protocols. Furthermore, even if some patients underwent less frequent dressing, they were adequately selected since the incidence of infection did not change considerably. In fact, in patients who underwent more than 20% of dressing in a range of 8–10 days, proven infections were 0.314 per 1000 days of CVC, similar to the incidence in the whole cohort.

Although we comprehensively examined the factors that led to the significant reduction in CLABSI, our study has several limitations. First, it is a retrospective, one-facility study. Given our cohort's low incidence of CLABSI, a much larger sample size is needed to perform multivariate analyses, considering all the variables examined. Future projects could explore some interesting data on the life of the catheter that have yet to be considered, such as the influence of different therapeutic protocols.

5. Conclusions

In conclusion, given our department's meager infection rate, this study provides important insights: it highlights the effectiveness of our nurse-driven protocol and demonstrates how meticulous attention and the introduction of new tools, such as a personal CVC logbook, contribute to positive patient outcomes. Targeted interventions with protocols produced by highly trained professionals, their sharing, and the intensive training of satellite hospital staff led to a significant drop in infectious complications among pediatric hematological oncology patients with CVC. This example will provide readers with a practical tool for implementing similar protocols in their settings.

Supplementary Materials: The following supporting information can be downloaded at: https://www.mdpi.com/article/10.3390/nursrep14040197/s1, Figure S1. CLABSI incidence in the subpopulation with lower dressing frequency. [1] For each threshold value on the x-axis, we included the subset of patients whose percentage of dressings falling within the 8–10 days range exceeded the threshold. Subsequently, we calculated the incidence of infection for this subset. Incomplete data were removed from the analysis; Table S1: Comparison of variables between CLABSI and non-infection and CVC removed because of infection and other causes.

Author Contributions: Conceptualization, A.L. and N.M.; methodology, M.S., D.V. and N.D.V.; software, F.T.; validation, N.D.V., S.T. and L.Z.; formal analysis, F.T.; investigation, M.S. and D.V; resources, A.L.; data curation, S.T., L.Z. and N.D.V.; writing—original draft preparation, F.T. and M.S.; writing—review and editing, N.M.; visualization, A.L.; supervision, N.M.; project administration, A.L.; funding acquisition, N.M. All authors have read and agreed to the published version of the manuscript.

Funding: This work was supported by the Ministry of Health, Rome, Italy, in collaboration with the Institute for Maternal and Child Health IRCCS Burlo Garofolo, Trieste, Italy.

Institutional Review Board Statement: The study was conducted according to the Declaration of Helsinki and approved by the Institutional Review Board of the Institute for Maternal and Child Health—IRCCS Burlo Garofolo (reference No. IRB RC 32/2023).

Informed Consent Statement: Written informed consent was obtained from all the parents and custodians of the patients involved in the study.

Data Availability Statement: The original contributions presented in the study are included in the article. Further inquiries can be directed to the corresponding author.

Public Involvement Statement: No public involvement in any aspect of this research.

Guidelines and Standards Statement: This manuscript was drafted against the STROBE guidelines for a cross-sectional study.

Use of Artificial Intelligence: AI or AI-assisted tools were not used in drafting any aspect of this manuscript.

Conflicts of Interest: The authors declare no conflicts of interest.

References

1. Cohen, N.; Rosenberg, T.; Rimon, A.; Friedman, S. Early removal of a permanent catheter during the acute management of the unstable pediatric hemato-oncology patient with suspected catheter-related bloodstream infection: A multi-disciplinary survey and review of the literature. *Eur. J. Pediatr.* **2023**, *182*, 795–802. [CrossRef] [PubMed]
2. Hord, J.D.; Lawlor, J.; Werner, E.; Billett, A.L.; Bundy, D.G.; Winkle, C.; Gaur, A.H.; Children's Hospital Association Childhood Cancer and Blood Disorders Network. Central line associated blood stream infections in pediatric hematology/oncology patients with different types of central lines. *Pediatr. Blood Cancer* **2016**, *63*, 1603–1607. [CrossRef]
3. Cellini, M.; Bergadano, A.; Crocoli, A.; Badino, C.; Carraro, F.; Sidro, L.; Botta, D.; Pancaldi, A.; Rossetti, F.; Pitta, F.; et al. Guidelines of the Italian Association of Pediatric Hematology and Oncology for the management of the central venous access devices in pediatric patients with onco-hematological disease. *J. Vasc. Access* **2022**, *23*, 3–17. [CrossRef] [PubMed]
4. Baskin, K.M.; DO, S.L.A.M.; Saad, T.F.; Journeycake, J.M.; Schaefer, C.M.; Modi, B.P.; Vrazas, J.I.; Gore, B.; Drews, C.B.B.; Doellman, B.D.; et al. Evidence-based strategies and recommendations for preservation of central venous access in children. *J. Parenter. Enter. Nutr.* **2019**, *43*, 591–614. [CrossRef] [PubMed]

5. Ullman, A.J.; Marsh, N.; Mihala, G.; Cooke, M.; Rickard, C.M. Complications of central venous access devices: A systematic review. *Pediatrics.* **2015**, *136*, e1331–e1344. [CrossRef] [PubMed]
6. Joo, E.J.; Kang, C.I.; Ha, Y.E.; Park, S.Y.; Kang, S.J.; Joung, M.K.; Kang, W.K.; Chung, D.R.; Peck, K.R.; Song, J.H. Clinical outcome of catheter salvage in neutropenic cancer patients with catheter-related infection. *Scand. J. Infect. Dis.* **2011**, *43*, 258–263. [CrossRef] [PubMed]
7. Garaventa, A.; Castagnola, E.; Dallorso, S.; Dini, G.; Trucco, D.; Vianello, O.; Carrega, G.; Cuneo, P.; Buffa, P.; Magillo, P. Sepsis in children with malignant neoplasia, equipped with a Broviac-type venous catheter. *Pediatr. Med. Chir.* **1995**, *17*, 147–150. [PubMed]
8. Pinon, M.; Bezzio, S.; Tovo, P.A.; Fagioli, F.; Farinasso, L.; Calabrese, R.; Marengo, M.; Giacchino, M. A prospective 7-year survey on central venous catheter-related complications at a single pediatric hospital. *Eur. J. Pediatr.* **2009**, *168*, 1505–1512. [CrossRef] [PubMed]
9. O'Grady, N.P.; Alexander, M.; Burns, L.A.; Dellinger, E.P.; Garland, J.; Heard, S.O.; Lipsett, P.A.; Masur, H.; Mermel, L.A.; Pearson, M.L.; et al. Guidelines for the prevention of intravascular catheter-related infections. *Clin. Infect. Dis.* **2011**, *52*, e162–e193. [CrossRef] [PubMed]
10. Fratino, G.; Molinari, A.C.; Parodi, S.; Longo, S.; Saracco, P.; Castagnola, E.; Haupt, R. Central venous catheter-related complications in children with oncological/hematological diseases: An observational study of 418 devices. *Ann. Oncol.* **2005**, *16*, 648–654. [CrossRef] [PubMed]
11. The Italian Data Protection Authority—General Authorisation to Process Personal Data for Scientific Research Purposes [3786078]. Authorization No. 9/2014. Available online: https://www.garanteprivacy.it/home/docweb/-/docweb-display/docweb/3786078 (accessed on 23 September 2024).
12. O'Grady, N.P. Healthcare infection control practices advisory committee. Guidelines for the prevention of intravascular catheter-related infections. *Am. J. Infect. Control* **2011**, *39*, S1–S34. [CrossRef] [PubMed]
13. van den Bosch, C.H.; Frakking, F.N.; Loeffen, Y.G.; van Tinteren, H.; van Der Steeg, A.F.; Wijnen, M.H.; van der Bruggen, J.T. The applicability of the central line-associated bloodstream infection (CLABSI) criteria for the evaluation of bacteremia episodes in pediatric oncology patients. *Eur. J. Haematol.* **2024**, *112*, 832–839. [CrossRef] [PubMed]
14. Taison, B.; O'Grady, N.P. Prevention of central line–associated bloodstream infections. *Infect. Dis. Clin.* **2017**, *31*, 551–559.
15. Cesaro, S.; Cavaliere, M.; Pegoraro, A.; Gamba, P.; Zadra, N.; Tridello, G. A comprehensive approach to the prevention of central venous catheter complications: Results of 10-year prospective surveillance in pediatric hematology-oncology patients. *Ann. Hematol.* **2016**, *95*, 817–825. [CrossRef] [PubMed]
16. R Core Team. *R: A Language and Environment for Statistical Computing*; R Foundation for Statistical Computing: Vienna, Austria, 2020.
17. Sjoberg, D.D.; Whiting, K.; Curry, M.; Lavery, J.A.; Larmarange, J. Reproducible summary tables with the gtsummary package. *R J.* **2021**, *13*, 570–580. [CrossRef]
18. Therneau, T. *A Package for Survival Analysis in R*; R Package Version 3.5-7; R Foundation for Statistical Computing: Vienna, Austria, 2023.
19. Carraro, F.; Cicalese, M.P.; Cesaro, S.; De Santis, R.; Zanazzo, G.; Tornesello, A.; Giordano, P.; Bergadano, A.; Giacchino, M. Guidelines for the use of long-term central venous catheter in children with hemato-oncological disorders. On behalf of supportive therapy working group of Italian Association of Pediatric Hematology and Oncology (AIEOP). *Ann. Hematol.* **2013**, *92*, 1405–1412. [CrossRef] [PubMed]
20. GaVeCeLT. Visual Exit Site Score. 2014. Available online: https://gavecelt.it/nuovo/sites/default/files/uploads/visual_exit_site_score.pdf (accessed on 23 September 2024).
21. Lafuente Cabrero, E.; Terradas Robledo, R.; Civit Cuñado, A.; García Sardelli, D.; Hidalgo López, C.; Giro Formatger, D.; Lacueva Perez, L.; Esquinas López, C.; Tortosa Moreno, A. Risk factors of catheter-associated bloodstream infection: Systematic review and meta-analysis. *PLoS ONE* **2023**, *18*, e0282290. [CrossRef] [PubMed]
22. Alwazzeh, M.J.; Alnimr, A.; Al Nassri, S.A.; Alwarthan, S.M.; Alhajri, M.; AlShehail, B.M.; Almubarak, M.; Alghamdi, N.S.; Wali, H.A. Microbiological trends and mortality risk factors of central line-associated bloodstream infections in an academic medical center 2015–2020. *Antimicrob. Resist. Infect. Control.* **2023**, *12*, 128. [CrossRef] [PubMed]
23. Dandoy, C.E.; Hausfeld, J.; Flesch, L.; Hawkins, D.; Demmel, K.; Best, D.; Osterkamp, E.; Bracke, T.; Nagarajan, R.; Jodele, S.; et al. Rapid cycle development of a multifactorial intervention achieved sustained reductions in central line-associated bloodstream infections in haematology oncology units at a children's hospital: A time series analysis. *BMJ Qual. Saf.* **2016**, *25*, 633–643. [CrossRef] [PubMed]

nursing reports

MDPI

Article

Innovation Support Reduces Quiet Quitting and Improves Innovative Behavior and Innovation Outputs among Nurses in Greece

Ioannis Moisoglou [1], Aglaia Katsiroumpa [2], Ioanna Prasini [3], Parisis Gallos [2], Maria Kalogeropoulou [2] and Petros Galanis [2,]*

1 Faculty of Nursing, University of Thessaly, 41500 Larisa, Greece; iomoysoglou@uth.gr
2 Clinical Epidemiology Laboratory, Faculty of Nursing, National and Kapodistrian University of Athens, 11527 Athens, Greece; aglaiakat@nurs.uoa.gr (A.K.); parisgallos@nurs.uoa.gr (P.G.); mariakalo@nurs.uoa.gr (M.K.)
3 Palliative Care Unit Galilee, 19004 Spata, Greece; iprasini@galilee.gr
* Correspondence: pegalan@nurs.uoa.gr; Tel.: +30-2107461471

Abstract: Background: Innovation is a crucial issue in healthcare services since it can affect job-related variables such as productivity, satisfaction, and burnout. The aim of our study was to examine the impact of innovation support on quiet quitting, innovative behavior, and innovation outputs among nurses. Methods: We conducted a cross-sectional study in Greece during April 2024. We employed a convenience sample of nurses. We followed the reporting of observational studies in epidemiology (STROBE). We used the following instruments: (a) the innovation support inventory (ISI) to measure innovation support; (b) the quiet quitting scale (QQS) to measure quiet quitting; (c) the innovative behavior inventory (IBI) to measure innovative behavior; and (d) the innovation outputs (IO) scale to measure innovation outputs. Our study questionnaire was anonymous, and nurses gave their informed consent to participate. The Ethics Committee of the Faculty of Nursing, National and Kapodistrian University of Athens, approved our study protocol, while we followed the guidelines of the Declaration of Helsinki. Results: Our study population included 328 nurses with a mean age of 42.3 years (standard deviation: 9.7). Among them, 89.9% were females. Our multivariable analysis identified a negative relationship between innovation support and quiet quitting. Moreover, we found that managerial support and cultural support improved several aspects of innovative behavior, such as idea generation, idea search, idea communication, implementation starting activities, involving others, and overcoming obstacles. Additionally, managerial support improved innovation outputs. Conclusions: Our findings suggested the positive impact of innovation support on quiet quitting, innovative behavior, and innovation outputs among nurses. Organizations and nurses' managers should establish an innovative working environment to improve nurses' passion, motives, and productivity.

Keywords: innovation; behavior; nurses; quiet quitting scale; support; innovative behavior inventory; innovation outputs

1. Introduction

Nurses who provide patient care face particular challenges in modern healthcare settings. These challenges include the increasing number of elderly patients with comorbidities, the requirement to enhance patient safety, the ongoing evolution of new health technologies, the constant need to integrate new scientific knowledge into daily clinical practice, the scarcity of available resources, and, in particular, the understaffing of services. In this highly demanding working environment, the development of innovative behavior by nurses can contribute to effective, efficient, and quality patient care.

A generally accepted definition of innovation is "the intentional introduction and application within a role, group, or organization of ideas, processes, products, or procedures, new to the relevant unit of adoption, designed to significantly benefit the individual, the group, the organization, or wider society" [1]. As healthcare organizations are complex, there is plenty of space to implement innovative actions. Among the four key roles of nurses, the American Nurses Association (ANA) includes that of nurses as innovators [2]. Nurses' innovative behaviors include idea generation, idea search, idea communication, implementation initiation activities, overcoming obstacles, innovation outputs, and engaging others [3]. Over time, nurses act as agents of innovation, positively influencing both the quality of healthcare and policy issues related to their profession. In particular, the implementation of innovative nursing protocols has contributed to the reduction of nosocomial infections, medication errors, and the better management of chronic diseases [4–6]. Nurses have shown a positive attitude and have adopted health information technology applications, such as the electronic health record or the use of mobile phone applications, in order to improve the quality of care provided to their patients [7–9]. In terms of health policies, innovative initiatives by nurses have contributed to the implementation of changes to improve nursing education [10].

For nurses to develop innovative behaviors, as well as to receive support and promotion of such work behaviors, the importance of their work environment has been recognized. Elements of the nurses' work environment, such as the foundation of quality, good working relationships between nurses and physicians, support from the supervisor and the organization, and the organizational culture, enhance the manifestation of innovative behavior [11–13]. The most crucial aspect in the growth of nurses' innovative behavior is the support they receive from their immediate supervisor, particularly in terms of leadership. An inclusive leadership style, where an individual has the ability to lead a diverse group of people while showing respect for each person's unique characteristics without prejudice, was found to have a significantly positive effect on innovative behavior [14]. One leadership style that provides opportunities for nurses to express new ideas and take initiatives is that of transformational leadership. A study has shown that transformational leadership was the most influential and also a predictor of innovative work behavior in nurses, compared to other leadership styles [15]. The supervisor's endorsement of innovation and the nurses' innovative behavior both impact the quality of nursing care and the well-being of the nurses [16,17]. In addition, the supervisor's demonstration of an ethical, humanistic, empathic, and mutually beneficial approach, as well as adopting a servant leadership strategy, encourages nurses to engage in innovative behavior [18].

An alarming trend that emerged during the COVID-19 pandemic is the behavior of quiet quitting. The concept of quiet quitting refers to a situation where an employee does not formally resign from his/her job but instead reduces level of performance. Employees only meet the basic criteria of the job without exerting extra effort, working longer hours, or arriving earlier, and without going above and beyond what is expected [19]. A comprehensive survey conducted in the United States by Gallup, a prominent job analysis and consulting agency, revealed that 50% of American corporate employees had chosen to quiet quit [20]. The primary factors contributing to employees quiet quitting work behavior include the employer's insufficient dedication to the advancement of employees' careers, management's failure to acknowledge the worth of their subordinates, a growing disengagement of employees from their work, a lack of recognition for the significance of employees' autonomy, and a decline in organizational trust among employees [21]. The development of a reliable and valid questionnaire made it possible to study this phenomenon in all sectors [22,23]. Initial research in the healthcare industry revealed the magnitude of the problem, indicating that nurses are more likely to engage in quiet quitting compared to other healthcare professionals, with a rate exceeding 60% [24]. Quiet quitting can be influenced by burnout and bullying, which are recognized as contributing factors. On the other hand, emotional intelligence and moral resilience decrease the chance of this behavior. Nurses who opt for quiet quitting are more inclined to express their turnover intention from their position [25]. The choice of quiet quitting by nurses is a work behavior that can be a barrier to innovation and efficiency in an organization, as these employees have no commitment to the organization, their thoughts are on leaving their job, and they do not show willingness to go beyond their job.

To the best of our knowledge, there are no studies that investigated the relationship between innovation support and quiet quitting, while the study of the relationship between innovation support and innovative behavior and innovation outputs among nurses is limited [13,26,27]. In particular, two studies in Turkey [13,26] and one study in Iran [27] revealed the positive impact of innovation support on innovative behavior and innovation outputs among nurses. All studies included nurses working in hospitals. Thus, our aim was to explore the impact of innovation support on quiet quitting, innovative behavior, and innovation outputs in a sample of nurses. In this context, our research hypotheses were the following:

H1. *Is there an association between innovation support and quiet quitting?*

H2. *Is there an association between innovation support and innovative behavior?*

H3. *Is there an association between innovation support and innovation outputs?*

2. Materials and Methods

2.1. Study Design

We conducted an online cross-sectional study in Greece during April 2024. Our inclusion criteria were the following: (a) nurses who understand the Greek language and (b) nurses who have been working at least three years in a clinical setting. We excluded nurses that do not understand the Greek language and do not work in clinical settings. We followed the reporting of observational studies in epidemiology (STROBE) [28].

2.2. Sample and Data Collection

We obtained a convenience sample of nurses through social media. In particular, we created an online version of our study questionnaire with Google Forms. Then, we posted the questionnaire on nurses' groups on Facebook and LinkedIn. We posted the questionnaire three times during a month to remind nurses to participate in our study. Our study questionnaire was anonymous, and nurses gave their informed consent to participate. In particular, we informed nurses about the aim and design of our study through the online questionnaire. After that, we asked nurses if they wanted to participate in our study. Nurses with a positive answer can then proceed to answer our questionnaire.

Minimum sample size was 262 nurses, assuming a low effect size ($f^2 = 0.05$) between predictors (i.e., managerial support, organizational support, and cultural support) and dependent variables (i.e., quiet quitting, innovative behavior, and innovation outputs), power of analysis as 95%, alpha level as 5%, and number of independent variables as 8 (i.e., three predictors and five confounders) [29].

2.3. Instruments

We measured demographic and job characteristics of nurses as follows: gender (females or males), age (continuous variable), understaffed department (no or yes), shift work (no or yes), and work experience (continuous variable). Additionally, we used the following instruments:

Innovation support inventory (ISI) [30]: The ISI includes 12 items and three factors: (a) "managerial support" with five items (item example: "My manager motivates me to come to him/her with new ideas"), (b) "organizational support" with three items (item example: "The way of remuneration in our organization motivates employees to suggest new things and procedures"), and (c) "cultural support" with four items (item example: "Most people in Greece come up with new, original ideas at work"). Answers are on a 5-point Likert scale from 1 (totally disagree) to 5 (totally agree). The score for each factor ranges from 1 to 5. Higher values represent more innovation. We used the valid Greek version of the ISI [31]. In our study, Cronbach's alpha for "managerial support", "organizational support", and "cultural support" was 0.825, 0.701, and 0.727, respectively.

Quiet quitting scale (QQS) [23]: The QQS includes nine items and three factors: (a) "detachment" with four items (item example: "I do the basic or minimum amount of work without going above and beyond"), (b) "lack of initiative" with three items (item example: "I do not express opinions and ideas about my work because I think that work conditions are not going to change"), and (c) "lack of motivation" with two items (item example: "I do not find motives in my job"). Answers are on a 5-point Likert scale from 1 (strongly disagree) to 5 (strongly agree). The score for each factor ranges from 1 to 5. Higher values represent higher levels of quiet quitting. We used the valid Greek version of the QQS [24]. Scale developers suggest a cut-off point of 2.06 to distinguish quiet quitters from non quiet quitters [22]. In our study, Cronbach's alpha for "detachment", "lack of initiative", and "lack of motivation" was 0.788, 0.729 and 0.861, respectively.

Innovative behavior inventory (IBI) [30]: The IBI includes 20 items and six factors: (a) "idea generation" with three items (item example: "I try new ways of doing things at work"), (b) "idea search" with three items (item example: "I try to get new ideas from colleagues or business partners"), (c) "idea communication" with four items (item example: "When I have a new idea, I try to persuade my colleagues of it"), (d) "implementation starting activities" with three items (item example: "I develop suitable plans and schedules for the implementation of new ideas"), (e) "involving others" with three items (item example: "I try to involve key decision makers in the implementation of an idea), and (f) "overcoming obstacles" with four items (item example: "I do not give up even when others say it cannot be done"). Answers are on a 5-point Likert scale from 1 (fully disagree) to 5 (fully agree). Score on each factor ranges from 1 to 5. Higher values represent more innovation. We used the valid Greek version of the IBI [31]. In our study, Cronbach's alpha for "idea generation", "idea search", "idea communication", "implementation starting activities", "involving others", and "overcoming obstacles" was 0.723, 0.860, 0.873, 0.818, 0.790, and 0.885, respectively.

Innovation outputs (IO) scale [30]: The IO includes three items and one factor. Item examples are the following: "I was often successful at work in implementing my ideas and putting them in practice" and "Many things I came up with are used in our organization". Answers are on a 5-point Likert scale from 1 (totally disagree) to 5 (totally agree). Score ranges from 1 to 5. Higher values represent better innovation outputs. We used the valid Greek version of the IO [31]. In our study, Cronbach's alpha for the IO was 0.706.

2.4. Ethical Issues

The Ethics Committee of the Faculty of Nursing, National and Kapodistrian University of Athens (reference number: 498, 1 April 2024) approved our study protocol. Additionally, our study followed the guidelines of the Declaration of Helsinki [32].

2.5. Statistical Analysis

We use numbers and percentages to present categorical variables. Moreover, we use mean, standard deviation (SD), median, minimum value, and maximum value to present continuous variables. We applied the Kolmogorov–Smirnov test and Q-Q plots to assess the distribution of continuous variables. We found that all continuous variables followed normal distribution. Innovation support was the independent variable, while quiet quitting, innovative behavior, and innovation outputs were the dependent variables. Since our dependent variables were continuous variables that followed normal distribution, we performed linear regression analysis. First, we conducted univariate regression analysis to examine the impact of innovation support without taking into consideration confounders. Then, we considered our demographic and job characteristics as potential confounders in the relationship between innovation support and quiet quitting, innovative behavior, and innovation outputs. In that way, we finally constructed multivariable linear regression models by eliminating confounders. We present unadjusted and adjusted coefficients beta, 95% confidence intervals (CI), *p*-values, and R2. *p*-values less than 0.05 were considered statistically significant. Since age and work experience were highly correlated (Pearson's correlation coefficient: 0.919; $p < 0.001$), we included only age in the multivariable models to avoid multicollinearity. We used the IBM SPSS 21.0 (IBM Corp.), released in 2012, and IBM SPSS Statistics for Windows, version 21.0 (IBM Corp., Armonk, NY, USA) for the analysis.

3. Results

3.1. Demographic and Job Characteristics

Our study population included 328 nurses. Among them, 89.9% (n = 295) were females and 10.1% (n = 33) were males. The mean age of our nurses was 42.3 years (SD: 9.7) with a range from 22 to 60 years. In our sample, 81.1% (n = 266) reported that they have been working in understaffed departments, and 70.1% (n = 230) have been working in shifts. The mean years of work experience was 17.7 (SD: 10.2), with a range from 3 to 36 years.

3.2. Study Scales

Detailed descriptive statistics for the study scales are shown in Table 1. Nurses reported higher levels of cultural support (mean: 2.94; SD: 0.66) and managerial support (mean: 2.61; SD: 0.79) than organizational support (mean: 1.98; SD: 0.76).

Table 1. Descriptive statistics for the study scales (N = 328).

Scale	Mean	Standard Deviation	Median	Minimum Value	Maximum Value
Innovation support inventory					
Managerial support	2.61	0.79	2.60	1	5
Organizational support	1.98	0.76	2.00	1	5
Cultural support	2.94	0.66	3.00	1	5
Quiet quitting scale					
Detachment	2.00	0.73	2.00	1	4.5
Lack of initiative	2.39	0.85	2.33	1	4.7
Lack of motivation	2.90	1.03	3.00	1	5
Innovative behavior inventory					
Idea generation	3.60	0.63	3.67	1.3	5
Idea search	3.98	0.69	4.00	1	5
Idea communication	3.60	0.73	3.75	1	5
Implementation starting activities	3.26	0.79	3.33	1	5
Involving others	3.64	0.69	3.67	1	5
Overcoming obstacles	3.56	0.76	3.50	1.3	5
Innovation outputs	3.46	0.65	3.67	1.3	5

Lack of motivation (mean: 2.90; SD: 1.03) was higher than lack of initiative (mean: 2.39; SD: 0.85) and detachment (mean: 2.00; SD: 0.73). Among our nurses, 66.2% (n = 217) could be considered quiet quitters since they had a score on QQS above the cut-off point of 2.06.

Regarding innovative behavior, nurses reported higher values on "idea search" (mean: 3.98; SD: 0.69) and "involving others" (mean: 3.64; SD: 0.69), and then on "idea generation" (mean: 3.60; SD: 0.63), "idea communication" (mean: 3.60; SD: 0.73), "overcoming obstacles" (mean: 3.56; SD: 0.76), and "implementation starting activities" (mean: 3.26; SD: 0.79).

The mean value of "innovation outputs" was 3.46 (SD: 0.65) with a range from 1.3 to 5.

3.3. Quiet Quitting

Our multivariable linear regression models identified a negative relationship between innovation support and quiet quitting (Table 2). In particular, managerial support reduced detachment (adjusted coefficient beta = −0.173; 95% CI = −0.281 to −0.065; *p*-value = 0.002), lack of initiative (adjusted coefficient beta = −0.314; 95% CI = −0.435

to −0.194; *p*-value < 0.001) and lack of motivation (adjusted coefficient beta = −0.331; 95% CI = −0.469 to −0.192; *p*-value < 0.001).

Table 2. Linear regression models with quiet quitting as the dependent variable (N = 328).

Dependent Variable *Independent Variables*	Univariate Model Unadjusted Coefficient Beta	95% CI for Beta	*p*-Value	Multivariable Model [a] Adjusted Coefficient Beta	95% CI for Beta	*p*-Value
Detachment [b]						
Managerial support	−0.136	−0.235 to −0.036	0.008	−0.173	−0.281 to −0.065	0.002
Organizational support	0.047	−0.057 to 0.152	0.373	0.012	−0.132 to 0.189	0.563
Cultural support	−0.032	−0.153 to 0.088	0.599	−0.036	−0.159 to 0.087	0.565
Lack of initiative [c]						
Managerial support	−0.335	−0.446 to −0.223	<0.001	−0.314	−0.435 to −0.194	<0.001
Organizational support	−0.190	−0.311 to −0.069	0.002	−0.038	−0.167 to 0.090	0.560
Cultural support	−0.116	−0.256 to 0.025	0.105	−0.037	−0.175 to 0.100	0.592
Lack of motivation [d]						
Managerial support	−0.460	−0.592 to −0.327	<0.001	−0.331	−0.469 to −0.192	<0.001
Organizational support	−0.411	−0.552 to −0.270	<0.001	−0.187	−0.334 to −0.039	0.014
Cultural support	−0.409	−0.573 to −0.244	<0.001	−0.288	−0.446 to −0.130	<0.001

[a] Multivariable models are adjusted for gender, age, understaffed department, shift work, and work experience. [b] R^2 for the multivariable model = 3.1%; *p*-value for ANOVA = 0.017. [c] R^2 for the multivariable model = 11.6%; *p*-value for ANOVA < 0.001. [d] R^2 for the multivariable model = 19.9%; *p*-value for ANOVA < 0.001.

Additionally, organizational support (adjusted coefficient beta = −0.187; 95% CI = −0.334 to −0.039; *p*-value = 0.014) and cultural support (adjusted coefficient beta = −0.288, 95% CI = −0.446 to −0.130; *p*-value < 0.001) reduced lack of motivation.

3.4. Innovative Behavior

Linear regression models with innovative behavior as the dependent variable are shown in Table 3. We found a positive relationship between innovation support and innovative behavior. In particular, managerial support improved several aspects of innovative behavior, such as idea generation (adjusted coefficient beta = 0.163; 95% CI = 0.072 to 0.253; and *p*-value < 0.001), idea search (adjusted coefficient beta = 0.119; 95% CI = 0.016 to 0.222; and *p*-value = 0.023), idea communication (adjusted coefficient beta = 0.207; 95% CI = 0.107 to 0.306; and *p*-value < 0.001), implementation starting activities (adjusted coefficient beta = 0.221; 95% CI = 0.112 to 0.330; and *p*-value < 0.001), involving others (adjusted coefficient beta = 0.154; 95% CI = 0.057 to 0.252; and *p*-value = 0.002), and overcoming obstacles (adjusted coefficient beta = 0.216; 95% CI = 0.107 to 0.324; and *p*-value < 0.001).

Table 3. Linear regression models with innovative behavior as the dependent variable (N = 328).

Dependent Variable *Independent Variables*	Univariate Model Unadjusted Coefficient Beta	95% CI for Beta	*p*-Value	Multivariable Model [a] Adjusted Coefficient Beta	95% CI for Beta	*p*-Value
Idea generation [b]						
Managerial support	0.195	0.111 to 0.280	<0.001	0.163	0.072 to 0.253	<0.001
Organizational support	0.134	0.044 to 0.224	0.004	0.021	−0.075 to 0.117	0.670
Cultural support	0.218	0.117 to 0.320	<0.001	0.181	0.078 to 0.284	0.001
Idea search [c]						
Managerial support	0.127	0.032 to 0.221	0.009	0.119	0.016 to 0.222	0.023
Organizational support	0.070	−0.029 to 0.170	0.164	0.013	−0.097 to 0.122	0.821
Cultural support	0.101	−0.013 to 0.215	0.083	0.081	−0.036 to 0.198	0.175

Table 3. *Cont.*

Dependent Variable *Independent Variables*	Univariate Model Unadjusted Coefficient Beta	95% CI for Beta	*p*-Value	Multivariable Model [a] Adjusted Coefficient Beta	95% CI for Beta	*p*-Value
Idea communication [d]						
Managerial support	0.245	0.147 to 0.343	<0.001	0.207	0.107 to 0.306	<0.001
Organizational support	0.184	0.080 to 0.288	0.001	0.048	−0.057 to 0.154	0.369
Cultural support	0.211	0.091 to 0.331	0.001	0.149	0.036 to 0.262	0.010
Implementation starting activities [e]						
Managerial support	0.267	0.162 to 0.373	<0.001	0.221	0.112 to 0.330	<0.001
Organizational support	0.219	0.108 to 0.331	<0.001	0.081	−0.036 to 0.197	0.173
Cultural support	0.222	0.093 to 0.351	0.001	0.147	0.023 to 0.272	0.020
Involving others [f]						
Managerial support	0.183	0.090 to 0.276	<0.001	0.154	0.057 to 0.252	0.002
Organizational support	0.165	0.067 to 0.263	0.001	0.082	−0.022 to 0.186	0.122
Cultural support	0.093	−0.021 to 0.207	0.110	0.028	−0.083 to 0.139	0.624
Overcoming obstacles [g]						
Managerial support	0.267	0.165 to 0.368	<0.001	0.216	0.107 to 0.324	<0.001
Organizational support	0.221	0.114 to 0.329	<0.001	0.104	−0.012 to 0.219	0.079
Cultural support	0.108	−0.018 to 0.234	0.094	0.028	−0.096 to 0.152	0.652

[a] Multivariable models are adjusted for gender, age, understaffed department, shift work, and work experience. [b] R^2 for the multivariable model = 9.8%; *p*-value for ANOVA < 0.001. [c] R^2 for the multivariable model = 2.3%; *p*-value for ANOVA = 0.045. [d] R^2 for the multivariable model = 20.2%; *p*-value for ANOVA < 0.001. [e] R^2 for the multivariable model = 16.5%; *p*-value for ANOVA < 0.001. [f] R^2 for the multivariable model = 12.3%; *p*-value for ANOVA < 0.001. [g] R^2 for the multivariable model = 11.3%; *p*-value for ANOVA < 0.001.

Moreover, we found that cultural support has a positive impact on idea generation (adjusted coefficient beta = 0.181; 95% CI = 0.078 to 0.284; and *p*-value = 0.001), idea communication (adjusted coefficient beta = 0.149; 95% CI = 0.036 to 0.262; and *p*-value = 0.010), and implementation starting activities (adjusted coefficient beta = 0.147; 95% CI = 0.023 to 0.272; and *p*-value = 0.020).

3.5. Innovation Outputs

Managerial support improved innovation outputs (adjusted coefficient beta = 0.230; 95% CI = 0.144 to 0.317; and *p*-value < 0.001), while organizational support and cultural support did not affect innovation outputs (Table 4).

Table 4. Linear regression models with innovation outputs as the dependent variable (N = 328).

Dependent Variable *Independent Variables*	Univariate Model Unadjusted Coefficient Beta	95% CI for Beta	*p*-Value	Multivariable Model [a] Adjusted Coefficient Beta	95% CI for Beta	*p*-Value
Innovation outputs [b]						
Managerial support	0.254	0.169 to 0.340	<0.001	0.230	0.144 to 0.317	<0.001
Organizational support	0.160	0.067 to 0.252	0.001	0.033	−0.059 to 0.126	0.476
Cultural support	0.085	−0.022 to 0.193	0.119	0.015	−0.084 to 0.113	0.771

[a] Multivariable model is adjusted for gender, age, understaffed department, shift work, and work experience.
[b] R^2 for the multivariable model = 22.3%; *p*-value for ANOVA < 0.001.

4. Discussion

This study investigated the role of innovative support in the emergence of quiet quitting as a work behavior and the effect of this support on the development of innovative behavior and the occurrence of innovation outcomes. The study findings indicated that the majority of participants are quiet quitters (experience detachment, lack of initiative, and lack of motivation), exhibit innovative behavior, and providing support for innovation decreases the chances of quiet quitting, promotes innovative behavior, and improves innovative results. Research on quiet quitting in the international health sector is fairly sparse, but our findings align with previous studies. A study conducted with 1760 healthcare professionals revealed that the proportion of nurses choosing quiet quitting was 66.4%, which was the greatest compared to other medical staff and healthcare professionals [24]. In another study, almost 77% of nurses were shown to demonstrate quiet quitting [33]. Detachment, lack of initiative, and lack of motivation are the three factors that compose quiet quitting. These factors can hinder an employee's ability to exhibit innovative behavior. The expression of personal initiative by nurses is associated with both idea generation and concept implementation [34]. By implementing the transformational leadership style, nurse supervisors have the ability to positively impact the psychological empowerment of nurses. This, in turn, has an influence on both intrinsic motivation and information sharing behavior, ultimately leading to an enhancement in innovative work behavior [35]. While all four attributes of transformational leadership (idealized influence, inspiration, intellectual stimulation, and individualized consideration) contribute positively to the growth of employees and the organization, it is intellectual stimulation in particular that fosters greater innovation and creativity among followers [36]. Also, there is a direct correlation between the growth in nurses' work engagement and their level of innovative behavior [37].

The participants in the current study had elevated scores in terms of innovative behavior. Aside from leadership support, particularly from supervisors, numerous other aspects in the nurses' work environment have a key role in fostering innovative behavior. Research findings indicate that higher levels of education and possession of certifications have a beneficial impact on an individual's innovative behavior [38]. Hence, the hospital administration's facilitation of educational and ongoing training opportunities for nurses might be considered as measures aimed at fostering innovation. Moreover, by enabling nurses to access information and fostering a culture of learning inside the organization, it not only establishes a structure for ongoing improvement and professional growth to enhance the quality of care but also encourages nurses to engage in innovative behavior [39,40]. The level of professional autonomy among nurses plays a significant role in fostering innovation within a health organization. Nurses who have a high degree of autonomy are able to generate innovative outcomes and contribute additional value through their innovative practices in delivering patient care and overall health services [41].

The present study also highlighted the impact of cultural support on reduced lack of motivation and the positive impact on idea generation, idea communication, and initiation of implementation activities. Most research focuses limitedly on the influence of managerial and organizational support on innovation. The significance and influence of national culture are somewhat undervalued, despite the fact that national culture serves as the framework within which organizations evolve. The findings of our study align with the existing body of international research, which has emphasized the impact of national culture on organizational culture [42,43]. Consumer innovativeness and innovation adoption behavior are frequently influenced by the cultural context of a country [44]. Efforts are already being made in the health sector to create a brand-new, comprehensive ecosystem for health innovation that influences how the public and commercial sectors collaborate in mutually beneficial partnerships to provide equal access as the main goal [45].

The health services industry is a dynamic setting marked by the growing occurrence of chronic illnesses, the need for ongoing enhancement of service safety, and the constant development of biomedical technology. The implementation of innovative approaches by nurses effectively tackles these issues and ensures the provision of optimal care [46–48]. The continuous backing from nursing leadership has the potential to augment the innovative endeavors of nurses [49]. Continual support for nurses is necessary due to their provision of services in a challenging work environment characterized by elevated levels of dissatisfaction, burnout, and quiet quitting [24,50]. An inadequate level of occupational wellbeing among nurses can hinder the emergence of creative conduct. Nurse leadership has the potential to amplify innovation, creativity, and well-being within the healthcare sector [51].

Our study had several limitations. First, we cannot establish a causal relationship between innovation support, quiet quitting, innovative behavior, and innovation outputs since we conducted a cross-sectional study. Second, we employed a convenience sample through social media to collect our data. Thus, our sample cannot be representative of the nurse's population in Greece. Although we achieved the minimum required sample size, further studies with random and more representative samples should be conducted not only in Greece but worldwide. Third, we eliminated several confounders in the relationship between innovation support and quiet quitting, innovative behavior, and innovation outputs. However, several other variables can act as confounders on this relationship and should be investigated in the future to get more valid results. Finally, although we used valid instruments to measure innovation support, quiet quitting, innovative behavior, and innovation outputs, the self-reported nature of these can introduce information bias in our study.

5. Conclusions

Innovation is a crucial component for improving a healthcare organization. The nurses' innovative behavior, as front-line healthcare providers, can enhance the quality of care and thus increase the organization's efficiency. This study emphasized the innovative behavior of nurses and the pivotal impact of management on the cultivation of this behavior and its results. Furthermore, healthcare organizations must not only promote innovation but also tackle the issue of quiet quitting, which was identified as having a significant impact in this study and may hinder the development of innovative behavior among nurses.

Author Contributions: Conceptualization, P.G. (Petros Galanis) and I.M.; methodology, P.G. (Petros Galanis), I.M., A.K., I.P., P.G. (Parisis Gallos) and M.K.; software, P.G. (Petros Galanis) and P.G. (Parisis Gallos); validation, A.K., I.P., M.K. and P.G. (Parisis Gallos); formal analysis, P.G. (Petros Galanis), A.K. and I.M.; investigation, P.G. (Petros Galanis), I.M., A.K., I.P., M.K. and P.G. (Parisis Gallos); resources, P.G. (Petros Galanis), I.M., A.K., I.P., M.K. and P.G. (Parisis Gallos); data curation, I.M., A.K., I.P. and P.G. (Parisis Gallos); writing—original draft preparation, P.G. (Petros Galanis), I.M., A.K., I.P., M.K. and P.G. (Parisis Gallos); writing—review and editing, P.G. (Petros Galanis), I.M., A.K., I.P., M.K. and P.G. (Parisis Gallos); supervision, P.G. (Petros Galanis); project administration, P.G. (Petros Galanis) and I.M. All authors have read and agreed to the published version of the manuscript.

Funding: This research received no external funding.

Institutional Review Board Statement: The study was conducted in accordance with the Declaration of Helsinki and approved by the Ethics Committee of Faculty of Nursing, National and Kapodistrian University of Athens, Greece (reference number; 498, 1 April 2024).

Informed Consent Statement: Informed consent was obtained from all subjects involved in the study.

Data Availability Statement: Our data are available from the corresponding author on reasonable request.

Public Involvement Statement: No public involvement in any aspect of this research.

Guidelines and Standards Statement: This manuscript was drafted against the (STROBE) for a cross-sectional study, descriptive research.

Use of Artificial Intelligence: AI or AI-assisted tools were not used in drafting any aspect of this manuscript.

Acknowledgments: We acknowledge all the participants who made this study possible.

Conflicts of Interest: The authors declare no conflicts of interest.

References

1. Anderson, N.; De Dreu, C.K.W.; Nijstad, B.A. The Routinization of Innovation Research: A Constructively Critical Review of the State-of-the-Science. *J. Organ. Behav.* **2004**, *25*, 147–173. [CrossRef]
2. Williams, T.E.; Baker, K.; Evans, L.; Lucatorto, M.A.; Moss, E.; O'Sullivan, A.; Seifert, P.C.; Siek, T.; Thomas, T.W.; Zittel, B. Registered Nurses as Professionals, Advocates, Innovators, and Collaborative Leaders: Executive Summary. *Online J. Issues Nurs.* **2016**, *21*, 1–11. [CrossRef] [PubMed]
3. Abd, S.; Mahgoub, E.-F.; Shazly, M.M.; El-Sayed, M. Relationship between Work Environment and Innovative Behavior among Staff Nurses. *Egypt. J. Health Care* **2019**, *10*, 64–76. [CrossRef]
4. Shaw, R.J.; McDuffie, J.R.; Hendrix, C.C.; Edie, A.; Lindsey-Davis, L.; Nagi, A.; Kosinski, A.S.; Williams, J.W. Effects of Nurse-Managed Protocols in the Outpatient Management of Adults with Chronic Conditions: A Systematic Review and Meta-Analysis. *Ann. Intern. Med.* **2014**, *161*, 113–121. [CrossRef] [PubMed]
5. Adams, D.; Bucior, H.; Day, G.; Rimmer, J.A. HOUDINI: Make That Urinary Catheter Disappear-Nurse-Led Protocol. *J. Infect. Prev.* **2012**, *13*, 44–46. [CrossRef]
6. Ruggiero, J.; Smith, J.; Copeland, J.; Boxer, B. Discharge Time Out: An Innovative Nurse-Driven Protocol for Medication Reconciliation. *Medsurg Nurs.* **2015**, *24*, 165–172.
7. Kutney-Lee, A.; Brooks Carthon, M.; Sloane, D.M.; Bowles, K.H.; McHugh, M.D.; Aiken, L.H. Electronic Health Record Usability: Associations with Nurse and Patient Outcomes in Hospitals. *Med. Care* **2021**, *59*, 625–631. [CrossRef]
8. Mayer, M.A.; Blanco, O.R.; Torrejon, A. Use of Health Apps by Nurses for Professional Purposes in Catalonia, Spain: Web-Based Survey Study. *JMIR Mhealth Uhealth* **2019**, *7*, e15195. [CrossRef]
9. Walker-Czyz, A. The Impact of an Integrated Electronic Health Record Adoption on Nursing Care Quality. *J. Nurs. Adm.* **2016**, *46*, 366–372. [CrossRef]
10. Eaton, M.K. Professional Advocacy: Linking Virginia's Story to Public Policy-Making Theory, Learning From the Past and Applying It to Our Future. *Policy Polit. Nurs. Pract.* **2012**, *13*, 105–112. [CrossRef]
11. Nazir, S.; Qun, W.; Hui, L.; Shafi, A. Influence of Social Exchange Relationships on Affective Commitment and Innovative Behavior: Role of Perceived Organizational Support. *Sustainability* **2018**, *10*, 4418. [CrossRef]
12. Xiang, D.; Ge, S.; Zhang, Z.; Twumwaah Budu, J.; Mei, Y. Relationship among Clinical Practice Environment, Creative Self-Efficacy, Achievement Motivation, and Innovative Behavior in Nursing Students: A Cross-Sectional Study. *Nurse Educ. Today* **2023**, *120*, 105656. [CrossRef] [PubMed]
13. Emiralioğlu, R.; Sönmez, B. The Relationship of Nursing Work Environment and Innovation Support with Nurses' Innovative Behaviours and Outputs. *J. Nurs. Manag.* **2021**, *29*, 2132–2141. [CrossRef] [PubMed]
14. Qi, L.; Liu, B.; Wei, X.; Hu, Y. Impact of Inclusive Leadership on Employee Innovative Behavior: Perceived Organizational Support as a Mediator. *PLoS ONE* **2019**, *14*, e0212091. [CrossRef]
15. Kamal Ahmed, A.; Abdeldayem Ata, A.; Naiem Abd-Elhamid, Z. Relationship between the Leadership Behaviors, Organizational Climate, and Innovative Work Behavior among Nurses. *Am. J. Nurs. Res.* **2019**, *7*, 870–878. [CrossRef]
16. Asurakkody, T.A.; Shin, S.Y. Innovative Behavior in Nursing Context: A Concept Analysis. *Asian Nurs. Res. (Korean Soc. Nurs. Sci.)* **2018**, *12*, 237–244. [CrossRef]
17. Mohamed El-Saidy, T.; Mohamed Baker, M.; Mohamed Khalefa El-saidy, T. Development of Nurse Manager Innovative Behavior and Its Effect on the Quality of Care for Elderly Patients. *Int. J. Nov. Res. Healthc. Nurs.* **2020**, *7*, 277–288.
18. Kül, S.; Sönmez, B. The Effect of Nurse Managers' Servant Leadership on Nurses' Innovative Behaviors and Job Performances. *Leadersh. Organ. Dev. J.* **2021**, *42*, 1168–1184. [CrossRef]
19. Scheyett, A. Quiet Quitting. *Soc. Work.* **2022**, *68*, 5–7. [CrossRef]
20. Harter, J. Is Quiet Quitting Real? Available online: https://www.gallup.com/workplace/398306/quiet-quitting-real.aspx (accessed on 2 August 2023).
21. Mahand, T.; Caldwell, C. Quiet Quitting-Causes and Opportunities. *Bus. Manag. Res.* **2023**, *12*, 9–19. [CrossRef]
22. Galanis, P.; Katsiroumpa, A.; Vraka, I.; Siskou, O.; Konstantakopoulou, O.; Moisoglou, I.; Gallos, P.; Kaitelidou, D. Quiet Quitting among Employees: A Proposed Cut-off Score for the "Quiet Quitting" Scale. *Arch. Hell. Med.* **2024**, *41*, 381–387.
23. Galanis, P.; Katsiroumpa, A.; Vraka, I.; Siskou, O.; Konstantakopoulou, O.; Moisoglou, I.; Gallos, P.; Kaitelidou, D. The Quiet Quitting Scale: Development and Initial Validation. *AIMS Public Health* **2023**, *10*, 828–848. [CrossRef] [PubMed]
24. Galanis, P.; Katsiroumpa, A.; Vraka, I.; Siskou, O.; Konstantakopoulou, O.; Katsoulas, T.; Moisoglou, I.; Gallos, P.; Kaitelidou, D. Nurses Quietly Quit Their Job More Often than Other Healthcare Workers: An Alarming Issue for Healthcare Services. *Int. Nurs. Rev.* **2024**. [CrossRef]
25. Moisoglou, I.; Katsiroumpa, A.; Vraka, I.; Kalogeropoulou, M.; Gallos, P.; Prasini, I.; Galanis, P. Quiet Quitting Threatens Healthcare Organizations and Services: Alarming Evidence from a Cross-Sectional Study with Nurses in Greece. *Int. J. Caring Sci.* **2024**, *17*, 1115–1122.
26. Sönmez, B.; İspir, Ö.; Önal, M.; Emiralioğlu, R. Turkish Psychometric Properties of the Innovative Behavior Inventory and Innovation Support Inventory: A Model Analysis on Nurses. *Nurs. Forum* **2019**, *54*, 254–262. [CrossRef] [PubMed]
27. Hashemian, M.; Hashemian Moghadam, A.; Hosseini, M.; Azizpour, I.; Mirzaei, A. Examining the Relationship between Workplace Fun and Innovative Behavior among Nurses: The Mediating Effect of Innovation Support and Affective Commitment. *J. Nurs. Manag.* **2024**, *2024*, 9629172. [CrossRef]

28. Vandenbroucke, J.P.; Von Elm, E.; Altman, D.G.; Gøtzsche, P.C.; Mulrow, C.D.; Pocock, S.J.; Poole, C.; Schlesselman, J.J.; Egger, M. Strengthening the Reporting of Observational Studies in Epidemiology (STROBE): Explanation and Elaboration. *Epidemiology* **2007**, *18*, 805–835. [CrossRef]
29. Lorah, J. Effect Size Measures for Multilevel Models: Definition, Interpretation, and TIMSS Example. *Large Scale Assess. Educ.* **2018**, *6*, 8. [CrossRef]
30. Lukes, M.; Stephan, U. Measuring Employee Innovation: A Review of Existing Scales and the Development of the Innovative Behavior and Innovation Support Inventories across Cultures. *Int. J. Entrep. Behav. Res.* **2017**, *23*, 136–158. [CrossRef]
31. Moisoglou, I.; Katsiroumpa, A.; Kolisiati, A.; Tsiachri, M.; Tsakalaki, A.; Galanis, P. Innovative Behavior Inventory and Innovation Support Inventory: Translation and Validation in Greek. *Res. Sq.* 2024, *preprint*. [CrossRef]
32. Association, W.M. World Medical Association Declaration of Helsinki: Ethical Principles for Medical Research Involving Human Subjects. *JAMA* **2013**, *310*, 2191–2194. [CrossRef]
33. Galanis, P.; Moisoglou, I.; Katsiroumpa, A.; Malliarou, M.; Vraka, I.; Gallos, P.; Kalogeropoulou, M.; Papathanasiou, I.V. Impact of Workplace Bullying on Quiet Quitting in Nurses: The Mediating Effect of Coping Strategies. *Healthcare* **2024**, *12*, 797. [CrossRef] [PubMed]
34. Zappalà, S.; Toscano, F.; Polevaya, M.V.; Kamneva, E.V. Personal Initiative, Passive-Avoidant Leadership and Support for Innovation as Antecedents of Nurses' Idea Generation and Idea Implementation. *J. Nurs. Scholarsh.* **2021**, *53*, 96–105. [CrossRef] [PubMed]
35. Masood, M.; Afsar, B. Transformational Leadership and Innovative Work Behavior among Nursing Staff. *Nurs. Inq.* **2017**, *24*, e12188. [CrossRef]
36. Bass, B.M. Two Decades of Research and Development in Transformational Leadership. *Eur. J. Work Organ. Psychol.* **2010**, *8*, 9–32. [CrossRef]
37. Wang, Y.X.; Yang, Y.J.; Wang, Y.; Su, D.; Li, S.W.; Zhang, T.; Li, H.P. The Mediating Role of Inclusive Leadership: Work Engagement and Innovative Behaviour among Chinese Head Nurses. *J. Nurs. Manag.* **2019**, *27*, 688–696. [CrossRef]
38. Dy Bunpin, J.J.; Chapman, S.; Blegen, M.; Spetz, J. Differences in Innovative Behavior among Hospital-Based Registered Nurses. *J. Nurs. Adm.* **2016**, *46*, 122–127. [CrossRef]
39. Zhong, Z.; Hu, D.; Zheng, F.; Ding, S.; Luo, A. Relationship between Information-Seeking Behavior and Innovative Behavior in Chinese Nursing Students. *Nurse Educ. Today* **2018**, *63*, 1–5. [CrossRef]
40. Kamel, F.F.; Abd, M.; Aref, E. Staff Nurses Perception Toward Organizational Culture and Its Relation to Innovative Work Behavior at Critical Care Units. *Am. J. Nurs. Sci.* **2017**, *6*, 251–260. [CrossRef]
41. Sönmez, B.; Yıldırım, A. The Mediating Role of Autonomy in the Effect of Pro-Innovation Climate and Supervisor Supportiveness on Innovative Behavior of Nurses. *Eur. J. Innov. Manag.* **2019**, *22*, 41–58. [CrossRef]
42. Chen, Y.; Podolski, E.J.; Veeraraghavan, M. National Culture and Corporate Innovation. *Pac.-Basin Financ. J.* **2017**, *43*, 173–187. [CrossRef]
43. Prim, A.L.; Filho, L.S.; Zamur, G.A.C.; Di Serio, L.C. The Relationship between National Culture Dimensions and Degree of Innovation. *Int. J. Innov. Manag.* **2017**, *21*, 1730001. [CrossRef]
44. Lim, H.; Park, J.S. The Effects of National Culture and Cosmopolitanism on Consumers' Adoption of Innovation: A Cross-Cultural Comparison. *J. Int. Consum. Mark.* **2013**, *25*, 16–28. [CrossRef]
45. WHO. *Governing Health Innovation for the Common Good*; Council brief No. 1; WHO: Geneva, Switzerland, 2021.
46. Whitmore, C.; Bird, M.; McGillion, M.H.; Carter, N.; Chen, R.; Pierazzo, J.; Carroll, S.L. Impact of Nurse Scientist-Led Digital Health Interventions on Management of Chronic Conditions. *Nurs. Outlook* **2020**, *68*, 745–762. [CrossRef] [PubMed]
47. Lee, A.Y.L.; Wong, A.K.C.; Hung, T.T.M.; Yan, J.; Yang, S. Nurse-Led Telehealth Intervention for Rehabilitation (Telerehabilitation) Among Community-Dwelling Patients With Chronic Diseases: Systematic Review and Meta-Analysis. *J. Med. Internet Res.* **2022**, *24*, e40364. [CrossRef] [PubMed]
48. Temmink, D.; Francke, A.L.; Hutten, J.B.F.; Van Der Zee, J.; Abu-Saad, H.H. Innovations in the Nursing Care of the Chronically Ill: A Literature Review from an International Perspective. *J. Adv. Nurs.* **2000**, *31*, 1449–1458. [CrossRef]
49. Richey, K.; Waite, S. Leadership Development for Frontline Nurse Managers Promotes Innovation and Engagement. *Nurse Lead.* **2019**, *17*, 37–42. [CrossRef]
50. Galanis, P.; Moisoglou, I.; Katsiroumpa, A.; Vraka, I.; Siskou, O.; Konstantakopoulou, O.; Meimeti, E.; Kaitelidou, D. Increased Job Burnout and Reduced Job Satisfaction for Nurses Compared to Other Healthcare Workers after the COVID-19 Pandemic. *Nurs. Rep.* **2023**, *13*, 1090–1100. [CrossRef]
51. Barr, T.L.; Nathenson, S.L. A Holistic Transcendental Leadership Model for Enhancing Innovation, Creativity and Well-Being in Health Care. *J. Holist. Nurs.* **2022**, *40*, 157–168. [CrossRef]

nursing reports

Article

Determining the Innovativeness of Nurses Who Engage in Activities That Encourage Innovative Behaviors

Marion Leary [1,*], George Demiris [1,2], J. Margo Brooks Carthon [1,2], Pamela Z. Cacchione [1,2,3], Subhash Aryal [4] and Jose A. Bauermeister [1]

1 School of Nursing, University of Pennsylvania, Philadelphia, PA 19104, USA; gdemiris@nursing.upenn.edu (G.D.); jmbrooks@nursing.upenn.edu (J.M.B.C.); pamelaca@nursing.upenn.edu (P.Z.C.); bjose@nursing.upenn.edu (J.A.B.)
2 Leonard Davis Institute of Healthcare Economics, University of Pennsylvania, Philadelphia, PA 19104, USA
3 Penn Presbyterian Medical Center, Philadelphia, PA 19104, USA
4 School of Nursing, Johns Hopkins University, Baltimore, MD 21205, USA; biostat13579@gmail.com
* Correspondence: mleary@nursing.upenn.edu; Tel.: +1-215-776-4235

Abstract: Background: We sought to understand the innovativeness of nurses engaging in innovative behaviors and quantify the associated characteristics that make nurses more able to innovate in practice. We first compared the innovativeness scores of our population; then we examined those who self-identified as an innovator versus those who did not to explore differences associated with innovativeness between these groups. Methods: A cross-sectional survey study of nurses in the US engaging in innovative behaviors was performed. We performed an exploratory factor analysis (EFA) to determine the correlates of innovative behavior. Results: Three-hundred and twenty-nine respondents completed the survey. Respondents who viewed themselves as innovators had greater exposure to HCD/DT workshops in the past year (55.8% vs. 36.6%, $p = 0.02$). The mean innovativeness score of our sample was 120.3 ± 11.2 out of a score of 140. The mean innovativeness score was higher for those who self-identified as an innovator compared with those who did not (121.3 ± 10.2 vs. 112.9 ± 14.8, $p =< 0.001$). The EFA created four factor groups: Factor 1 (risk aversion), Factor 2 (willingness to try new things), Factor 3 (creativity and originality) and Factor 4 (being challenged). Conclusion: Nurses who view themselves as innovators have higher innovativeness scores compared with those who do not. Multiple individual and organizational characteristics are associated with the innovativeness of nurses.

Keywords: universal design; organizational innovation; healthcare reform; creativity

1. Introduction

Incorporating innovative behaviors in the profession of nursing is a relatively new notion, with most literature examining the use of innovation methodologies in practice dating back just 10–15 years [1,2]. In the last five years though, we have seen a groundswell of support encouraging individuals and organizations to consider incorporating innovation into education and practice [3–7]. This transformation has occurred because of the ever-changing healthcare environment that struggles with "wicked problems" (those that are notoriously difficult to solve) and emerging health concerns, as well as the need to understand and create new models of care and emerging technologies [3,8]. Because nurses are situated in the problem space with patients and communities, they can more deeply contextualize the problem areas and innovative solutions needed. But not all nurses see themselves as innovators or have the support to innovate. Therefore, determining what combination of individual and organizational characteristics enhances a nurse's innovativeness will be key to nurses leading in this space.

Innovativeness is a personal characteristic defined as "a behavior which is dependent upon the perceived attributes of the innovation" [9]. It is also an awareness of the need

Nurs. Rep. **2024**, *14*, 849–870. https://doi.org/10.3390/nursrep14020066 https://www.mdpi.com/journal/nursrep

to innovate [10]. Few studies within nursing have examined innovativeness [11]. There is still a paucity of data regarding what factors contribute specifically to the innovativeness of nurses and whether nurses are inherently innovative, as some have suggested, or if it is a behavior that can be developed, as called for by the Future of Nursing 2020–2030 report [5,11–14]. Educational institutions, programs for continuing education, and healthcare settings have a distinct opportunity to develop nurses as leaders in innovation, as fostering innovation in healthcare has the potential to improve outcomes for patients and health systems alike [15,16]. By understanding the characteristics of nurses engaging in innovative behaviors, including whether they self-identify as an innovator, health system leaders could use these data to assess and cultivate more balanced, innovative teams. However, without reliable data on the characteristics contributing to nurses' innovativeness, it will not be possible to properly quantify and cultivate those innovative behaviors in practice [17].

The purpose of this study was to expand the limited findings in this area by examining the characteristics of nurses in the US who show interest in innovation and engage in activities that encourage innovative behavior. We sought to understand the innovativeness of these nurses and quantify the associated characteristics that make nurses more able to innovate in practice. We also sought to determine differences between those nurses who self-identified as innovators and those who did not.

2. Materials and Methods

2.1. Study Design

This study was designed as a cross-sectional, observational survey study. We sought to measure participants' innovativeness using the Scales for the Measurement of Innovativeness tool and examine their association with individual and organizational characteristics. Based on these results, we compared those who self-identified as innovators with those who did not to show similarities and differences related to their innovativeness scores. We hypothesized that there would be differences between the innovativeness scores and characteristics of those who identified as innovators the scores of those who did not; with those identifying as an innovator having higher innovativeness scores and possessing greater characteristics associated with innovativeness (e.g., attending more innovation events).

2.2. Setting

Data collection for this study began on 12 December 2022, and ended on 22 January 2023. The study population included nurses, and the sample specifically targeted nurses engaging in innovative behaviors.

2.3. Partcipants

Eligible participants included nurses who engaged in innovative behaviors, were licensed, and worked in all settings in the US (e.g., clinical, educational, start-ups). Participants under 18 years of age, undergraduate nursing students, and nurses who do not read English were excluded from the study.

We sought to recruit a national sample of nurses who showed interest in innovation by engaging in activities supporting innovative behaviors in the last three years. Nurses were asked to complete the 10–15 min survey. No incentives to participate in the survey were offered. The snowballing technique was used, asking all participants to share the study description and survey link with their colleagues and on their social media platforms.

As noted, not all nurses have the opportunity to innovate. Therefore, to determine the characteristics that make a nurse more innovative, we sampled nurses who were actively engaging in innovative behaviors. Future work will look at comparing nurses engaging in innovative behaviors versus those not engaging in innovative behaviors to determine if they have different characteristics.

2.4. Variables

Participants' innovative behavior, individual sociodemographic (e.g., age, race, gender, income, education, institutional setting, years of practice), and organizational data (e.g., hospital location, Magnet status, job satisfaction) were collected via self-report using the Qualtrics survey platform. Variables included in the demographic and organizational surveys were chosen based on the conceptual models informing this study: the Individual Innovation in the Workplace theory and the Diffusion of Innovation theory [18,19]. Some items in the demographic and organizational survey were modeled on the survey used in the 2016 RN4CAST to examine institutional changes regarding education, staffing, work environment, and well-being [20]. Permission was obtained from the author (MM) for use on this project.

2.5. Data Sources/Measurement

All questionnaires were distributed and completed by participants via the Qualtrics website (Provo, UT, USA). At the beginning of the survey, a screening tool was completed by the respondent.

Once screening was completed, respondents who selected at least one innovative behavior were provided with study consent language. The participant consented by completing the survey and submitting it through the online portal (Qualtrics, Provo, UT, USA).

2.5.1. Scales for the Measurement of Innovativeness

The Scales for the Measurement of Innovativeness score was used to assess nurses' innovativeness. The original validated tool is a paper-based, self-report survey developed in 1977 to measure the willingness to change in an individual, not actual adoption behavior. This is an important distinction, as nurses may want to be innovative but may have constraints or barriers preventing them from innovating [9]. The Scales for the Measurement of Innovativeness has been used in previous studies to quantify the innovativeness of nurses [12,14]. Based on the Diffusion of Innovation theory, the scale was designed as a 7-point Likert scale [18]. The Scales for the Measurement of Innovativeness has a maximum score of 140 (20 questions ranked per the Likert scale 1–7); a higher score is associated with a higher degree of innovativeness and willingness to change [9]. We received permission from the publisher (Blackwell Publishing, Inc.) for this study to transfer the survey into an electronic format.

The Innovativeness score was calculated by scoring the 7-point Likert scale (Strongly Agree = 7, Agree = 6, Moderately Agree = 5, Undecided = 4, Moderately Disagree = 3, Disagree = 2, Strongly Disagree = 1) and totaling each of the individual respondents' scores for the 20 questions included in the Scale. Some questions from the survey were reverse scored to account for the directionality of the wording of the question, as recommended by Hurt & Cook [9]. The total sum was calculated to obtain a total possible score of 140 for each respondent.

2.5.2. Innovative Behavior

The innovative behavior items included information on whether a respondent participated in any innovation events such as hackathons, accelerators, incubators, design sprints, design thinking workshops, human-centered design courses, innovation fellowships, and challenges, reported as yes/no; the frequency of participation (e.g., 1–2 times over the past three years) was also captured. Questions specific to a respondent's ability or willingness to innovate were captured on a frequency scale of never to always or not at all to very.

2.5.3. Individual Characteristics

Demographic data included age, race, gender, income, education, institutional setting, years of practice, clinical level, and specialty area. Questions were captured as continuous variables for age and years of practice; the remaining demographic questions were captured as categorical variables (e.g., for Race: Asian, Black, White, Other). Other individual characteristics captured included satisfaction with one's current position as a nurse and institution, feeling supported, and number of years worked. The number of innovation events participated in and exposed to in the past year was also included.

2.5.4. Organizational Characteristics

Organizational data included items such as hospital location (urban/rural) and Magnet status (yes/no). Other variables regarding perceived facilitators of and barriers to innovativeness were collected. Questions related to satisfaction with opportunities to be creative and innovative and to lead, as well as whether their institution offered any HCD/DT or Innovation education, lectures, resources, and workshops were also collected.

2.6. Statistical Methods

We estimated descriptive statistics (mean, standard deviation) for our variables of interest. We then examined whether participants' individual and organizational characteristics differed based on whether a participant self-identified as an innovator. For these analyses, we compared groups using Student's *t*-tests or one-way ANOVAs with Tukey post hoc comparisons for continuous variables and Pearson's Chi-square tests for categorical variables. To adjust for Type I errors in multigroup comparisons we employed a Tukey post hoc comparison where appropriate [21,22]. We also used Pearson correlations to examine linear associations between continuous variables. We used complete case analysis as minimal missing data did not affect the models we used.

Using exploratory factor analysis (EFA), we confirmed the construct validity of the Scales for the Measurement of Innovativeness tool. Using Principal Axis Factoring with a varimax rotation, we assessed whether distinct factor scores would emerge with eigenvalue scores greater than one. The presence of distinct factor scores would suggest different components of what constitutes innovation according to the Scales for the Measurement of Innovativeness tool. After determining the extracted factors, we estimated the unique and shared explained variance across the 20 items. Consistent with best practices, factor loads greater than 0.4 indicated an item's contribution to a defined factor during the analysis. Using bivariate comparisons, we created standardized (z-score) factor scores from the EFA and subsequently examined whether nurses' individual and organizational characteristics differed across these factors.

2.7. Ethics Criteria

The study was approved by the University of Pennsylvania Institute Review Board (Protocol #852671).

3. Results

We received 662 survey responses. Of those, 305 (46.07%) began the screening survey but did not complete it. Three-hundred and forty-nine (52.72%) respondents passed the screening survey and agreed to participate, 4 (0.60%) completed the screening survey but subsequently chose not to participate and 2 (0.30%) completed the innovativeness survey but did not select that they agreed to participate and thus were removed from the analysis.

Of the 349 who passed the screening and agreed to participate, 15 did not start the survey and were removed. Ten respondents started the survey twice. Of the ten duplicate surveys, five were kept in the analysis. If the respondent had both an incomplete and complete survey, their incomplete survey was removed. If they had two completed surveys, their most recently completed were kept for analysis. A total of 329 surveys were analyzed (Figure 1).

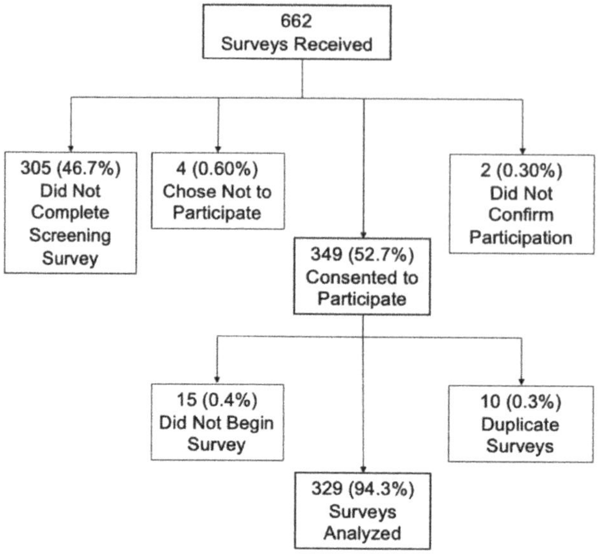

Figure 1. Enrollment schematic.

3.1. Individual Characteristics

The mean age of respondents was 47.17 ± 12.19 years. Most respondents—264/305 (86.56%)—were female, and 234/305 (76.72%) were white (Table 1). Most respondents had either a master's degree 122/306 (39.87%), or PhD or other Doctorate 87/306 (28.43%). The majority of respondents, 202/301 (67.11%), received their initial nursing education from a baccalaureate degree program (Table 1). On average, the respondents had worked in the nursing field for 21.49 ± 12.67 years. Less than half of the respondents, (129/300, 43.00%), worked in a hospital. The current positions of those who responded were quite diverse, with the most respondents in any category, 110/300 (36.67%), stating Other, which included positions such as "Founder", "Entrepreneur", "Consultant", and "Educator".

Table 1. Individual characteristics by participant's self-view as an innovator.

	Total Population	Views Self as an Innovator	Does Not View Self as an Innovator	t	df	*p*-Value
N	n = 329	n = 285	n = 41			
Age, years (m ± sd), n = 295	47.17 ± 12.18	47.69 ± 12.21	43.76 ± 11.62	1.88	1	0.06
Gender, n (%), n = 305				1.98	2	0.37
Female	264 (86.6)	226 (79.3)	38 (92.7)			
Male	33 (10.8)	30 (10.5)	3 (7.3)			
Other	8 (2.6)	8 (3.0)	0 (0)			
Race, n = 305				5.27	3	0.15
Asian	22 (7.2)	20 (7.0)	2 (4.9)			
Black	36 (11.8)	29 (10.1)	7 (17.1)			
Other	13 (4.3)	9 (3.2)	4 (9.8)			
White	234 (76.7)	206 (72.3)	28 (68.3)			
Hispanic or Latino, n = 306				0.61	1	0.66
Yes	15 (4.9)	14 (4.9)	1 (2.4)			

Table 1. *Cont.*

	Total Population	Views Self as an Innovator	Does Not View Self as an Innovator	t	df	*p*-Value
Highest Level of Education Completed in Nursing, n = 306						
Hospital Diploma	0 (0)	0 (0)	0 (0)			
Associate Degree Program	0 (0)	0 (0)	0 (0)			
Baccalaureate Degree Program	52 (17.0)	46 (16.1)	6 (14.6)	5.74	3	0.13
Master's Degree	122 (39.9)	111 (39.0)	11 (26.8)			
Doctor of Nursing Practice	45 (14.7)	35 (12.3)	10 (24.4)			
PhD or other Doctorate	87 (28.4)	73 (25.6)	14 (34.2)			
Licensure, n = 306						
LPN, RN	1 (0.3)	1 (0.4)	0 (0)			
RN	254 (83.0)	221 (77.5)	33 (80.4)	3.75	3	0.29
Other	12 (3.9)	12 (4.2)	0 (0)			
RN, Other	39 (12.8)	31 (10.9)	8 (19.5)			
From What Type of Program Did You Receive Your Initial Nursing Education, n = 301						
Associate Degree Program	49 (16.3)	42 (14.7)	7 (17.1)	1.64	3	0.65
Baccalaureate Degree Program	202 (67.1)	172 (65.4)	30 (73.2)			
Diploma Program	23 (7.6)	21 (7.4)	2 (4.9)			
Graduate Program	27 (9.0)	25 (8.8)	2 (4.9)			
Current Position, n (%), n = 300						
Staff Nurse	30 (10.0)	25 (8.8)	5 (12.2)			
Nurse Practitioner	19 (6.3)	16 (5.6)	2 (4.9)			
Clinical Nurse Specialist	12 (4.0)	8 (2.8)	4 (9.8)			
Nurse Anesthetist	1 (0.3)	0 (0)	1 (2.4)			
Nurse Midwife	2 (0.7)	1 (0.4)	1 (2.4)			
Nurse Manager	19 (6.3)	17 (6.0)	2 (4.9)	12.68	9	0.18
Nurse Practitioner	19 (6.3)	16 (5.6)	3 (7.3)			
Senior Nursing Administrator	25 (8.3)	19 (6.7)	6 (14.6)			
Faculty member/Researcher	67 (22.3)	58 (20.3)	9 (22.0)			
Director of Innovation	15 (5.0)	15 (5.3)	0 (0)			
Other	110 (36.7)	99 (34.7)	11 (26.8)			
Are you satisfied with your current position as a nurse, n = 303				0.55	1	0.46
Yes	222 (73.3)	190 (66.7)	32 (78.1)			
No	81 (26.7)	72 (33.3)	9 (21.9)			
Are you satisfied with your current institution, n = 303				3.38	1	0.66
Yes	223 (73.6)	188 (66.0)	35 (85.4)			
No	80 (26.4)	74 (26.0)	6 (14.6)			
Do you feel supported by your						
Nurse Colleagues, n = 296	257 (86.8)	221 (77.5)	36 (87.8)	0.41	1	0.52
Nurse Manager, n = 288	217 (75.4)	182 (73.9)	35 (89.7)	5.03	1	0.03
Executive Leadership, n = 298	190 (63.8)	160 (56.8)	30 (73.2)	2.53	1	0.11
How many years have you worked in Nursing? (m ± stdev), n = 297	21.5 ± 12.7	21.9 ± 9	19.2 ± 1.8	1.25	1	0.21
How many years have you worked as a clinician? (m ± stdev), n = 294	14.6 ± 11.0	14.9 ± 0.7	12.8 ± 1.6	1.16	1	0.25
How many years have you worked at your current institution? (m ± stdev), n = 296	8.9 ± 9.0	8.8 ± 0.6	9.7 ± 1.4	−0.55	1	0.58
Do you work in a hospital?, n = 300						
Yes	129 (43.0)	106 (37.2)	23 (56.1)	3.32	1	0.68
No	171 (57.0)	153 (53.7)	18 (43.9)			

Table 1. *Cont.*

	Total Population	Views Self as an Innovator	Does Not View Self as an Innovator	t	df	p-Value
Employment Status, n = 301						
Employed in healthcare	260 (86.4)	226 (79.3)	34 (82.9)	2.94	2	0.23
Employed, but not in healthcare	33 (11.0)	26 (9.1)	7 (17.1)			
How many innovation events have you participated in the last 1 year? n = 321						
1	111 (34.6)	93 (32.6)	18 (43.9)	4.18	3	0.24
2–3	119 (37.1)	103 (36.1)	16 (39.0)			
4–5	46 (14.3)	41 (14.4)	5 (12.2)			
6 or more	45 (14.0)	43 (15.4)	2 (5.0)			
Have you been exposed to human-centered design/design thinking in the past 1 year	Yes					
Activities, n = 325	209 (64.3)	184 (64.6)	25 (61.0)	0.23	1	0.63
Lectures, n = 324	224 (69.1)	200 (70.2)	24 (58.5)	2.47	1	0.12
Other, n = 308	227 (73.7)	71 (24.9)	10 (24.4)	0.00	1	0.99
Projects, n = 324	199 (61.4)	177 (62.1)	22 (53.7)	1.19	1	0.28
Resources, n = 324	211 (65.1)	189 (66.3)	22 (53.7)	2.72	1	0.10
Workshops, n = 323	174 (53.9)	159 (56.4)	15 (46.1)	5.65	1	0.02
Innovativeness score, n = 329	120.3 ± 11.2	121.3 ± 10.2	112.9 ± 14.8	4.64	1	<0.001

PhD, doctor of philosophy; LPN, licensed practical nurse; RN, registered nurse.

Most respondents, 285/326 (87.42%), viewed themselves as innovators. The majority of the respondents had been exposed to HCD and DT activities 209/323 (64.70%), lectures 224/325 (68.82%), projects 199/324 (61.42%), workshops 174/324 (53.70%), and other related innovative activities 227/324 (70.06%). In the last year, most respondents participated in 1–3 innovation events 230/321 (71.65%) (Table 1).

3.2. Organizational Characteristics

Of those who worked in a hospital, 126/298 (42.28%) were at a hospital with Magnet status. Most respondents, 212/296 (71.62%), considered their institution innovative, and 219/296 (73.98%) considered their institution supportive of innovative thinking by its nurses. However, of those where it was applicable, only 56/135 (41.48%) got protected time away from the bedside to work on projects. Just over half of the nurses who responded, 176/323 (54.48%), were very willing to implement innovation methodologies in their day-to-day work, but just 121/323 (37.46%) and 28/323 (8.67%) felt as though they were often or always able to implement innovation methodologies in their day-to-day work (Table 2).

Table 2. Organizational Characteristics by Participant's Self-view as an Innovator.

	Total Population	Views Self as an Innovator	Does Not View Self as an Innovator	t	df	p-Value
N	n = 329	n = 285	n = 41			
Type of Institution, n (%), n = 298						
Rural	20 (6.7)	19 (6.7)	1 (2.4)	6.44	3	0.09
Suburban	61 (20.5)	53 (18.6)	8 (19.5)			
Urban	193 (64.8)	161 (56.5)	32 (78.1)			
Other	24 (8.1)	24 (0.4)	0 (0)			
Magnet Status, n = 298						
Yes	126 (42.3)	106 (37.2)	20 (48.8)	3.06	2	0.22
No	56 (18.8)	46 (16.1)	10 (24.4)			
Not Applicable	116 (38.9)	105 (36.8)	11 (26.8)			

Table 2. *Cont.*

	Total Population	Views Self as an Innovator	Does Not View Self as an Innovator	t	df	*p*-Value
Do you consider your institution to be innovative n = 296				0.01	1	0.92
Yes	212 (71.4)	183 (64.2)	29 (70.7)			
No	85 (28.6)	73 (25.6)	12 (29.3)			
Does your institution support innovative thinking by its nurses? n = 296				0.42	1	0.52
Yes	219 (74.0)	187 (65.6)	32 (78.0)			
No	77 (26.0)	32 (11.2)	9 (21.9)			
Do you get protected time away from the bedside to work on other projects? n = 294				.56	2	0.76
Yes	56 (19.0)	47 (16.5)	9 (22.0)			
No	79 (26.9)	67 (23.5)	12 (29.3)			
Not applicable	159 (54.1)	139 (48.8)	20 (48.8)			
How willing are you to implement innovation methodologies in your day-to-day work? n = 323				16.53	4	0.002
Not at all	1 (0.3)	0 (0)	1 (2.4)			
Rarely	3 (0.9)	2 (0.7)	1 (2.4)			
Somewhat	35 (10.8)	28 (9.8)	7 (17.1)			
Mostly	108 (33.4)	89 (31.2)	19 (46.3)			
Very	176 (54.5)	163 (57.8)	13 (31.7)			
How often are you able implement innovation methodologies in your day-to-day work? n = 324				8.58	4	0.07
Never	6 (1.9)	4 (1.4)	2 (4.9)			
Rarely	32 (9.9)	26 (9.1)	2 (4.9)			
Sometimes	137 (42.3)	115 (40.4)	22 (53.7)			
Often	121 (37.4)	112 (39.3)	9 (22.0)			
Always	28 (8.6)	26 (9.1)	2 (4.9)			
How often do you encounter obstacles that impede you from being innovative in your day-to-day work? n = 323				4.28	4	0.37
Never	1 (0.3)	1 (0.4)	0 (0)			
Rarely	25 (7.7)	23 (8.1)	2 (4.9)			
Sometimes	128 (38.6)	112 (39.3)	16 (39.0)			
Often	140 (43.3)	124 (43.5)	16 (39.0)			
Always	29 (9.0)	22 (7.7)	7 (17.1)			
How satisfied are you with the following aspects of your job: Opportunities for advancement, n = 296				2.01	3	0.57
Very Satisfied	104 (35.1)	90 (35.3)	14 (34.2)			
Moderately Satisfied	101 (34.1)	84 (32.9)	17 (41.2)			
A little Dissatisfied	52 (17.6)	45 (16.7)	7 (17.1)			
Very Dissatisfied	39 (13.2)	36 (14.1)	3 (7.3)			
How satisfied are you with the following aspects of your job: Opportunities to be creative,	n = 298			15.43	3	0.001
Very Satisfied	122 (10.9)	112 (43.6)	10 (24.4)			
Moderately Satisfied	93 (31.2)	73 (28.4)	20 (48.8)			
A little Dissatisfied	43 (31.2)	33 (12.8)	10 (24.4)			
Very Dissatisfied	40 (13.4)	39 (15.2)	1 (2.4)			

Table 2. *Cont.*

	Total Population	Views Self as an Innovator	Does Not View Self as an Innovator	t	df	*p*-Value
How satisfied are you with the following aspects of your job: Opportunities to be innovative,	n = 300					
Very Satisfied	121 (40.3)	111 (42.9)	10 (24.4)	14.77	3	0.002
Moderately Satisfied	89 (29.7)	69 (26.7)	20 (48.8)			
A little Dissatisfied	50 (16.7)	40 (15.4)	10 (24.4)			
Very Dissatisfied	40 (13.3)	39 (66.1)	1 (2.4)			
How satisfied are you with the following aspects of your job: Opportunities to lead,	n = 298					
Very Satisfied	133 (44.6)	113 (44.0)	20 (48.8)	2.74	3	0.43
Moderately Satisfied	98 (32.9)	84 (32.7)	14 (34.1)			
A little Dissatisfied	39 (13.0)	33 (12.8)	6 (14.6)			
Very Dissatisfied	28 (9.4)	27 (10.5)	1 (0.24)			
How satisfied are you with the following aspects of your job: Time away from clinical responsibilities,	n = 285					
Very Satisfied	106 (37.2)	92 (37.2)	14 (36.8)	2.85	3	0.42
Moderately Satisfied	76 (26.7)	66 (26.7)	10 (26.3)			
A little Dissatisfied	45 (15.8)	36 (14.6)	9 (23.7)			
Very Dissatisfied	58 (20.4)	53 (2.0)	5 (13.2)			
How satisfied are you with the following aspects of your job: Work schedule,	n = 299					
Very Satisfied	168 (56.2)	145 (56.2)	23 (56.1)	2.47	3	0.48
Moderately Satisfied	90 (30.1)	77 (29.9)	13 (31.7)			
A little Dissatisfied	29 (9.7)	27 (46.6)	2 (4.9)			
Very Dissatisfied	12 (4.0)	9 (32.1)	3 (7.3)			
How satisfied are you with the following aspects of your job: Choice of nursing as a career,	n = 305					
Very Satisfied	208 (68.2)	179 (67.8)	29 (70.7)	1.60	3	0.66
Moderately Satisfied	76 (24.9)	65 (24.6)	11 (26.8)			
A little Dissatisfied	16 (5.3)	15 (5.7)	1 (2.4)			
Very Dissatisfied	5 (1.6)	5 (1.9)	0 (0)			
How would you rate: Relationship with co-workers,	n = 298					
Excellent	147 (49.3)	126 (49.0)	21 (51.2)	1.38	3	0.71
Good	124 (41.6)	107 (41.6)	17 (41.5)			
Fair	19 (6.4)	16 (6.2)	3 (7.3)			
Poor	8 (2.7)	8 (3.1)	0 (0)			
How would you rate: Adequacy of resources,	n = 298					
Excellent	95 (31.9)	77 (30.0)	18 (43.9)	4.54	3	0.21
Good	135 (45.3)	117 (45.5)	18 (43.9)			
Fair	53 (17.8)	49 (19.1)	4 (9.8)			
Poor	15 (5.0)	14 (5.4)	1 (2.4)			
How would you rate: Support from supervisors,	n = 296					
Excellent	128 (43.2)	104 (40.8)	24 (58.5)	6.83	3	0.08
Good	96 (32.4)	83 (32.5)	13 (31.7)			
Fair	46 (15.5)	43 (16.9)	3 (7.3)			
Poor	26 (8.8)	25 (9.8)	1 (2.4)			

Table 2. *Cont.*

	Total Population	Views Self as an Innovator	Does Not View Self as an Innovator	t	df	p-Value
How would you rate: Overall work environment,	n = 298					
Excellent	116 (38.9)	99 (38.5)	17 (41.5)	1.24	3	0.74
Good	123 (41.3)	105 (40.9)	18 (43.9)			
Fair	54 (18.1)	49 (19.1)	5 (12.2)			
Poor	5 (1.7)	4 (1.6)	1 (2.4)			
Has your institution offered any of the following:	Yes					
HCD/DT education, n = 283	107 (37.8)	94 (33.0)	13 (31.7)	0.76	1	0.38
HCD/DT lectures, n = 283	102 (36.0)	90 (31.6)	12 (29.3)	0.96	1	0.33
HCD/DT resources, n = 282	119 (42.2)	106 (37.2)	13 (31.7)	1.80	1	0.18
HCD/DT workshops, n = 283	100 (35.3)	87 (30.5)	13 (31.7)	0.28	1	0.60
Innovation education, n = 284	166 (58.5)	145 (50.9)	21 (51.2)	1.03	1	0.31
Innovation lectures, n = 284	156 (54.9)	137 (48.1)	19 (46.3)	1.43	1	0.23
Innovation resources, n = 282	174 (61.7)	152 (53.3)	22 (53.7)	1.31	1	0.25
Innovation workshops, n = 283	139 (49.1)	120 (42.1)	19 (46.3)	0.15	1	0.70

HCD/DT, human-centered design/design thinking.

Few institutions offered resources 119/282 (42.20%), education 107/283 (37.81%), workshops 100/283 (35.34%), or lectures 102/283 (36.04%) specific to HCD and DT. Many institutions offered innovation resources 174/282 (61.70%), education 166/284 (58.45%), workshops 139/283 (49.12%), and lectures 156/285 (54.74%) (Table 2).

3.3. *Self-Identified as an Innovator*

Differences in respondent characteristics based on whether the respondents viewed themselves as innovators (n = 285) or not (n = 41) showed no statistically significant difference in demographic characteristics (Table 1). However, we observed significant differences in participants' self-identification as innovators. Respondents who self-identified as innovators had greater exposure to HCD/DT workshops in the past year (56.38% vs. 46.13%, $p = 0.02$). Additionally, those who self-identified as innovators were more willing to implement innovation methodologies in their day-to-day work (57.80% vs. 31.71%, $p = 0.002$), more satisfied with their opportunities to be creative (43.58% vs. 24.39%, $p = 0.001$) and their opportunities to be innovative (42.86% vs. 24.39% $p = 0.002$) (Table 2).

3.4. *Innovativeness Score*

The total sample's mean innovativeness score was 120.3 ± 11.2 out of a score of 140. We found the mean difference in the total innovativeness score was higher for those who viewed themselves as innovators compared with those who did not (121.3 ± 10.2 vs. 112.9 ± 14.8, p =< 0.001) (Table 1). We also found the innovativeness scores to be higher for those who work in healthcare compared with those who do not (120.9±10.3 vs. 115.1±12.5, $p = 0.003$) and for respondents who had been exposed to HCD/DT workshops (121.5 ± 9.9 vs. 118.8 ± 12.5, $p = 0.04$) (Table 3). Additionally, a Student's t-test showed differences in innovativeness scores regarding whether respondents felt their institutions supported innovative thinking by its nurses, (121.3 ± 9.6 vs. 117.7 ± 12.8, $p = 0.01$) and whether respondents' institutions offered HCD/DT education (122.7 ± 9.2 vs. 118.9 ± 11.4, $p = 0.003$), lectures (122.8 ± 9.2 vs. 118.9 ± 11.3, $p = 0.003$), resources (122.6 ± 9.1 vs. 119.0 ± 10.8, $p = 0.004$), HCD/DT education (122.7 ± 9.2 vs. 118.9 ± 11.4, $p = 0.003$), lectures (122.8 ± 9.2 vs. 118.9 ± 11.3, $p = 0.003$), resources (122.6 ± 9.1 vs. 119.0 ± 10.8, $p = 0.004$), and workshops (122.2 ± 10.2 vs. 119.3 ± 10.9, $p = 0.03$) and innovation lectures (122.1 ± 9.6 vs. 118.1 ± 11.7, $p = 0.002$), and workshops(121.7 ± 10.0 vs. 118.9 ± 11.6, $p = 0.03$) (Table 4).

Table 3. Individual characteristics and innovativeness scores.

	Total Population	Innovativeness Score	t	df	*p*-Value
N	n = 329				
Age, yrs (m ± sd), n = 295	47.2 ± 12.2	r = 0.22			<0.001
Gender, n (%), n = 305			67.53	2, 302	0.43
Female	264 (86.6)	120.5 ± 10.2			
Male	33 (10.8)	118.4 ± 14.2			
Other	8 (2.6)	117.4 ± 12.8			
Race, n = 305			0.29	3, 301	0.41
Asian	22 (7.2)	118.7 ± 11.3			
Black	36 (11.8)	117.9 ± 10.2			
Other	13 (4.3)	119.2 ± 10.4			
White	234 (76.7)	120.8 ± 10.8			
Ethnicity, n = 306			−0.28	298	0.78
Hispanic or Latino	15 (4.9)	121.1 ± 12.5			
Highest Level of Education Completed in Nursing, n = 306			5.84	3, 302	0.60
Hospital Diploma	0 (0)	0 ± 0			
Associate Degree Program	0 (0)	0 ± 0			
Baccalaureate Degree Program	52 (17.0)	119.8 ± 10.4			
Master's Degree	122 (39.9)	120.3 ± 9.7			
Doctor of Nursing Practice	45 (14.7)	122.0 ± 10.6			
PhD or other Doctorate	87 (28.4)	119.4 ± 12.3			
Licensure, n = 306			0.90	3, 302	0.53
LPN, RN	1 (0.3)	135 ± 0			
RN	254 (83.0)	120.1 ± 10.9			
Other	12 (3.9)	121.8 ± 9.2			
RN, Other	39 (12.8)	120.0 ± 10.0			
From What Type of Program Did You Receive Your Initial Nursing Education, n = 301			11.11	3, 297	0.91
Associate Degree Program	49 (16.3)	119.8 ± 13.3			
Baccalaureate Degree Program	202 (67.1)	120.1 ± 10.2			
Diploma Program	23 (7.6)	120.7 ± 11.7			
Graduate Program	27 (9.0)	121.5 ± 7.7			
Current Position, n = 300			17.29	9, 290	0.28
Staff Nurse	30 (10.0)	119.4 ± 11.9			
Nurse Practitioner	19 (6.3)	118.7 ± 11.0			
Clinical Nurse Specialist	12 (4.0)	117.4 ± 12.2			
Nurse Anesthetist	1 (0.3)	134 ± 0			
Nurse Midwife	2 (0.7)	108.5 ± 9.2			
Nurse Manager	19 (6.3)	118.2 ± 12.3			
Nurse Practitioner	19 (6.3)	118.7 ± 11.0			
Senior Nursing Administrator	25 (8.3)	119.5 ± 9.3			
Faculty member/Researcher	67 (22.3)	120.4 ± 11.7			
Director of Innovation	15 (5.0)	125.7 ± 7.7			
Other	110 (36.7)	121.0 ± 8.9			
Are you satisfied with your current position as a nurse, n = 305			−0.76	301	0.45
Yes	222 (73.3)	120.5 ± 10.3			
No	81 (26.7)	119.4 ± 12.0			
Are you satisfied with your current institution, n = 305			−0.59	301	0.55
Yes	223 (73.6)	120.4 ± 10.4			
No	80 (26.4)	119.6 ± 11.8			

Table 3. *Cont.*

	Total Population	Innovativeness Score	t	df	*p*-Value
Do you feel supported by your		Yes vs. No			
Nurse Colleagues, n = 296	257 (86.8)	120.8 ± 10.3 vs. 117.1 ± 13.2	−2.01	294	0.05
Nurse Manager, n = 288	217 (75.4)	120.3 ± 10.5 vs. 119.5 ± 11.9	−0.54	286	0.56
Executive Leadership, n = 298	190 (63.8)	120.7 ± 10.2 vs. 119.3 ± 11.5	−1.13	296	0.26
How many years have you worked in Nursing? (m ± stdev), n = 297	21.5 ± 12.7	r = 0.17	2.94	1	0.004
How many years have you worked as a clinician? n = 294	14.6 ± 11.0	r = 0.18	3.05	1	0.002
How many years have you worked at your current institution? n = 296	8.9 ± 9.0	r = 0.08	1.35	1	0.18
Do you work in a hospital? n = 300					
Yes	129 (43)	120.9 ± 9.4	1.10	298	0.27
No	171 (57)	119.6 ± 12.1			
Employment Status, n = 301					
Employed in healthcare	260 (86.4)	120.9 ± 10.3	2.99	291	0.003
Employed, but not in healthcare	33 (11.0)	115.1 ± 12.5			
How many innovation events have you participated in the last 1 year? n = 321					
1 [a]	111 (34.6)	118.6 ± 11.2	8.34	3, 317	0.004
2–3 [b]	119 (37.1)	119.4 ± 10.8			
4–5	46 (14.3)	122.5 ± 12.8			
6 or more	45 (14.0)	125.0 ± 8.3			
Have you been exposed to human-centered design/design thinking in the past 1 year:	Yes	Yes vs. No			
Activities, n = 325	209 (64.3)	121.4 ± 10.7 vs. 118.3 ± 11.9	−2.41	323	0.17
Lectures, n = 324	224 (69.1)	120.7 ± 12.4 vs. 119.3 ± 12.4	−0.97	322	0.33
Other, n = 308	227 (73.7)	122.5 ± 8.7 vs. 119.8 ± 11.3	−1.93	306	0.06
Projects, n = 324	199 (61.4)	120.7 ± 11.0 vs. 119.6 ± 11.6	−0.81	322	0.42
Resources, n = 324	211 (65.1)	121.0 ± 10.9 vs. 118.9 ± 11.7	−1.62	322	0.11
Workshops, n = 323	174 (53.9)	121.5 ± 9.9 vs. 118.8 ± 12.5	−2.11	321	0.04
Do you view yourself as an innovator? n = 326		Yes vs. No			
Yes	285 (87.4)	121.3 ± 10.2 vs. 112.9 ± 14.8	−4.64	324	0.001

Overall, there is a difference in the means but no difference in pairwise analysis; a Tukey test found differences in "How many innovation events have you participated in the last 1 year?" [a], 1 vs. 6 or more ($p = 0.006$) and [b], 2–3 vs. 6 or more ($p = 0.02$). Yrs, years; PhD, doctor of philosophy; LPN, licensed practical nurse; RN, registered nurse; m, mean; stdev, standard deviation.

Table 4. Organizational characteristics and innovativeness scores. (**A**) mean and standard deviation results; (**B**) correlation results.

(A)	Total Population	Innovativeness Score (m/sd)	t	df	*p*-Value
	n = 329				
Type of Institution, n = 298					
Rural	20 (6.7)	121.8 ± 8.1	7.4	3, 294	0.10
Suburban	61 (20.5)	118.9 ± 12.3			
Urban	193 (64.8)	120.2 ± 10.5			
Other	24 (8.1)	125 ± 8.4			
Magnet Status, n = 298					
Yes	126 (42.3)	119.2 ± 11.1	0.35	180	0.72
No	56 (18.8)	119.8 ± 12.3			
Not Applicable	116 (38.9)	n/a			

Table 4. *Cont.*

(A)	Total Population	Innovativeness Score (m/sd)	t	df	p-Value
Do you consider your institution to be innovative, n = 297					
Yes	212 (71.4)	120.9 ± 9.8	−1.29	295	0.20
No	85 (28.6)	119.1 ± 12.6			
Does your institution support innovative thinking by its nurses? n = 296					
Yes	219 (74.0)	121.3 ± 9.6	−2.58	294	0.01
No	77 (26.0)	117.7 ± 12.8			
Do you get protected time away from the bedside to work on other projects? n = 294					
Yes	56 (19.0)	120.8 ± 10.0	−0.99	133	0.33
No	79 (26.9)	118.8 ± 12.4			
Not applicable	159 (54.1)	n/a			
Has your institution offered any of the following:	Yes	Yes vs. No			
HCD/DT education, n = 283	107 (37.8)	122.7 ± 9.2 vs. 118.9 ± 11.4	−2.9672	281	0.003
HCD/DT lectures, n = 283	102 (36.0)	122.8 ± 9.2 vs. 118.9 ± 11.3	−2.9808	281	0.003
HCD/DT resources, n = 282	119 (42.2)	122.6 ± 9.1 vs. 119.0 ± 10.8	−2.9141	280	0.004
HCD/DT workshops, n = 283	100 (35.3)	122.2 ± 10.2 vs. 119.3 ± 10.9	−2.1655	281	0.03
Innovation education, n = 284	166 (58.5)	121.7 ± 10.0 vs. 118.3 ± 11.5	−2.6285	282	0.09
Innovation lectures, n = 284	156 (54.9)	122.1 ± 9.6 vs. 118.1 ± 11.7	−3.1240	282	0.002
Innovation resources, n = 282	174 (61.7)	121.1 ± 10.0 vs. 119.1 ± 11.8	−1.5120	280	0.13
Innovation workshops, n = 283	139 (49.1)	121.7 ± 10.0 vs. 118.9 ± 11.6	−2.1994	281	0.03
Other, n = 255	56 (22.0)	121.9 ± 9.8 vs. 119.7 ± 11.3	−1.3170	253	0.19

(B)	Total Population	Innovativeness Score (Correlation Coefficient)	p-Value
	n = 329		
How willing are you to implement innovation methodologies in your day-to-day work?	n = 323		
Not at all	1 (0.3)		
Rarely	3 (0.9)	r = 0.32	0.001
Somewhat	35 (10.8)		
Mostly	108 (33.4)		
Very	176 (54.5)		
How often are you able implement innovation methodologies in your day-to-day work?	n = 324		
Never	6 (1.9)		
Rarely	32 (9.9)	r = 0.20	0.0003
Sometimes	137 (42.3)		
Often	121 (37.4)		
Always	28 (8.6)		
How often do you encounter obstacles that impede you from being innovative in your day-to-day work?	n = 323		
Never	1 (0.3)		
Rarely	25 (7.7)	r = −0.09	0.13
Sometimes	128 (38.6)		
Often	140 (43.3)		
Always	29 (9.0)		

Table 4. *Cont.*

(B)	Total Population	Innovativeness Score (Correlation Coefficient)	*p*-Value
How satisfied are you with the following aspects of your job: Opportunities for advancement	n = 296		
Very Satisfied	104 (35.1)	r = 0.09	0.12
Moderately Satisfied	101 (34.1)		
A little Dissatisfied	52 (17.6)		
Very Dissatisfied	39 (13.2)		
How satisfied are you with the following aspects of your job: Opportunities to be creative	n = 298		
Very Satisfied	122 (10.9)	r = 0.10	0.08
Moderately Satisfied	93 (31.2)		
A little Dissatisfied	43 (31.2)		
Very Dissatisfied	40 (13.4)		
How satisfied are you with the following aspects of your job: Opportunities to be innovative	n = 300		
Very Satisfied	121 (40.3)	r = 0.10	0.09
Moderately Satisfied	89 (29.7)		
A little Dissatisfied	50 (16.7)		
Very Dissatisfied	40 (13.3)		
How satisfied are you with the following aspects of your job: Opportunities to lead,	n = 298		
Very Satisfied	133 (44.6)	r = 0.08	0.16
Moderately Satisfied	98 (32.9)		
A little Dissatisfied	39 (13.0)		
Very Dissatisfied	28 (9.4)		
How satisfied are you with the following aspects of your job: Time away from clinical responsibilities	n = 285		
Very Satisfied	106 (37.2)	r = 0.01	0.83
Moderately Satisfied	76 (26.7)		
A little Dissatisfied	45 (15.8)		
Very Dissatisfied	58 (20.4)		
How satisfied are you with the following aspects of your job: Work schedule	n = 299		
Very Satisfied	168 (56.2)	r = 0.13	0.03
Moderately Satisfied	90 (30.1)		
A little Dissatisfied	29 (9.7)		
Very Dissatisfied	12 (4.0)		
How satisfied are you with the following aspects of your job: Choice of nursing as a career	n = 305		
Very Satisfied	208 (68.2)	r = 0.02	0.02
Moderately Satisfied	76 (24.9)		
A little Dissatisfied	16 (5.3)		
Very Dissatisfied	5 (1.6)		
How would you rate: Relationship with co-workers, n = 298			
Excellent	147 (49.3)	r = 0.14	0.01
Good	124 (41.6)		
Fair	19 (6.4)		
Poor	8 (2.7)		

Table 4. *Cont.*

(B)	Total Population	Innovativeness Score (Correlation Coefficient)	*p*-Value
How would you rate: Adequacy of resources, n = 298			
Excellent	95 (31.9)	r = 0.06	0.32
Good	135 (45.3)		
Fair	53 (17.8)		
Poor	15 (5.0)		
How would you rate: Support from supervisors, n = 296			
Excellent	128 (43.2)	r = 0.07	0.25
Good	96 (32.4)		
Fair	46 (15.5)		
Poor	26 (8.8)		
How would you rate: Overall work environment, n = 298			
Excellent	116 (38.9)	r = 0.12	0.04
Good	123 (41.3)		
Fair	54 (18.1)		
Poor	5 (1.7)		

n, number; m/sd, mean/standard deviation; t, t-statistic; df, degrees of freedom; HCD/DT, human-centered design/design thinking; vs., versus.

A one-way ANOVA was used to compare the innovativeness scores with how many innovation events a respondent participated in over the past year. We found that the more innovation events a respondent participated in, the higher that person's innovativeness score would be (one event, 118.6 ± 11.2 vs. 2–3, 119.4 ± 10.8 vs. 4–5, 122.5 ± 12.8 vs. six or more, 125.0 ± 8.3, $p = 0.004$). Tukey's test for multiple comparisons found a statistically significant difference in the innovativeness scores between the two groups; one innovation event compared with six or more innovation events ($p = 0.006$) and 2–3 events compared with six or more innovation events ($p = 0.02$) (Table 3).

3.5. Exploratory Factor Analysis

An EFA was performed. The total variance explained was 56.66% (Table 5). Four factors emerged in the rotated factor matrix, with Factor 1 having an eigenvalue of 6.38, which accounted for 31.88% of the variance. Factor 2 had an eigenvalue of 2.46, accounting for 12.29% of the variance. Factor 3 had an eigenvalue of 1.47, accounting for 7.37% of the variance. Factor 4 had an eigenvalue of 1.03, accounting for 5.13% of the variance (Table 6).

Table 5. Total variance explained.

Total Variance Explained						
Factor	Initial Eigenvalues			Extraction Sums of Squared Loadings		
	Total	% of Variance	Cumulative %	Total	% of Variance	Cumulative %
1	6.38	31.88	31.88	5.87	29.37	29.37
2	2.46	12.29	44.17	1.93	9.64	39.01
3	1.47	7.37	51.54	1.09	5.46	44.47
4	1.03	5.13	56.66	0.54	2.68	47.15

Table 6. Exploratory factor analysis—rotated factor matrix.

n = 329	Mean (SD)	Factor 1 (Risk Aversion)	Factor 2 (Willingness to Try New Things)	Factor 3 (Creativity and Originality)	Factor 4 (Being Challenged)
I often find myself skeptical of new ideas. *	5.77 (1.06)	0.71			
I rarely trust new ideas until I can see whether the vast majority of people around me accept them. *	5.91 (1.05)	0.62			
I am reluctant about adopting new ways of doing things until I see them working for people around me. *	5.88 (1.16)	0.61			
I am aware that I am usually one of the last people in my group to accept something new. *	6.28 (0.95)	0.60			
I am suspicious of new inventions and new ways of thinking. *	5.76 (1.25)	0.60			
I must see other people using new innovations before I will consider them. *	5.98 (1.03)	0.59			
I tend to feel that the old way of living and doing things is the best way. *	6.01 (0.99)	0.49			
I am generally cautious about accepting new ideas.	4.59 (1.75)	0.43			
I enjoy trying out new ideas.	6.63 (0.73)		0.66		
I enjoy taking part in the leadership responsibilities of the groups I belong to.	6.24 (0.92)		0.62		
I seek out new ways to do things.	6.53 (0.78)		0.60		
I feel that I am an influential member of my peer group.	6.12 (0.99)		0.60		
My peers often ask me for advice or information.	6.36 (1.07)		0.56		
I am receptive to new ideas.	6.42 (0.77)		0.56		
I frequently improvise methods for solving a problem when an answer is not apparent.	6.10 (0.99)		0.46		
I am an inventive kind of person.	5.91 (1.14)			0.76	
I consider myself to be creative and original in my thinking and behavior.	6.19 (0.97)		0.43	0.65	
I find it stimulating to be original in my thinking and behavior.	6.40 (0.80)		0.46	0.46	
I am challenged by unanswered questions.	5.76 (1.40)				0.89
I am challenged by ambiguities and unsolved problems.	5.43 (1.70)				0.67

The items above were scored on a 7-point Likert scale ranging from 7–1; some items were reverse scored 1–7 as noted above with an asterisk (*).

3.6. Description of Factors

Factor 1 (risk aversion) included eight survey questions about risk aversion and reluctance to accept new ideas. Factor 2 (willingness to try new things and being an influencer and leader) included nine items related to survey questions that focused on willingness to try new things and being an influencer and leader in relation to new ideas. Factor 3 (creativity and originality) included three items focused on survey questions about creativity and originality in thinking and behavior. Factor 4 (being challenged) included two items related to survey questions focused on being challenged by unanswered questions and ambiguity.

3.7. Comparison across the Factors

We examined the associations between our four factors and the individual and organization characteristics (see Supplementary Material; Figure 2).

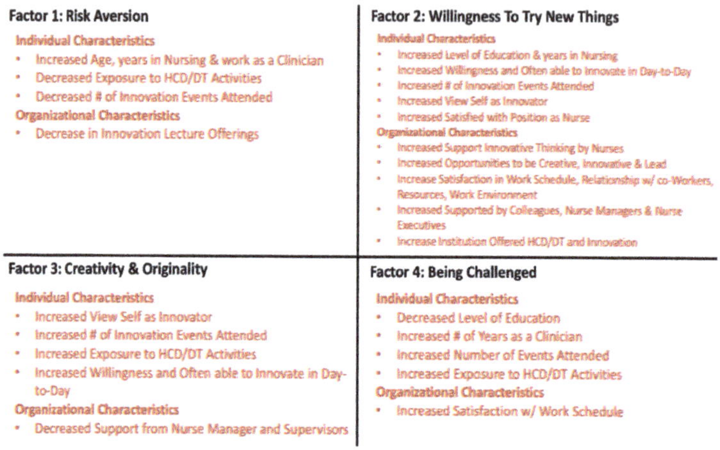

Figure 2. Correlates of innovative behavior.

3.7.1. Factor 1

For Factor 1 (risk aversion), A one-way ANOVA comparing how many innovation events respondents had participated in over the last year ($p = 0.04$), and their willingness to implement innovative methodologies in day-to-day work ($p = 0.0001$) were all positively associated with increased risk aversion. Though the one-way ANOVA showed a statistically significant difference in at least two groups for each variable, a Tukey test for multiple comparisons did not show differences in the pairwise analysis, respectively. A Student's *t*-test found that whether respondents were exposed to HCD/DT activities in the last year or not was associated with risk aversion ($p = 0.03$). Additionally, a Student's *t*-test found a difference in the level of risk aversion related to whether or not a respondent's institution had offered innovation lectures in the past year (0.08 ± 0.78 vs. -0.15 ± 0.97, $p = 0.03$) (see Supplementary Material).

3.7.2. Factor 2

For Factor 2 (willingness to try new things and being an influencer and leader), a one-way ANOVA was performed and found a positive association with how many innovation events the respondent participated in over the last year ($p =< 0.001$), how often they could implement innovative methodologies in day-to-day work ($p = 0.0006$), and their willingness to implement innovative methodologies ($p = 0.002$). Though the one-way ANOVA showed a statistically significant difference in at least two groups for each variable, a Tukey test for multiple comparisons did not show differences in the pairwise analysis, respectively (see Supplementary Material).

A Student's *t*-test found that whether respondents viewed themselves as innovators (0.05 ± 0.76 vs. -0.40 ± 1.3, $p = 0.002$) and whether their institutions supported innovative thinking by their nurses (0.08 ± 0.63 vs. -0.16 ± 1.0, $p = 0.01$) were associated with willingness to try new things and being an influencer and leader about new ideas.

Whether an institution offered innovation resources (12 ± 0.61 vs. -0.12 ± 0.94, $p = 0.01$), education (0.10 ± 0.64 vs. -0.008 ± 0.91, $p = 0.05$), workshops (0.12 ± 0.60 vs.

−0.08 ± 0.89, p = 0.03), lectures (0.13 ± 0.61 vs. −0.11 ± 0.91, p = 0.01) and HCD/DT education (0.20 ± 0.55 vs. −0.08 ± 0.86, p = 0.003), lectures (0.18±0.56 vs. −0.07±0.85, p = 0.01), and resources (0.20 ± 0.56 vs. −0.07 ± 0.69, p = 0.001) were all positively associated with willingness to try new things and being an influencer and leader about new ideas.

3.7.3. Factor 3

For Factor 3 (creativity and originality), a Student's t-test showed that respondents were more willing to be creative and original in their thinking if they viewed themselves as innovators (0.11 ± 0.74 vs. −0.69 ± 1.0, p =< 0.001), and if in the last year, the respondent has been exposed to HCD/DT workshops (0.10 ± 0.68 vs. −0.09 ± 0.96, p = 0.04) and other HCD/DT events (0.21 ± 0.80 vs. −0.04 ± 0.80, p = 0.02).

A one-way ANOVA found that how many innovation events the respondent had participated in over the last year (p = 0.01) was also positively associated with creativity and originality in thinking. Tukey's test for multiple comparisons found a more significant difference in the Factor 3 score in one group regarding how many innovation events the respondent had participated in over the last year, six or more events compared with one event (p = 0.02) (Tables S1 and S2 in the Supplemental Material).

3.7.4. Factor 4

For Factor 4 (being challenged), a one-way ANOVA found a significant difference in the respondents' association with being challenged based on how many innovation events the respondents participated in over the last year (p =< 0.001). Though the Tukey test for multiple comparisons did not show differences in the pairwise analysis, the one-way ANOVA showed statistically significant differences in at least two groups for each variable (Tables S1 and S2 in the Supplemental Material).

4. Discussion

We were interested in understanding the innovativeness of nurses who engaged in innovative behaviors to quantify the characteristics and traits that make nurses more willing to be innovative in their practice. Understanding these will allow the tailoring of curricula for students, clinical education for nurses, and support work with health systems to create an environment more conducive to nurse-led innovation. Therefore, we sought to understand the individual and organizational characteristics of nurses who viewed themselves as innovators in comparison to those who did not, while also quantifying their innovativeness using the Scales for the Measurement of Innovativeness survey.

We also performed an EFA to confirm the survey items' contribution to one of the four identified factors: Risk Aversion (Factor 1), Willingness to Try New Things and Being an Influencer and Leader (Factor 2), Creativity and Originality (Factor 3) and Being Challenged (Factor 4). From the survey results and the EFA, we were able to identify the correlates of innovative behavior (Figure 2).

4.1. Individual and Organizational Characteristics

As noted, there was a paucity of data regarding the characteristics that contribute to the innovativeness of nurses. Our results showed that there are individual and organizational characteristics that contribute to nurses' innovativeness. Nurses who viewed themselves as innovators had higher average innovativeness scores and were more satisfied with their opportunities to be creative and innovative at their institutions.

Three main results emphasize these findings: (1) the number of innovation events participated in by respondents has a significant effect on their innovativeness scores, as those who attended six or more innovation events had higher innovativeness scores than those who attended 1–3 innovation events; (2) respondents who are more satisfied with aspects of their organizations had higher innovativeness scores than those who were not; and (3) respondents whose institutions offered various HCD/DT and innovation activities also had higher innovativeness scores compared with respondents whose institutions did not offer those activities. As noted, research focused on innovation has acknowledged specific individual and organizational characteristics that support innovative behavior; for individuals, a belief in one's ability to be innovative and a focus on creativity; for organizations, supportive leadership as well as promoting awareness of and access to innovation [19,23,24].

Our findings showed that if nurses are exposed to innovation methodologies and activities, nurses are more willing to innovate. A recent study provided further evidence and found that nurses who attended innovation events, such as hackathons, were more confident when participating in innovative behaviors than those who had not [25].

Therefore, health system leaders invested in innovation should seek to create opportunities to encourage nurses to attend more HCD/DT and innovation events and offer these activities within their hospitals and health systems. Providing access to these may make nurses more willing to implement and create new ideas to solve the problems they see in their practices and be leaders in their institutions. Nevertheless, we found that only some institutions offered resources specific to HCD and DT. However, many offered resources specific to innovation. This is an important consideration, as we found in our previously published paper that nurses published papers regarding their use of HCD/DT methodologies in their practice less often than their physician counterparts [2]. Whether that means they are not using HCD/DT in practice or just not publishing their work needs further investigation. Regardless, future work should determine how hospitals and health systems define innovation, how they think about HCD and DT, and the rate at which they offer these activities to their nurses.

The work environment plays a prominent role in the innovativeness of nurses. We found that respondents who worked at institutions that supported innovative thinking by their nurses had higher innovativeness scores than nurses who worked at institutions that they felt did not support innovative thinking by nurses. There was also a relationship between innovativeness scores, how often respondents were able to implement innovation in their day-to-day work, and how satisfied they were with their overall work environment. Organizations that support nurses in their ability to innovate foster nurses with higher innovativeness scores and who are more willing to innovate. However, in our population, very few respondents (8.6%) felt as though they could "always" implement innovation methodologies in their day-to-day work, even though the majority of respondents (54.5%) were "very" willing to innovate.

Additionally, many respondents "often" felt obstacles at their institutions impeded them from being innovative. This is a crucial point to consider, as one may be willing to innovate but lack the resources, structure, and institutional support to innovate. For example, most nurses in our survey who worked in a clinical role stated that they did not get protected time away from the bedside to work on other projects.

This is concerning. As noted, respondents whose organizations supported innovative thinking by their nurses had higher innovativeness scores. With the current nursing climate of burnout and understaffing, some institutions may not see the value in allowing their nurses time away from their clinical responsibilities to work on innovation projects or attend innovation and HCD/DT activities [26]. Institutions should consider the future ramifications of this type of thinking, as our results show that it could have a detrimental effect on the innovativeness of their nurses.

Moreover, how supported by a Nurse Manager a respondent felt was significantly different for those who viewed themselves as innovators than for those who did not, with those identifying as innovators feeling less supported. Leadership is essential in how supported nurses feel and their abilities to innovate. Hospital and health system leaders should consider addressing how they support their leadership through innovation to have a nursing staff that thinks differently and feels supported to transform care.

4.2. Scales for the Measurement of Innovativeness

To understand the innovativeness of nurses, we sought to determine the reliability and face validity of the Scales for the Measurement of Innovativeness tool in our population. We found that the Scales for the Measurement of Innovativeness survey was highly reliable in our population of nurses engaging in innovative behaviors. In addition, face validity suggests that respondents understood the questions being asked of them regarding their innovativeness and found the questions appropriate.

From our EFA, we discovered four domains to guide our contextualization of nurses' innovativeness: Factor 1 included questions related to risk aversion and reluctance to accept new ideas. Factor 2 included questions connected with a willingness to try new things and being an influencer and leader in relation to new ideas. Factor 3 included questions regarding creativity and originality in thinking and behavior. Factor 4 focused on being challenged by unanswered questions and ambiguity.

Interestingly, counter to our previous results showing a positive relationship between participation at innovation events and innovativeness scores, there was a negative correlation between the number of innovation events respondents participated in and risk aversion and reluctance to accept new ideas for Factor 1, meaning that those who are risk averse and reluctant to accept new ideas participated in fewer innovation events. Therefore, encouraging nurses who may tend more toward risk aversion to attend events such as hackathons, where participants are encouraged to take risks and be creative in a safe and supportive environment, may help to decrease reluctance to innovate in their clinical practices. Future work should explore this hypothesis further.

The EFA also showed that, for nurses to be innovative, organizational factors play a significant role. Consequently, we need to consider how the environment of hospitals and health systems enables or dissuades nurses from leading in innovation. As was shown, nurses engaging in innovative behaviors are willing to innovate. However, if the environment is not conducive to encouraging innovation by nurses, innovative behaviors could be stifled.

4.3. Limitations

There are several limitations to this study. This study only surveyed nurses in the US; therefore, the heterogeneity of this group may not be generalizable to other nurses residing outside of the US. This was a cross-sectional study and, as such, may not represent the experiences of nurses over time. Building on this program of study, a longitudinal study should be considered in the future. Additionally, whether willingness to innovate translates to implementation needs to be determined.

As this study only examined nurses actively engaging in innovation behaviors that support innovation, we may have unintentionally excluded nurses who innovate in their clinical practice but have yet to participate in innovative behaviors such as hackathons, innovation workshops, or design sprints. Future studies should examine the innovativeness of all nurses, not just those engaging in innovative behaviors. This will allow us to understand the innovativeness of the nursing profession in general.

5. Conclusions

Compared to those who do not, nurses who view themselves as innovators have higher innovativeness scores. There are multiple individual and organizational characteristics that support the innovativeness of nurses, including how many innovation events one has participated in within the past year, exposure to HCD/DT workshops, whether one feels there is institutional support for innovative thinking by nurses, and whether the institution offered certain HCD/DT and innovation activities. Understanding how to incorporate these characteristics into the curricula of nursing schools and workplace culture will allow more nurses to be prepared to innovate and feel confident doing so. Academic institutions and healthcare organizations have a responsibility to support and foster the innovativeness of nurses for the good of the profession as well as the health and well-being of our patients and communities.

Supplementary Materials: The following supporting information can be downloaded at: https://www.mdpi.com/article/10.3390/nursrep14020066/s1, Table S1: Exploratory Factor Analysis across Individual Characteristics; Table S2: Exploratory Factory Analysis across Organizational Characteristics.

Author Contributions: Conceptualization, M.L., J.A.B., G.D. and S.A.; methodology, M.L., J.A.B., G.D. and S.A.; validation, M.L., J.A.B. and S.A.; formal analysis, M.L., J.A.B. and S.A.; investigation, M.L.; data curation, M.L., J.A.B. and S.A.; writing—original draft preparation, M.L.; writing—review and editing, M.L., J.A.B., G.D., S.A., P.Z.C. and J.M.B.C.; visualization, M.L., J.A.B., G.D. and S.A; supervision, M.L., J.A.B., G.D. and S.A. All authors have read and agreed to the published version of the manuscript.

Funding: This research received no external funding.

Institutional Review Board Statement: The study was conducted in accordance with the Declaration of Helsinki and approved by the Institutional Review Board (or Ethics Committee) of the University of Pennsylvania (protocol code #852671 and 8 December 2022).

Informed Consent Statement: Informed consent was obtained from all subjects involved in the study. Respondents who passed the screening survey were provided with study consent language. The participants consented by completing the survey and submitting it through the online portal (Qualtrics, Provo, UT, USA).

Data Availability Statement: The data presented in this study are available on request from the corresponding author.

Public Involvement Statement: There was no public involvement in any aspect of this research.

Guidelines and Standards Statement: This manuscript was drafted against the Strengthening the Reporting of Observational Studies in Epidemiology (STROBE) guidelines for reporting observational studies.

Use of Artificial Intelligence: A language editing application was used to check the grammar, spelling and for any unintentional plagiarism.

Acknowledgments: We want to thank the nurses who took the time to participate in this study—and who engage in innovative behaviors.

Conflicts of Interest: M.L. is the PI and Co-I on grants related to the use of Human-centered Design and Design Thinking in healthcare.

References

1. Altman, M.; Huang, T.T.; Breland, J.Y. Peer reviewed: Design thinking in health care. *Prev. Chronic Dis.* **2018**, *15*, E117. [CrossRef] [PubMed]
2. Leary, M.; Cacchione, P.C.; Demiris, G.; Brooks Carthon, J.M.; Bauermeister, J.A. An Integrative Review of Human-centered Design and Design Thinking for the Creation of Health Interventions. *Nurs. Forum* **2022**, *57*, 1137–1152. [CrossRef] [PubMed]
3. American Nurses Association. ANA Enterprise Strategic Plan. Available online: https://www.nursingworld.org/~4abeff/globalassets/ana-enterprise/about-us/descriptions-enterprise-strategies-and-objectives.pdf (accessed on 1 July 2022).
4. BDO. Unleashing Nurse-Led Innovation. Available online: https://www.bdo.com/insights/industries/healthcare/unleashing-nurse-led-innovation (accessed on 13 February 2021).
5. The Future of Nursing 2020–2030: Charting a Path to Achieve Health Equity. Available online: https://nap.nationalacademies.org/catalog/25982/the-future-of-nursing-2020-2030-charting-a-path-to (accessed on 29 April 2023).
6. Hassmiller, S.B.; Daniel, G.A. *Taking Action: Top 10 Priorities to Promote Health Equity and Well-Being in Nursing;* Sigma Theta Tau: Indianapolis, IN, USA, 2023.
7. O'Hara, S.; Ackerman, M.H.; Raderstorf, T.; Kilbridge, J.F.; Melnyk, B.M. Building and sustaining a culture of innovation in nursing Academics, Research, Policy, and Practice: Outcomes of the National Innovation Summit. *J. Prof. Nurs.* **2022**, *43*, 5–11. [CrossRef] [PubMed]
8. American Hospital Association. Innovation/New Models of Care. 2023. Available online: https://www.aha.org/topics/innovationnew-models-care (accessed on 29 April 2023).
9. Hurt, H.T.; Joseph, K.; Cook, C.D. Scales for the measurement of innovativeness. *Hum. Commun. Res.* **1977**, *4*, 58–65. [CrossRef]

10. Asurakkody, T.A.; Shin, S.Y. Innovative Behavior in Nursing Context: A Concept Analysis. *Asian Nurs. Res.* **2018**, *12*, 237–244. [CrossRef] [PubMed]
11. Dy Bunpin, J.J., 3rd; Chapman, S.; Blegen, M.; Spetz, J. Differences in Innovative Behavior Among Hospital-Based Registered Nurses. *J. Nurs. Adm.* **2016**, *46*, 122–127. [CrossRef] [PubMed]
12. Clement-O'Brien, K.; Polit, D.F.; Fitzpatrick, J.J. Innovativeness of nurse leaders. *J. Nurs. Manag.* **2011**, *19*, 431–438. [CrossRef] [PubMed]
13. Kennedy, B.; Curtis, K.; Waters, D. Is there a relationship between personality and choice of nursing specialty: An integrative literature review. *BMC Nurs.* **2014**, *13*, 40. [CrossRef] [PubMed]
14. Stilgenbauer, D.J.; Fitzpatrick, J.J. Levels of Innovativeness among Nurse Leaders in Acute Care Hospitals. *J. Nurs. Adm.* **2019**, *49*, 150–155. [CrossRef] [PubMed]
15. Kimble, L.; Massoud, M.R. What do we mean by innovation in healthcare. *Eur. Med. J.* **2017**, *1*, 89–91. [CrossRef]
16. World Health Organization. *Nursing and Midwifery*; World Health Organization; Available online: https://www.who.int/news-room/fact-sheets/detail/nursing-and-midwifery (accessed on 18 March 2022).
17. Selznick, B.S.; Mayhew, M.J. Measuring undergraduates' innovation capacities. *Res. High. Educ.* **2018**, *59*, 744–764. [CrossRef]
18. Rogers, E.M.; Singhal, A.; Quinlan, M.M. Diffusion of innovations. In *An Integrated Approach to Communication Theory and Research*; Routledge: Oxfordshire, UK, 2010; pp. 432–448.
19. Scott, S.G.; Bruce, R.A. Determinants of innovative behavior: A path model of individual innovation in the workplace. *Acad. Manag. J.* **1994**, *37*, 580–607. [CrossRef]
20. Sloane, D.M.; Smith, H.L.; McHugh, M.D.; Aiken, L.H. Effect of Changes in Hospital Nursing Resources on Improvements in Patient Safety and Quality of Care: A Panel Study. *Med. Care* **2018**, *56*, 1001–1008. [CrossRef] [PubMed]
21. García-Pérez, M.A. Use and misuse of corrections for multiple testing. *Methods Psychol.* **2023**, *8*, 100120. [CrossRef]
22. Rothman, K.J. No adjustments are needed for multiple comparisons. *Epidemiology* **1990**, *1*, 43–46. [CrossRef] [PubMed]
23. Siregar ZM, E.; Suryana, E.A.; Senen, S.H. Factors influencing innovative work behavior: An individual factors perspective. *Int. J. Sci. Technol. Res.* **2019**, *8*, 324–327.
24. Li, X.; Zheng, Y. The Influential Factors of Employees' Innovative Behavior and the Management Advices. *J. Serv. Sci. Manag.* **2014**, *7*, 446–450. [CrossRef]
25. Kagan, O.; Sciasci, N.G.; Koszalinski, R.S.; Kagan, D.H.; Leary, M.; Nadel, H. Nurses' confidence in starting a new venture, startup or project in the context of nurse-led hackathons: Results of prehackathon survey. *Nurs. Outlook* **2023**, *71*, 101961. [CrossRef] [PubMed]
26. Nurse.org. This Is the State of Nursing. 2022. Available online: https://media.nurse.org/docs/State+of+Nursing+-+2023.pdf (accessed on 17 March 2023).

nursing reports

MDPI

Article

When Infections Are Found: A Qualitative Study Characterizing Best Management Practices for Central Line-Associated Bloodstream Infection and Catheter-Associated Urinary Tract Infection Performance Monitoring and Feedback

Alice A. Gaughan [1], Sarah R. MacEwan [1,2], Megan E. Gregory [1,3,4], Jennifer L. Eramo [1], Laura J. Rush [1], Courtney L. Hebert [1,3] and Ann Scheck McAlearney [1,3,5,*]

1 The Center for the Advancement of Team Science, Analytics, and Systems Thinking in Health Services and Implementation Science Research (CATALYST), College of Medicine, The Ohio State University, Columbus, OH 43202, USA; Alice.Gaughan@osumc.edu (A.A.G.); Sarah.MacEwan@osumc.edu (S.R.M.); Megan.Gregory@ufl.edu (M.E.G.); Jennifer.Eramo@osumc.edu (J.L.E.); Laura.Rush@osumc.edu (L.J.R.); Courtney.Hebert@osumc.edu (C.L.H.)

2 Division of General Internal Medicine, College of Medicine, The Ohio State University, Columbus, OH 43202, USA

3 Department of Biomedical Informatics, College of Medicine, The Ohio State University, Columbus, OH 43210, USA

4 Department of Health Outcomes & Biomedical Informatics, College of Medicine, University of Florida, Gainesville, FL 32608, USA

5 Department of Family and Community Medicine, College of Medicine, The Ohio State University, Columbus, OH 43201, USA

* Correspondence: Ann.McAlearney@osumc.edu; Tel.: +1-614-293-8973

Abstract: Healthcare-associated infections (HAIs) remain a significant patient safety problem that can lead to illness and death, despite the implementation of clinical bundles to prevent HAIs. Management practices can support HAI prevention, but their role in HAI performance monitoring and feedback is not well understood. To address this knowledge gap, we previously conducted semi-structured interviews with staff at 18 hospitals to examine the role of management practices around the prevention of central line-associated bloodstream infections (CLABSIs) and catheter-associated urinary tract infections (CAUTIs). Interview transcripts were analyzed to identify themes related to HAI performance monitoring and feedback. The current analysis focuses on 10 higher-performing hospitals that were successful in preventing CLABSIs and CAUTIs. These institutions had robust practices including timely event analysis, leadership engagement, and multidisciplinary participation in HAI reviews. Across these sites, we found common goals including investigating HAIs without blame and identifying opportunities for improvement. Management practices such as timely analysis of HAIs, collaboration between facility leadership and multidisciplinary team members, and a focus on identifying the failure of a procedure or protocol, rather than the failure of staff members, are all approaches that can support infection prevention efforts. These management practices may be especially important as hospitals attempt to address increases in CLABSI and CAUTI rates that may have occurred during the coronavirus pandemic.

Keywords: infection prevention; healthcare-associated infections; best practices; management practices; qualitative methods; HAI performance monitoring and feedback

1. Introduction

Healthcare-associated infections (HAIs), including central line-associated bloodstream infections (CLABSIs) and catheter-associated urinary tract infections (CAUTIs) contribute to increased patient morbidity and mortality while adding unnecessary costs to healthcare [1–3]. Since HAIs are largely preventable, clinical bundles have been created and promulgated to reduce the occurrence of HAIs. Clinical bundles for device-related HAIs like CLABSIs and CAUTIs include both tools and policies related to the insertion, maintenance, and removal of those devices [4,5]. Despite this clinical focus, success in HAI reduction has been variable, suggesting that other factors, such as management practices, may have a role in infection prevention [6]. Improving our understanding of the procedures and/or protocols implemented as part of the HAI performance monitoring and feedback process can inform management practices, identify opportunities to improve clinical practice, and prevent future infections.

The importance of investigating the cause of each HAI is supported by the principles and practices of a patient safety culture which highlights the value of opportunities to learn from failure, especially when the goal is to minimize high-risk patient safety errors [7]. While the value of investigating HAIs is evident, little is known about the details of how this is achieved in hospitals that are more successful at preventing HAIs. This study, therefore, examines various approaches to the CLABSI and CAUTI performance monitoring and feedback process to characterize those management practices that may improve patient safety outcomes related to these infections.

2. Materials and Methods

2.1. Study Design

We conducted site visits at hospitals in the United States (US) between September 2017 and November 2019 to study management practices around HAI prevention. As part of this work, we explored the HAI performance monitoring and feedback processes at these hospitals, with a primary focus on central line-associated bloodstream infections (CLABSIs) and catheter-associated urinary tract infections (CAUTIs). The Standards for Reporting Qualitative Research (SRQR) checklist was used when writing this report [8].

2.2. Study Sites and Participants

Hospital performance data, including infection rates for CLABSIs and CAUTIs, are collected by the Centers for Medicare & Medicaid Services and shared through Hospital Care Compare on Medicare.gov [9]. Using the publicly available Hospital Care Compare data focused on hospital performance for CLABSIs and CAUTIs, we aimed to recruit a collection of hospitals designated as better than the national benchmark; average or no different than national benchmark; or worse than the national benchmark.

Over 40 hospitals with different levels of success in preventing CLABSIs and CAUTIs were invited to participate in the study by emailing information to chief hospital executives at each site. Using a purposive sampling approach, we aimed to recruit hospitals with a variety of organizational characteristics including HAI performance. In advance of the site visit, hospital leadership was provided with a list of desired key informants (executives, clinical leaders, infection prevention staff, and nurses) for interviews during the in-person site visit. Clinical leaders assisted with recruiting staff for interviews.

As previously described, the larger study sample included 18 hospitals that varied with respect to their CLABSI and CAUTI rates compared to the national average (i.e., better, average, or worse) based on Hospital Care Compare data [10]. Other hospital characteristics such as geographic region and association with an academic institution were also considered to increase variety in our study sample. In the larger study [11] and across all hospitals, we held in-person interviews with 471 key informants including hospital administrators, frontline staff (e.g., physicians and nurses), and leaders from departments such as infectious diseases, infection control, and epidemiology. This sub-analysis focused on the 10 higher-performing hospitals rated as better or no different than the national benchmark for CLABSIs and CAUTIs and included a total of 245 informants across all roles described above.

2.3. Data Collection

One-on-one and group interviews were conducted in person using a semi-structured interview guide that included questions about management practices surrounding their hospital's efforts in HAI prevention. Topics covered in the interviews included the following: Goal Setting and Support; Strategic Alignment/Communication and Information Sharing; Systematic Education; Interprofessional Collaboration; Meaningful Use of Data; and Recognition for Success. The focus of this smaller study centered around when an occurrence of a CLABSI or CAUTI was reported (e.g., what was done and by whom). Study team members conducted interviews in staff breakrooms and hospital conference rooms. Interviewers included thirteen members of the research team who were MS-, ScD-, or PhD-trained health services and healthcare management researchers. Interviewees did not know their interviewer prior to their interview. All interviews were audio-recorded, transcribed verbatim, and de-identified.

2.4. Data Analysis

Interview transcripts were studied using deductive and inductive thematic analysis [12]. Three research team members who were MS- or PhD-trained health services researchers coded a small sample of transcripts using a preliminary coding dictionary developed from topics in the interview guide. Coders met at a minimum of weekly to discuss code definitions and make adjustments to the coding dictionary to ensure the consistency of coding. When the coding dictionary was finalized, the remaining transcripts were split among coders and codes were applied across all transcripts. Coders continued to meet as needed to resolve questions about the application of codes through collective consensus. This approach allowed for the consistent categorization of data based on general themes derived from the interview guide. The development of themes from codes was part of our iterative analytic process and occurred during our weekly coding and analysis meetings. HAI performance monitoring was one theme identified from the coded transcripts through our deductive analysis. Our inductive analysis involved the constant comparative method and enabled us to identify emergent themes around best practices for HAI performance monitoring and feedback. Comparison of themes across sites allowed us to characterize differences in management practices between sites that were higher- or lower-performing with respect to HAI prevention. The data presented in this study are focused on the perspectives of individuals at hospitals with average or better performance with respect to CLABSI and CAUTI rates compared to the national average. ATLAS.ti qualitative analysis software (ATLAS.ti Scientific Software Development GmbH, Berlin, Germany) was used to support the analysis of transcripts from the 10 higher-performing sites.

2.5. Ethical Considerations

The Institutional Review Board of our institution approved this study. Verbal informed consent was obtained from all subjects participating in the study.

3. Results

3.1. Hospital Characteristics

A majority of the interviewees who discussed management practices around HAI performance monitoring and feedback were from 10 hospitals that had been identified a priori as higher-performing: "better" with respect to HAI prevention or "average" in both CLABSI and CAUTI performance but had recently accelerated their infection prevention efforts. Interviewees at most of the lower-performing hospitals (i.e., the other eight hospital sites in our study) failed to provide examples of management practices related to HAI performance monitoring and feedback. The characteristics of the 10 higher-performing hospitals included in this sub-analysis are presented in Table 1.

Table 1. Hospital characteristics of the 10 higher-performing sites selected for sub-analysis.

Site	CAUTI Performance [1]	CLABSI Performance [1]	Hospital Size [2]	Academic Teaching Hospital	Region
1	Better	Average	Extra Large	Yes	Midwest
2	Average	Better	Medium	No	South
3	Average	Better	Large	Yes	Northeast
4	Average	Better	Medium	Yes	Northeast
5	Average	Average	Small	Yes	Midwest
6	Average	Average	Small	No	Midwest
7	Better	Average	Large	Yes	Midwest
8	Better	Better	Large	Yes	Northeast
9	Better	Better	Extra Large	Yes	South
10	Average	Better	Small	No	South

[1] CAUTI and CLABSI performance data were acquired from the Centers for Medicare & Medicaid Services (CMS) Hospital Care Compare data. [2] Hospital size was defined by the number of beds: Small = less than 300 beds; Medium = 300 to 499 beds; Large = 500 to 899 beds; and Extra Large = 900 or more beds.

3.2. *Best Practices in HAI Monitoring and Feedback*

Across hospitals, comments by interviewees at higher-performing sites revealed a common theme that robust practices were in place around HAI performance monitoring and feedback. Interviewees described the practices including specific management practice elements, ways of promoting safety culture, and the roles of those leading HAI performance monitoring and feedback. We discuss each management practice and associated subthemes in more detail in the subsections that follow.

3.2.1. Management Practice Elements of HAI Performance Monitoring and Feedback

At each of these hospitals, interviewees described HAI performance monitoring and review processes that involved three management practice elements: (1) a timely review of the HAI, often in real time and during regularly scheduled meetings; (2) active awareness and engagement of hospital leadership; and (3) multidisciplinary participation in HAI reviews. One participant described the timely review of HAIs in their organization, which were initiated when infections were communicated to the director of the medical ICU immediately upon detection: "In real time, every time they discover a CAUTI, CLABSI, whatever, they bring it to our attention then. And we discuss it weekly in our HAC [hospital-acquired condition] meeting". In a different hospital, a leader of Quality and Safety highlighted the importance of leadership engagement in HAI reviews by explaining, "A debriefing happens with the clinicians in real time, but it's a debriefing that gets shared or re-debriefed at all levels of the organization, all the way up to the senior management team. So, everybody has the same appreciation for where the processes fell down, and where they can be improved". A description of the third management practice was provided by a leader in Infection Prevention who explained how HAI performance monitoring and feedback processes involved multidisciplinary participation in their organization, "There are event reviews for CLABSI and CAUTI. It used to be just infection prevention and the nurses. And now we have the attending, the respiratory therapy if they need to be there, the dialysis team. So, all those participants participate in that event review". Additional representative quotations about these elements of HAI performance monitoring and feedback are presented in Table 2.

Table 2. Management practice elements of HAI performance monitoring and feedback.

Best Practices	Representative Quotes
Timely reviews	We get an email immediately, so we know as soon as infection prevention has confirmed it. It goes into our patient safety alert system. And then . . . the manager identifies hopefully somebody who was involved in that case, an RN, to review the infection.
	We learned that with CLABSI and CAUTI, you have to look at it every day. And nothing is assumed to just happen by chance.
Leadership engagement	We've always had the CLABSI event reviews . . . so there is more awareness and accountability. So, we get participation, and when it drifts away a little bit, we get a push from our executive sponsor to make sure that everyone is participating.
	We get an email sent to the leadership of that unit, as well as the hospital senior leadership. And, if it hasn't included the intensivists, then we will send it on to the intensivists too so that way they are aware. It goes into our patient safety alert system.
Multidisciplinary participation	It's multidisciplinary and that information is actually rolled out back to the front-line staff as well. So, if it happened on unit [name], the nursing director, the bedside nurse, hopefully the attending, and dialysis if they were involved, would all participate and do a drill down on what could we have done better to improve the outcome of this patient to prevent a CLABSI or a CAUTI.
	At huddle, we go over opportunities. We will offer discussions, you know. Sometimes people will interact or ask questions. . . . We also consult with our infection preventionist. You know, is there anything from your perspective that we missed, or we could have done better . . . ? Just to get the whole perspective.

3.2.2. Promoting Safety Culture in HAI Performance Monitoring and Feedback

Also salient across higher-performing hospitals was the promotion of safety culture in HAI performance monitoring and feedback which included stressing the importance of framing infection reviews as examinations of the failures of processes and procedures and not as ways to establish blame or punish staff. For example, an executive leader explained the focus on processes: "The nurse and the shift lead or assistant nurse manager or manager will present what they found in that 8 AM bed huddle, and that kind of makes everybody have that ownership of it. It's not one person, it's usually the process. Did we follow the process?" A medical director elaborated that the HAI performance monitoring and feedback process should not place blame on the individual, "You know, trying to make it less about whose fault is it and, you know, assigning blame, to: 'Let's fix the system. It is a system problem. Where can the system improve?' Rather than pointing at an individual doctor or nurse who you know wasn't following what they should've done. And how to improve different things like timeouts and those things". Additional representative quotations describing these practices are presented in Table 3.

Table 3. Promoting safety culture in HAI performance monitoring and feedback.

Best Practices	Representative Quotes
Focus on process	There's usually a huddle on reporting about how that occurred, what we could have done different, what we could have improved on, was there anything at all? So, I think that they are very good about, on an individual basis, kind of recapping the things that we could have done differently, and the areas that we may have missed, and ways to improve.
	We have a weekly round-up here. Where all of nursing, and it's a multidisciplinary meeting every Friday at 10 am, where we discuss let's say, any hospital-acquired infections. We do a drill down. It gets presented to the entire team. And the teams actually present their fallouts with the help of the infection control department. That's also a meeting where we have the opportunity to introduce new algorithms or introduce new practices. So, this round-up is a great forum for us.

Table 3. *Cont.*

Best Practices	Representative Quotes
Not assigning blame	Staff really, I feel, really want to do the right thing. They really do. I believe their hearts are really in the right place. So, with this [HAI review], I think it's, you know, we do the no blame, because usually it's sort of a few, it's a period of time that we miss something, right?
	These event reviews are fairly time-consuming. Nobody wants to do it. I wouldn't say they're punitive, but they're somewhat, it's an opportunity to improve. It's a no-blame environment. It's just like, what did we do wrong?

3.2.3. Using HAI Performance Monitoring and Feedback to Identify Opportunities for Improvement

Finally, the goal of identifying opportunities for improvement when HAIs occurred and in preventing future infections was described by interviewees from multiple disciplines across these higher-performing hospitals. We found that the presentation of these opportunities for improvement could be led or driven by individuals with different roles. For instance, a manager of quality and patient safety explained a HAI review process where infection prevention took the lead: "So, if we had a CAUTI, we would actually, the IP [infection preventionist] would come and tell us [the opportunity for improvement committee] about what she found, and the investigation, and who worked on it, and what we could do to improve it." A unit director of another hospital shared that their process for HAI review was driven by staff leadership at the unit level, "So, when one is identified on the unit, we will go back and talk with them, have a meeting with the attending and someone from infection prevention, members of their team who lead the unit. And then sometimes a staff nurse, but certainly staff leadership. And we go through a process that looks at … what was going on with the patient at the time, and did we have any opportunities there that were missed, pieces of the bundle basically, or anything unique to that case". Quotations providing examples of these different approaches to leading HAI performance monitoring and feedback processes are presented in Table 4.

Table 4. Role leading HAI performance monitoring and feedback.

Role	Representative Quotes
Infection Control	Between the manager and infection control, we each review the chart. What did we do right? What did we do wrong? Bring it to our attention, whether it was something as simple as you didn't change an outside Foley, to you didn't document good care, to whatever.
	We receive notification as soon as a CLABSI is identified from infection prevention. It gets sent to quality, it is sent to nursing, it is sent to physician leaders. And then our clinical nurse specialists do what they call a deep dive. So, they get in the patient's chart, and they start looking at all sorts of things which includes was the line changed when it was supposed to be? Was there a documented need for the line? Why is the line still there? Have you done a good job documenting? And any gaps or errors in which he or she can see about the case. And then our quality committees or our safety committee will often go through those details to understand, you know, to learn from that. Because we still have CLABSIs.
Unit Leadership	As a unit, what our leadership did was at our morning safety huddles and evening safety huddles was they would review what were the risk factors that this patient had for developing infection, and what were some of the modifiable things that we could have done as nursing to prevent that.
	We are having an open discussion on what was done, what can we do better. And when I was the quality rep [resentative], I took that information back and educated my staff. I can't answer for every unit or every person, but I know what I did. And I mean, we went two years without a CLABSI. And it was just holding people accountable.

4. Discussion

Our study revealed important core elements of management practices for CLABSI and CAUTI performance monitoring and feedback. These core elements included timely and rigorous HAI reviews, strong leadership engagement, and regular involvement of multidisciplinary staff. These findings provide greater nuance to existing guidance surrounding broader HAI performance monitoring and feedback [13]. Our study findings also highlight the importance of identifying opportunities for improvement in infection prevention, regardless of which member of the healthcare team leads the infection review process. These results demonstrate that there are multiple approaches to HAI performance monitoring and feedback that are in use at higher-performing hospitals, and these may be contributing to their lower infection rates. What appears to be most important is that the critical elements of the performance monitoring and feedback process are carried out in a way that is embraced by both hospital leaders and frontline staff [14–17].

Of note, prior studies have acknowledged that fostering a safety culture is an important element of successful infection prevention programs [7,18]. In alignment with this evidence, we found that interviewees from higher-performing hospitals did not assign blame to staff when evaluating CLABSIs and CAUTIs. Emphasizing the importance of safety culture may be another way to support productive HAI performance monitoring and feedback processes by framing investigations as an opportunity to inform process improvements that can then prevent future infections.

During the COVID-19 pandemic, the National Steering Committee for Patient Safety released an urgent call to improve patient safety because of the worrisome rise in HAIs [19–22] emphasizing the need for additional efforts in infection prevention. As the pandemic has transitioned to an endemic phase and CLABSI and CAUTI rates seem to be improving [23–25], patient safety is still of paramount importance. Focusing on management practices specific to performance monitoring and feedback used in high-performing hospitals may provide a useful structure through which to investigate deficits in practice and to identify core elements of these processes that can be strengthened to achieve improvements in patient safety outcomes. Identifying opportunities for improvement in infection prevention using best management practices in HAI performance monitoring and feedback remains critical to creating and maintaining quality and safety in the healthcare environment.

Our study has several limitations. As this work was part of a larger project investigating multiple management strategies for CLABSI and CAUTI prevention, it is possible that a study focused specifically on management practices related to performance monitoring and feedback processes at lower-performing sites may reveal additional information that did not emerge in our study. While we utilized CLABSI and CAUTI performance ratings to select higher- and lower-performing hospitals, it is important to acknowledge that performance ratings are assigned at the hospital level while management practices often vary at the unit level, depending on standard operating procedures or protocols for a particular unit or service. The potential relationship between performance ratings and management practices is therefore complex, such that we cannot directly attribute infection prevention performance to the management practices reported by our study participants.

5. Conclusions

Participants in our study described management practices around conducting timely reviews of HAIs, ensuring hospital leadership's engagement in the process, and securing the involvement of multidisciplinary members of the healthcare team, all of which may have contributed to their success in HAI prevention. Sharing the findings of these HAI reviews with hospital staff as learning opportunities can help foster a patient safety culture where investigating infections is never punitive and may help advance infection prevention efforts and, ideally, help hospitals achieve lower HAI rates.

Author Contributions: Conceptualization, A.A.G., S.R.M., M.E.G., C.L.H. and A.S.M.; methodology, A.A.G., S.R.M., M.E.G., C.L.H. and A.S.M.; formal analysis, A.A.G., S.R.M., M.E.G., C.L.H. and A.S.M.; investigation, A.A.G., S.R.M., M.E.G., C.L.H. and A.S.M.; resources, A.S.M.; data curation, A.A.G., S.R.M., M.E.G., C.L.H. and A.S.M.; writing—original draft preparation, A.A.G., S.R.M., M.E.G., J.L.E., L.J.R., C.L.H. and A.S.M.; writing—review and editing, A.A.G., S.R.M., M.E.G., J.L.E., L.J.R., C.L.H. and A.S.M.; visualization, A.A.G., S.R.M., M.E.G. and A.S.M.; supervision, A.S.M.; project administration, A.A.G. and A.S.M.; funding acquisition, A.S.M. All authors have read and agreed to the published version of the manuscript.

Funding: This research was funded by a grant from the Agency for Healthcare Research and Quality, grant# R01HS024958. The views expressed in this paper are solely those of the authors and do not represent any US government agency or any institutions with which the authors are affiliated. The funding source played no role in study design, data acquisition, analysis, or decision to report these data. The findings and conclusions in this report are those of the authors and do not represent the views of Agency for Healthcare Research and Quality or the US Federal Government.

Institutional Review Board Statement: The study was conducted in accordance with the Declaration of Helsinki and approved by the Institutional Review Board of The Ohio State University (2017H0017, approved 2 February 2017) for studies involving humans.

Informed Consent Statement: For this study, we received IRB approval from our institution and approval for a waiver of documentation of consent. All participants provided informed verbal consent. There is no identifiable information about participants.

Data Availability Statement: Due to participant privacy concerns, the data presented in this study are not publicly available. The data may be requested from the corresponding author.

Public Involvement Statement: There was no public involvement in any aspect of this research.

Guidelines and Standards Statement: This manuscript was drafted against the Consolidated Criteria for Reporting Qualitative Research (https://www.equator-network.org/, accessed on 2 February 2024).

Acknowledgments: The authors would like to thank Natalie Gaines, Jeanette Gardner, Lindsey Sova, Caroline Sugar, Meg Suttle, Jaclyn Volney, and Toby Weinert, all affiliated with the authors' institution, for their assistance with this project. The authors would also like to express their gratitude to the key informants and hospitals that participated in this study.

Conflicts of Interest: The authors declare no conflicts of interest.

References

1. McCleskey, S.G.; Shek, L.; Grein, J.; Gotanda, H.; Anderson, L.; Shekelle, P.G.; Keeler, E.; Morton, S.; Nuckols, T.K. Economic Evaluation of Quality Improvement Interventions to Prevent Catheter-Associated Urinary Tract Infections in the Hospital Setting: A Systematic Review. *BMJ Qual. Saf.* **2022**, *31*, 308–321. [CrossRef] [PubMed]
2. Oliveira, R.M.C.; de Sousa, A.H.F.; de Salvo, M.A.; Petenate, A.J.; Gushken, A.K.F.; Ribas, E.; Torelly, E.M.S.; Silva, K.C.C.D.; Bass, L.M.; Tuma, P.; et al. Estimating the Savings of a National Project to Prevent Healthcare-Associated Infections in Intensive Care Units. *J. Hosp. Infect.* **2024**, *143*, 8–17. [CrossRef] [PubMed]
3. Cassini, A.; Plachouras, D.; Eckmanns, T.; Abu Sin, M.; Blank, H.-P.; Ducomble, T.; Haller, S.; Harder, T.; Klingeberg, A.; Sixtensson, M.; et al. Burden of Six Healthcare-Associated Infections on European Population Health: Estimating Incidence-Based Disability-Adjusted Life Years through a Population Prevalence-Based Modelling Study. *PLoS Med.* **2016**, *13*, e1002150. [CrossRef]
4. Greene, M.T.; Krein, S.L.; Huis, A.; Hulscher, M.; Sax, H.; Sakamoto, F.; Sakihama, T.; Tokuda, Y.; Fowler, K.E.; Saint, S. Infection Prevention Practices in the United States, the Netherlands, Switzerland, and Japan: Results from National Surveys. *Infect. Control Hosp. Epidemiol.* **2021**, *42*, 1206–1214. [CrossRef] [PubMed]
5. Wasserman, S.; Messina, A. Bundles in Infection Prevention and Safety—ISID 2019. Available online: https://isid.org/wp-content/uploads/2018/02/ISID_InfectionGuide_Chapter16.pdf (accessed on 2 April 2024).
6. Scheck McAlearney, A.; Hefner, J.L.; Robbins, J.; Harrison, M.I.; Garman, A. Preventing Central Line-Associated Bloodstream Infections: A Qualitative Study of Management Practices. *Infect. Control Hosp. Epidemiol.* **2015**, *36*, 557–563. [CrossRef]
7. Braun, B.I.; Chitavi, S.O.; Suzuki, H.; Soyemi, C.A.; Puig-Asensio, M. Culture of Safety: Impact on Improvement in Infection Prevention Process and Outcomes. *Curr. Infect. Dis. Rep.* **2020**, *22*, 34. [CrossRef] [PubMed]
8. O'Brien, B.C.; Harris, I.B.; Beckman, T.J.; Reed, D.A.; Cook, D.A. Standards for Reporting Qualitative Research: A Synthesis of Recommendations. *Acad. Med.* **2014**, *89*, 1245. [CrossRef] [PubMed]
9. U.S. Centers for Medicare and Medicaid Services. Find Healthcare Providers: Compare Care Near You. Available online: https://www.medicare.gov/care-compare/?redirect=true&providerType=Hospital (accessed on 2 April 2024).

10. MacEwan, S.R.; Beal, E.W.; Gaughan, A.A.; Sieck, C.; McAlearney, A.S. Perspectives of Hospital Leaders and Staff on Patient Education for the Prevention of Healthcare-Associated Infections. *Infect. Control Hosp. Epidemiol.* **2022**, *43*, 1129–1134. [CrossRef] [PubMed]
11. McAlearney, A.S.; Gaughan, A.A.; DePuccio, M.J.; MacEwan, S.R.; Hebert, C.; Walker, D.M. Management Practices for Leaders to Promote Infection Prevention: Lessons from a Qualitative Study. *Am. J. Infect. Control* **2021**, *49*, 536–541. [CrossRef]
12. Terry, G.; Hayfield, N.; Clarke, V.; Braun, V. Thematic Analysis. In *The SAGE Handbook of Qualitative Research in Psychology*, 2nd ed.; SAGE: London, UK, 2017; pp. 17–37.
13. Storr, J.; Twyman, A.; Zingg, W.; Damani, N.; Kilpatrick, C.; Reilly, J.; Price, L.; Egger, M.; Grayson, M.L.; Kelley, E.; et al. Core Components for Effective Infection Prevention and Control Programmes: New WHO Evidence-Based Recommendations. *Antimicrob. Resist. Infect. Control* **2017**, *6*, 1–18. [CrossRef]
14. Engel, F.D.; Dos Santos Cunha, K.; Magalhães, A.L.P.; Meirelles, B.H.S.; de Mello, A.L.S.F. Management Actions for Prevention and Control of Healthcare-Associated Infections: A Grounded Theory Approach. *J. Nurs. Manag.* **2022**, *30*, 1355–1365. [CrossRef] [PubMed]
15. Hansen, S.; Remschmidt, C.; Schröder, C.; Behnke, M.; Gastmeier, P. Strengthening the Role of Hospital Leadership in Infection Control (LEAD-IC)—A Multimodal Educational Intervention in German Acute Care Hospitals. *BMC Med. Educ.* **2023**, *23*, 758. [CrossRef] [PubMed]
16. Sartini, M.; Patrone, C.; Spagnolo, A.M.; Schinca, E.; Ottria, G.; Dupont, C.; Alessio-Mazzola, M.; Bragazzi, N.L.; Cristina, M.L. The Management of Healthcare-Related Infections through Lean Methodology: Systematic Review and Meta-Analysis of Observational Studies. *J. Prev. Med. Hyg.* **2022**, *63*, E464–E475. [CrossRef] [PubMed]
17. Krauss, D.M.; Molefe, A.; Hung, L.; Hayes, K.; Gorman, C.; Latterner, M.; Henderson, S.; Miller, M. Emergent Themes from a Quality Improvement Programme for CLABSI/CAUTI Prevention in ICUs amid the COVID-19 Pandemic. *BMJ Open Qual.* **2022**, *11*, e001926. [CrossRef] [PubMed]
18. Hessels, A.J.; Guo, J.; Johnson, C.T.; Larson, E. Impact of Patient Safety Climate on Infection Prevention Practices and Healthcare Worker and Patient Outcomes. *Am. J. Infect. Control* **2023**, *51*, 482–489. [CrossRef] [PubMed]
19. Blot, S.; Ruppé, E.; Harbarth, S.; Asehnoune, K.; Poulakou, G.; Luyt, C.-E.; Rello, J.; Klompas, M.; Depuydt, P.; Eckmann, C.; et al. Healthcare-Associated Infections in Adult Intensive Care Unit Patients: Changes in Epidemiology, Diagnosis, Prevention and Contributions of New Technologies. *Intensive Crit. Care Nurs.* **2022**, *70*, 103227. [CrossRef] [PubMed]
20. HealthLeaders. Urgent Call Made to Improve Patient Safety. Available online: https://www.healthleadersmedia.com/clinical-care/urgent-call-made-improve-patient-safety (accessed on 2 April 2024).
21. Buetti, N.; Ruckly, S.; de Montmollin, E.; Reignier, J.; Terzi, N.; Cohen, Y.; Siami, S.; Dupuis, C.; Timsit, J.-F. COVID-19 Increased the Risk of ICU-Acquired Bloodstream Infections: A Case-Cohort Study from the Multicentric OUTCOMEREA Network. *Intensive Care Med.* **2021**, *47*, 180–187. [CrossRef] [PubMed]
22. Baker, M.A.; Sands, K.E.; Huang, S.S.; Kleinman, K.; Septimus, E.J.; Varma, N.; Blanchard, J.; Poland, R.E.; Coady, M.H.; Yokoe, D.S.; et al. The Impact of Coronavirus Disease 2019 (COVID-19) on Healthcare-Associated Infections. *Clin. Infect. Dis. Off. Publ. Infect. Dis. Soc. Am.* **2022**, *74*, 1748–1754. [CrossRef] [PubMed]
23. Mitchell, B.G.; Stewardson, A.J.; Kerr, L.; Ferguson, J.K.; Curtis, S.; Busija, L.; Lydeamore, M.J.; Graham, K.; Russo, P.L. The Incidence of Nosocomial Bloodstream Infection and Urinary Tract Infection in Australian Hospitals before and during the COVID-19 Pandemic: An Interrupted Time Series Study. *Antimicrob. Resist. Infect. Control* **2023**, *12*, 61. [CrossRef]
24. Bartles, R.; Moore, A.; Martin, R.; Clarkson, R.; Ebinger, L. Using a Comprehensive On-Site Assessment Process to Reduce Central Line-Associated Bloodstream Infection Rates. *J. Infus. Nurs. Off. Publ. Infus. Nurses Soc.* **2023**, *46*, 266–271. [CrossRef]
25. Teus, J.K.; Mithen, L.; Green, H.; Hutton, A.; Fernandez, R. Impact of Infection Prevention and Control Practices, including Personal Protective Equipment, on the Prevalence of Hospital-Acquired Infections in Acute Care Hospitals during COVID-19: A Systematic Review and Meta-Analysis. *J. Hosp. Infect.* **2024**, *147*, 32–39. [CrossRef] [PubMed]

nursing reports

MDPI

Article

Experiences for Geriatric Care from Nursing Students' Knowledge: A Qualitative Approach

Elsa Gil-Mateu [1,2], Silvia Reverté-Villarroya [1,2,*], Núria Albacar-Riobóo [1,2] and Josep Barceló-Prats [2,3]

[1] Nursing Department, Campus Terres de l'Ebre, Universitat Rovira Virgili, Avenue Remolins, 13-15, 43500 Tarragona, Spain; elsa.gil@urv.cat (E.G.-M.); nuria.albacar@urv.cat (N.A.-R.)
[2] Advanced Nursing Research Group, Universitat Rovira i Virgili, 43002 Tarragona, Spain; josep.barcelo@urv.cat
[3] Nursing Department, Campus Catalunya, Universitat Rovira Virgili, Avenue Catalunya, 35, 43002 Tarragona, Spain
* Correspondence: silvia.reverte@urv.cat

Abstract: (1) Background: Studies have shown that clinical experience has an impact on how students perceive geriatric care. The vulnerability of older people particularly allows students to reflect on and evaluate their learning. In this context, communication between tutors and students is important to guiding a contextualized view of the complexity of clinical situations. The principal objective was to explore the feelings, perceptions, and experiences of nursing students in geriatric care units during their practices. (2) Methods: This is a qualitative study using content analysis where the data collected were analyzed deductively. An intentional sample of 81 nursing degree students enrolled in the subject of clinical practices. During these sessions, a dynamic discussion forum was incorporated. (3) Results: There were 6 forums with a total of 591 participants, with an average of 98.5 per forum. Four categories emerged: humanization, geriatric nurse, aging, and learning. (4) Conclusions: A change of management oriented to the person-centered model would improve the quality in the residences and as well as in the expectations of the students towards geriatric nursing. Changing perspectives could be a way to confront and become aware of the fallacies of care that have been evidenced. This study was not registered.

Keywords: geriatric; nursing students; practice; qualitative analysis; teaching methods

1. Introduction

Nursing, as a discipline, is the result of the evolution of the activity of care within contemporary societies, giving a professionalized character to the set of tasks related to care. For this reason, this discipline has needed to develop its own body of scientific knowledge in order to define its nursing activities, to develop their teaching and research, as well as to improve their healthcare practice. The ultimate aim of all these contributions has been to increase the quality of care for the individual, the family, or the community. Consequently, caregiving is a complex practice that requires integrating diverse elements. According to Brykczynska, the essential points of care are compassion, competence, confidence, trust, and awareness. These are basic and inescapable virtues that are required to provide quality care for a human being. They are both personal and professional habits and are mutually necessary [1].

In this idea, training in all the capacities of the human being in order to be able to respond to the problems that life holds becomes the primary goal of education. So, the intersection between attitudes, knowledge, and skills is what they call competence. Acquiring new skills is not only an activity prior to work or what we do in isolation, but is carried out in the course of the work itself, becomes a fundamental piece in its acquisition and development, and consequently, in the process of professionalization. The student is competent because he feels and reflects, and acts accordingly on his knowledge, skills,

Nurs. Rep. **2024**, *14*, 733–743. https://doi.org/10.3390/nursrep14020056 https://www.mdpi.com/journal/nursrep

motives, and values, with flexibility and perseverance in solving problems presented by the practice. And this is what is called reflexive competence, a transversal competence [2,3].

In fact, it is in actual clinical practice—conceived as an open, dynamic, and changing space characterized by the complexity its situations— where the students find a setting conducive to carry out processes of reflection, deliberation, clinical reasoning, and decision-making [4–6].

Nursing in the 21st century is capable of addressing care from an ethical and moral standpoint, but reaching this level of maturity requires changes in curricular focus, institutions, and the profession itself. Nursing, therefore, can be considered a dualistic discipline. It is a science of health, but also of the human, trying to distance itself from reductionist tendencies [7]. There are different theories and models that attempt to address this need to find meaning in care.

Certain phenomenological theories propose discovering meaning in these human experiences by directing care towards the patient's world, which is known as "being with" the person [8,9]. For example, according to Watson, care is a moral idea, rather than a work-oriented attitude. Internalizing and mastering these concepts are what allow care workers to operate in the context of human complexity. Parse's model presents us with the "Human Becoming Theory" in which, according to the author, "becoming" refers to the possibilities within a human being or what we are in potentiality. For Benner, a person interprets their symptoms in relation to the impact these may have on what is important to them, which includes family, work, leisure, and relationships. Therefore, identifying what is important to the patient is the key to caring for them meaningfully. Benner associates the clinical judgement that determines action with Schön's practical reasoning, defining it as reasoning in transition, embedded in an interaction with the person and family that cannot be converted into mere procedures or techniques, but arises from an insight into each situation and the knowledge of how to deal with them [9]. According to this author, the basic competencies acquired by students with university training are completed with experience and permanent reflection. The overarching idea in all these models and paradigms is to understand the health–illness spectrum as a life experience that is expressed through narrative that provides nursing with a profound knowledge linking moment, care, person, and situation [10].

In the field of geriatric nursing, the growing demand for care caused by an increasingly ageing population is a challenge for healthcare services. The vulnerability of older people particularly allows students to reflect on and evaluate their learning. Studies have shown that clinical experience has an impact on how students perceive this field [10–12].

In this context, communication between tutors and students is important to guiding a contextualized view of the complexity of clinical situations, the analysis and elaboration of clinical reasoning, decision-making, and the exercise of care [13,14]. Teachers are thus expected to use reflective practice, promoting the use of technology, to help students contemplate positive as well as negative experiences in both clinical and academic settings. Present day students belong to a generation that understands information and communication technologies (ICTs) as part of their everyday environment [15,16]. Universities and organizations need to innovate and make constant improvements to adapt curricula to this increasingly virtual environment. As a result, active methodologies such as forums, the flipped-classroom, or conceptual maps are a strategic framework for student-centred learning, steering trainees towards action [16]. However, in the case of clinical training, it is difficult to obtain instruments that allow for an active methodology outside the classroom.

The overall objective of this study was to analyze the experiences that arise from nursing students in their clinical practices in geriatric care units. By encouraging students to go through a reflective process, perceptions and emotions emerge that empower them as agents of transformation within their future areas of work and can support their nursing practice.

2. Materials and Methods

2.1. Design

This is a qualitative study using a using content analysis [17]; the data collected were analyzed deductively. We recognize that findings are interpretative, and they have been constructed with the participants the of the study. This approach was considered the most appropriate to exploring the reality of students undergoing clinical training in geriatric services, allowing for needs analysis and the implementation of future strategies. An analysis was carried out for quantitative and qualitative variables of the participants and of forum interventions using means, standard deviations (SDs), and percentages.

2.2. Participants

A total and intentional population of 81 fourth-year nursing degree students enrolled in clinical practicums in geriatric care units during the academic years 2018–2019 and 2019–2020 were selected.

2.3. Data Collection

The data were collected between January 2019 and March 2020. During this period the students carried out their clinical practices. These practices were divided into cycles of 5 weeks each. In total there were 6 cycles of practices, and each cycle was accompanied by a virtual forum. Data were extracted from this forum. (Table 1)

Table 1. Virtual forum codes.

Forums	Code	Number of Students (n = 81)
January/February 2019	GG*1	12
February–March 2019	GG2	15
March–April 2019	GG3	14
April–May 2019	GG4	12
January–February 2020	GG5	14
February–March 2020	GC6	14

*GG = Geriatrics Group.

2.4. Intervention

Each student chose a different service. During clinical practice, tutors initiated a discussion forum and students were encouraged to participate in it during the course of their internship, the objective of the forum was to maintain a virtual community, where they can express their different experiences. Training was provided to tutors who actively participated in the forum. These tutors served as reference points for the students, motivating them, providing them with information, and addressing any issues that arose while keeping the virtual environment alive. The forums began with a presentation of their practice sites. The tutor responded or encouraged students to bring up topics of interest. The students had to respond with short interventions (4 or 5 lines), answering the tutor's question and following the students' thematic thread. At the end of each cycle, a face-to-face seminar was held, where all the information shared and generated in the virtual environment was reviewed [18].

2.5. Qualitative Analysis

An in-depth reading of the forums was carried out by S.R.-V. and E.G.-M and the text was coded into units of meaning. These were further coded, compared, contrasted, and ordered into subcategories and finally grouped into main categories representing the main themes of discourse. The data were validated by all study participants. The data were managed using the open-source Weft QDA 1.0.1 for Windows software and analyzed using content analysis [17]. The consolidated COREQ qualitative research reporting criteria were followed [19].

The codes, subcategories, and categories provided the structure of the discourse. In order to further validate the research, the content was analyzed by the students in their end-of-practicum seminars.

2.6. Ethics

The study obtained approval from the Pere Virgili Institute for Health Research's Drug Research Ethics Committee, with the code 121/2020. The introductory workshop of the practicum provided information on the study, the functioning of the forum, and its voluntary participation. All participants signed the corresponding informed consent voluntarily. Non-participation did not entail a change in the treatment or the follow-up to the student. To maximize confidentiality, no names were registered or encoded. The study was carried out in accordance with the precepts of the Declaration of Helsinki [20].

3. Results

A total of 81 students participated. Six forums were held with a total of 591 interventions, with an average of 98.5 per forum. In total, 70.6% of the students were women with an average age of 21.18 years (SD = 2.18).

In the data analysis, the following thematic categories emerged: humanization, geriatric nurse, ageing, and learning (Table 2).

Table 2. Qualitative Analysis.

Category	Definition	Subcategories
Humanization	To value the dignity and individuality of the person, based on a comprehensive approach where the biological, psychological, social, and spiritual dimensions interact.	Person-Centered Care Family Restraints Communication
Geriatric Nursing	Ability to put into practice the knowledge, skills, and attitudes of the nursing profession at the service of the resolution and prevention of a health problem.	Emotion management Geriatric Institutions Clinical safety
Ageing	The set of morphological, functional, and psychological changes that entail changes in the structure and function of the different systems, increasing the individual's vulnerability to environmental stress and disease.	Loneliness Stigma Fragility Abuse Finitude Polymedication
Learning	The process of acquiring knowledge, skills, values and attitudes through study, teaching, or experience.	Training Critical thinking

3.1. Categories

3.1.1. Humanization

Students reflect on humanized care, noting deficiencies in geriatric services. They discussed people-centered care, a practice that needs time, flexibility, knowledge of people, and their emotions, characteristics that they do not observe in clinical practices.

> *"Although I believe that patient care is becoming more humane and the ethical basis of care is being taken into account, there is still work to be done to establish a person-centred model of care for the older people."* (GG6)

> *"These are people who need comprehensive attention and care, centred on the person and not on the illness, and this requires time and personnel that are not available."* (GG4)

They discussed the role of the family in the humanized care model, and they talked about changes in family structures and increasing the proportion of older people living alone.

> *"I noted that the ageing of the population and changes in family structures have led to an increase in the need for health care resources for older people."* (GG2)

> *"We judge the family of geriatric patients, and this is a big mistake on our part. Each person has their own story and it is important to know their background in order to understand the situation they are in."* (GG3)

Restraints pose an ethical problem for students, presenting them with a theoretical and practical dilemma that is difficult to address.

> *"What I have observed in practice is that due to lack of time and staff, they prefer mechanical restraint first, but often even pharmacological restraint is used several times in the same shift. I personally believe that it should be eradicated as far as possible because I think it is inhumane."* (GG3)

Finally, communication becomes a therapeutic action inherent in humanized care. Communication skills are recognized as a valuable tool for improving a patient's prognosis, although there is an increasing lack of communication skills, particularly in the case of people with cognitive impairments and as a result of the mechanization of care.

> *"We need to explain what we do and how we do it, but most of the time we assume that patients already know what we are going to do because we have done it more than once or because we think they are not interested or will not understand it."* (GG4)

> *"Active listening is a practice that we should always adopt and there should be no excuses for not doing it, as it is the basis of communication and of much nursing care."* (GG5)

3.1.2. Geriatric Nursing

Certain moments in caregiving are stressful for students as they involve emotional processing and management.

> *"And what I wanted to ask is whether you all are also so affected by the unexpected death of a patient you had grown fond of. I think I lack the skills to not carry that home with me, I feel sad on these occasions..."* (GG5)

They addressed the problems of working conditions offered in geriatric institutions.

> *"As nursing students, seeing the state of geriatric care, it discourages us that once we have finished our degree and in the world of work, geriatric centres are one of our last preferences, not because of the type of patients, but because of the type of contracts, the excess workload, the lack of personnel, etc."* (GG6)

They were very critical on the issue of clinical safety, whether in medicine preparation, information transfer at shift changes, or in the management of protective isolations.

> *"The criteria for protective isolation are not met, we find doors to isolated rooms open, patients with multidrug-resistant bacteria walking down the corridor, isolation wards where one person is infected and another is not."* (GG2)

> *"Good prevention is key to reducing the volume of care and complications, allowing more attention to be devoted to preventing other conditions, improving care and hygiene. "* (GG4)

3.1.3. Ageing

The informants reflected on the social problems of ageing and talk about loneliness among older people.

> *"These are people who find themselves in a complicated social situation where they spend many hours alone, without company, which means that they cannot express themselves."* (GG4)

They also discussed the stigma around older people, especially highlighting diseases involving cognitive impairment.

> *"I have seen stigmatization towards the older people. There are gestures and actions, for example in Alzheimer's, and they don't give these the importance they deserve."* (GG3)

They also highlighted the apparent frailty of older people, noting that sometimes their own actions are not always correct.

> *"It is very important to give the patient autonomy, because we often unintentionally deny it, thinking t'hey are older, they can't manage alone'. I tend to think that because I see them as frail."* (GG6)

This raised the issue of the institutional mistreatment of older people in residential care settings.

> *"We also find a lot of news where there is talk of elder abuse, and they appear to be more vulnerable because of their illnesses."* (GG3)

Trainees were also concerned about the amount of medication received by people living in geriatric institutions.

> *"The issue of polymedication among the older people is huge. I think that we should try to prioritise and minimise the administration of medication."* (GG4)

Finally, they were struck by the issue of death and the finitude of this stage of life.

> *"Many of the patients I have had who have been suffering have often commented on wanting to end the situation or have expressed a wish to die."* (GG2)

3.1.4. Learning

Students debated the low social value placed on geriatric care as a speciality, although they appreciated the learning opportunity.

> *"We all agree that geriatrics is a greatly undervalued speciality, but I think that doesn't take away from the good moments. In addition to having learned a lot about ulcers and care, I have also been able to see the evolution of the different patients, the way patients and professionals interact."* (CG6)

> *"As professionals, we have to continue updating the knowledge we already have, as well as expanding it. During this course, I have realised that you can always learn more in any area of care, from techniques to how to manage certain behaviours."* (GG3)

All this acquired training enabled students to develop critical thinking, in other words, to reflect on and understand their daily work.

> *"I've been deepening my knowledge of wound care, a field that I think is very broad and of real importance for our profession. All this knowledge has allowed me to develop optimal critical thinking, being able to decide for myself and apply previously learned techniques."* (GG1)

4. Discussion

The informants, like some authors, demonstrated that humanization is a complex process involving all dimensions of a person and ranging from policy to culture, healthcare organization, training of health and social care professionals, and the development of care plans [21,22]. Respect for privacy, a person's autonomy, management of emotions, spirituality, and adequate communication were all mentioned as important factors in humanizing care.

A person-centred model, therefore, arises, where the aim is to generate home-like environments, focusing on the preferences and needs of older people and on the ability of the professionals involved to learn about these preferences, patients' life histories, and diversity [23].

The students recognize the necessity of working within this model of care, where the aim is to work with people and not with diseases. They see the need to include the family as part of care, although they note that changes in the social structure of families and carers make this challenging to achieve. Previous studies confirm these structural changes and uphold the role of family and social networks as institutions conducive to active ageing [24,25].

In order to implement this model, existing research emphasizes the need for changes in working conditions and staffing ratios. López et al. [26] concluded that good care is related to both work and personal resources. They also noted that professional strain must be reduced for the promotion of quality care. Institutions do not always respond to the demands of professionals, as demonstrated in the study by Dwyer [27] where nurses felt devalued by the system. The students associate this lack of personnel with the mechanical and pharmacological restraint of residents, emphasising the need to eradicate this practice. According to them, and in line with the literature [28,29], health can be said to improve when patient care is based on a person-centred, non-restraint model.

Delving into reflective thinking when students were in their clinical practices allowed them to reflect on the role of institutions in working on the people-centered model. This model has been called for a long time in care models, so the paradigm of transformation defends a more humanized practice, identifying what is meaningful for the person. Students identify structural factors that make it difficult to work along these lines.

Thus, although the current demand for geriatric nurses is well documented, mechanized care, clinical safety concerns, and the professional burnout highlighted make students consider this speciality among their last professional preferences. This attitude, which is also evidenced in the literature [30,31], indicates that a change in the management model is vital to improving the quality of care. Other studies [32,33] have shown that this attitude is also related to the emotions associated with ageing. This is reflected in the students 'conversations where the end of life and close relationships with the residents can provoke sadness.

This encounter with ageing makes them reflect on issues such as frailty, polymedication, and the overall complexity of caring for the older people. These results are consistent with studies [21,34] showing that although geriatrics is a speciality that recognizes social dimensions and claims to promote a holistic approach, the training of professionals is focused on pharmaceutical interventions, and more centred on cure than on care, despite professionals themselves recognizing that the best treatments are not pharmacological.

This leads students to consider elder abuse, which Leibing [21] defines as structural violence. Previous authors [26,35–39] provide reasons why the older people are more vulnerable to abuse.

Students reflect on the vulnerability of the older people; they say they have difficulty addressing issues such as the end of life. Studies by Reverté et al. or Osorio et al. conclude that these situations create anxiety [40,41]. Consequently, the results of this study underline the need to promote attitudes aimed at alleviating this anxiety about ageing and to educate students in good emotional management to cope with the end of life. Some authors [42–44] have pointed out that support integrated into clinical practice along with critical reflection improve students' knowledge, understanding, and attitudes towards older people [45–48].

The clinical practices are the moment when the student arrives at a professional situation and faces an intense life experience, related to the illness, pain, suffering, and death of patients. These experiences impact their personality. The implementation of an easily accessible virtual space without time restrictions, in small groups, where lived situations can be shared and exposed, accompanies them in their learning and helps them to develop the reflective thinking and reduce the anxiety described in some studies [4,49].

The need to be critical and reflective is considered one of the challenges and solutions for teaching–learning processes in clinical practice environments. Active methodologies, such as forums, are a resource for exchanging knowledge among participants; they are educational strategies that allow the development of critical thinking in the practicums, where the tutor and the students need virtual spaces to dialogue and seek ethical, competent, and reflective actions [18].

Finally, forums offer a method for accompanying clinical practice with a space for sharing experiences. It is a space to contribute, with a deep reflection, about the experiences, as the described categories show. As we have seen, this type of tool allows students to deal with complex issues that arise from the training, to improve their experience, and thus to promote and maintain an interest in geriatric nursing.

5. Study Limitations

The study was aimed at senior nursing students. The study sample was intentionally collected, and although participation was voluntary and the study was reported, this could have limited the results. Also, the fact that the female sex predominates is a factor that could have influenced the characteristics of the participations.

6. Conclusions

This study demonstrates that changes in institutional practice towards a more person-centred model of care would both improve the quality of nursing homes as well as the expectations of students towards geriatric nursing as a professional option. Changing perspectives would raise awareness and help address the shortcomings in care that students have brought to light. This requires nursing practice to engage in a process of reflection to integrate people's beliefs and values, apply knowledge and clinical judgement, organize resources, and evaluate the quality of its interventions.

This study has made it possible to explore trainees' feelings and perceptions on caring for older people, so that teachers can understand their attitudes and concerns and address any misconceptions. This approach has allowed students to reflect on and understand the experience of professional clinical practice. Their experiences have brought up different feelings regarding their inability to look after a patient's best interests. Understanding how and why such emotions arise can help to improve nursing practice, particularly in geriatric nursing, and to ultimately improve care for older people, their families and their communities.

Author Contributions: Conceptualization, S.R.-V. and E.G.-M.; methodology, S.R.-V. and E.G.-M.; software, S.R.-V.; validation, S.R.-V., E.G.-M., J.B.-P. and N.A.-R.; formal analysis, S.R.-V. and E.G.-M.; investigation, S.R.-V. and E.G.-M.; resources, S.R.-V. and E.G.-M.; data curation, S.R.-V. and E.G.-M.; writing—original draft preparation, E.G.-M.; writing—review and editing, S.R.-V.; supervision, J.B.-P. and N.A.-R.; project administration S.R.-V. and E.G.-M. All authors have read and agreed to the published version of the manuscript.

Funding: This research received no external funding.

Institutional Review Board Statement: The study was conducted in accordance with the Declaration of Helsinki and approved by the Virgili Institute for Health Research's Drug Research Ethics Committee, with the code 121/2020.

Informed Consent Statement: Written informed consent was obtained from all subjects involved in this study to publish this paper.

Data Availability Statement: The data presented in this study are available on request from the corresponding author.

Public Involvement Statement: Final year nursing degree students participated in this study.

Guidelines and Standards Statement: This manuscript was drafted against the Strengthening the Reporting of Observational Studies in Epidemiology (STROBE) and the guidelines were followed in this observational study.

Acknowledgments: We thank the students of the Universitat Rovira Virgili who participated in the study.

Conflicts of Interest: The authors declare no conflicts of interest.

References

1. Brykcynska, G. *Caring: The Compassion and Wisdom of Nuring*, 1st ed.; Jolley, M., Ed.; Routledge: London, UK, 1996.
2. Martínez-Momblán, M.A.; Colina-Torralva, J.; De la Cueva-Ariza, L.; Guix-Comellas, E.M.; Romero-García, M.; Delgado-Hito, P. Analysis of the evolution of competences in the clinical practice of the nursing degree. *Rev. Lat.-Am. Enferm.* **2020**, *28*, e3231. [CrossRef]
3. Sangrá, A.; Guitert, M.; Behar, P.A. Monográfico. Competencias y metodologías innovadoras para la educación digital. *Rev. Ibereoamericana Educ. A Distancia* **2023**, *26*, 9–16. [CrossRef]
4. Suarez-Garcia, J.M.; Maestro-Gonzalez, A.; Zuazua-Rico, D.; Sánchez-Zaballos, M.; Mosteiro-Diaz, M.P. Stressors for Spanish nursing students in clinical practice. *Nurse Educ. Today* **2018**, *64*, 16–20. [CrossRef] [PubMed]
5. Iorga, M.; Dondas, C.; Zugun-Eloae, C. Depressed as Freshmen, Stressed as Seniors: The Relationship between. Depression, Perceived Stress and Academic Results among Medical Students. *Behav. Sci.* **2018**, *8*, 70. [CrossRef] [PubMed]
6. Salifu, D.A.; Gross, J.; Salifu, M.A.; Ninnoni, J.P. Experiences and perceptions of the theory-practice gap in nursing in a resource-constrained setting: A qualitative description study. *Nurs. Open* **2019**, *6*, 72–83. [CrossRef] [PubMed]
7. Buitrago Malaver, L.A.; Arias López, B.E. Los aportes del enfoque biográfico narrativo para la generación de conocimiento en Enfermería. *Index Enferm.* **2018**, *27*, 62–66. Available online: http://scielo.isciii.es/scielo.php?script=sci_arttext&pid=S1132-1296 2018000100013&lng=es (accessed on 7 October 2022).
8. Raile Alligood, M.; Marriner Tomey, A. *Modelos y Teorías de Enfermería*, 7th ed.; Elsevier: Barcelona, Spain, 2011.
9. Acebedo-Urdiales, S.; Rodero-Sánchez, V.; Vives-Relats, C.; Aguarón-García, M.J. La mirada de Watson, Parse y Benner para el análisis complejo y la buena práctica. *Index Enferm.* **2007**, *16*, 40–44. Available online: https://scielo.isciii.es/scielo.php?script=sci_arttext&pid=S1132-12962007000100009 (accessed on 7 October 2022). [CrossRef]
10. Baumbusch, J.; Dahlke, S.; Phinney, A. Nursing students' knowledge and beliefs about care of older adults in a shifting context of nursing education. *J. Adv. Nurs.* **2012**, *68*, 2550–2558. [CrossRef] [PubMed]
11. Fulmer, T. A retrospective/prospective on the future of geriatric nursing. *Geriatr. Nurs.* **2020**, *41*, 29–31. [CrossRef]
12. Che, C.C.; Chong, M.C.; Hairi, N.N. What influences student nurses' intention to work with older people? A cross-sectional study. *Int. J. Nurs. Stud.* **2018**, *85*, 61–67. [CrossRef]
13. Schön, D.A. *La Formación de Profesionales Reflexivos. Hacia un Nuevo Diseño de la ENSEÑANZA y el aprendizaje en las Profesiones*, 2nd ed.; Ediciones Paidós Ibérica: Barcelona, Spain, 1992.
14. Cerecero, I. 10 Modelos Relacionados Con La Práctica Reflexiva. *Rev. Panam. Pedagog.* **2019**, *28*, 155–181. [CrossRef]
15. Goodchild, T. Does technology really enhance nurse education? *Nurse Educ. Today* **2018**, *66*, 69–72. [CrossRef] [PubMed]
16. Silva, J.; Maturana Castillo, D. Una propuesta de modelo para introducir metodologías activas en educación superior. *Innovación Educ.* **2017**, *17*, 117–131. Available online: http://www.scielo.org.mx/scielo.php?script=sci_arttext&pid=S1665-26732017000100 117&lng=es&tlng=es (accessed on 10 January 2024).
17. Bardin, L. *Análisis de Contenido*, 2nd ed.; Akal: Madrid, Spain, 1996.

18. Gil-Mateu, E.; Reverté-Villarroya, S.; Albacar-Riobóo, N.; Barceló-Prats, J. A Hybrid Methodology for the Evaluation of Clinical Practice in Final-Year Nursing Students. *Nurs. Rep.* **2023**, *13*, 1004–1015. Available online: https://www.mdpi.com/2039-4403/13/3/88 (accessed on 10 January 2024). [CrossRef] [PubMed]
19. Tong, A.; Sainsbury, P.; Craig, J. Consolidated criteria for reporting qualitative research (COREQ): A 32-item checklist for interviews and focus groups. *Int. J. Qual. Health Care* **2007**, *19*, 349–357. [CrossRef]
20. World Medical Asociation (AMM). *Declaración de Helsinki de la AMM—Principios EÉticos para las Investigaciones Médicas en Seres Humanos*; World Medical Association, Inc.: Fortaleza, Brasil, 2013; pp. 1–8. Available online: https://www.wma.net/es/policies-post/declaracion-de-helsinki-de-la-amm-principios-eticos-para-las-investigaciones-medicas-en-seres-humanos/ (accessed on 25 November 2023).
21. Leibing, A. Geriatrics and humanism: Dementia and fallacies of care. *J. Aging Stud.* **2019**, *51*, 100796. [CrossRef]
22. Rodríguez Sánchez, M.I.; Rodríguez Cabello, M.P.; Martínez Martín, M.L. Care model without physical restraints in nursing homes. Narrative review. *Gerokomos* **2021**, *32*, 238–244. Available online: http://scielo.isciii.es/scielo.php?script=sci_arttext&pid=S1134-928X2021000500238&lng=es (accessed on 3 March 2023).
23. Zabalegui, A. Cuidado centrado en el paciente, una función intrínseca a la Enfermería. *Nursing* **2017**, *34*, 6. Available online: https://www.elsevier.es/es-revista-nursing-20-articulo-cuidado-centrado-el-paciente-una-S0212538217301310 (accessed on 20 September 2022). [CrossRef]
24. Instituto Internacionals de Estudios Sobre la Familia. El Papel de la Familia en el Envejecimiento Activo. *Volume 2. Madrid.* 2015. Available online: https://fiapam.org/wp-content/uploads/2013/06/Informe20132.pdf (accessed on 12 December 2023).
25. Brullet, C. Cambios familiares y nuevas políticas sociales en España y Cataluña. El cuidado de la vida cotidiana a lo largo del ciclo de vida. *Educar* **2010**, *45*, 51–79. Available online: https://raco.cat/index.php/Educar/article/view/214608 (accessed on 15 December 2023). [CrossRef]
26. López, J.; Pérez-Rojo, G.; Noriega, C.; Velasco, C. Personal and work-related factors associated with good care for institutionalized older adults. *Int. J. Environ. Res. Public Health* **2021**, *18*, 820. [CrossRef]
27. Dwyer, D. Experiences of registered nurses as managers and leaders in residential aged care facilities: A systematic review. *Int. J. Evid. Based Heal.* **2011**, *9*, 388–402. [CrossRef] [PubMed]
28. Urrutia Beascoa, A.M. Modelo de Cuidado Centrado en la Persona con Reducción del uso de Sujeciones FÍSICAS y Químicas: Conceptualización e Implantación. Ph.D. Thesis, Universidad Complutense de Madrid, Madrid, Spain, 2017. Available online: https://hdl.handle.net/20.500.14352/22638 (accessed on 10 January 2024).
29. Comité Interdisciplinar de Sujeciones. Documento de Consenso Sobre Sujeciones Mecánicas y Farmacológicas. *Madrid; 2014.* Available online: https://www.segg.es/media/descargas/Documento_de_Consenso_sobre_Sujeciones.pdf (accessed on 5 January 2024).
30. Molina Pérez, C. ¿Es suficiente un cambio de modelo de cuidados en el ámbito hospitalario? *Cuad. Gerontológicos* **2019**, *25*, 12–18. Available online: https://sngg.es/uploads/files/revista_25.pdf (accessed on 3 January 2024).
31. Garbrah, W.; Välimäki, T.; Kankkunen, P. Facilitating students' interest in older people nursing: Gerontological nurse teachers under scrutiny. *Nurse Educ. Pract.* **2021**, *50*, 102929. [CrossRef]
32. Dai, F.; Liu, Y.; Ju, M.; Yang, Y. Nursing students' willingness to work in geriatric care: An integrative review. *Nurs. Open* **2021**, *8*, 2061–2077. [CrossRef] [PubMed]
33. Chai, X.; Cheng, C.; Mei, J.; Fan, X. Student nurses' career motivation toward gerontological nursing: A longitudinal study. *Nurse Educ. Today* **2019**, *76*, 165–171. [CrossRef] [PubMed]
34. Webster, F.; Bremner, S.; Oosenbrug, E.; Durant, S.; McCartney, C.J.; Katz, J. From Opiophobia to Overprescribing: A Critical Scoping Review of Medical Education Training for Chronic Pain. *Pain Med.* **2017**, *18*, 1467–1475. [CrossRef] [PubMed]
35. Ropero Padilla, C. El Maltrato Hacia los Ancianos. Propuesta y Diseño de un Protocolo Para la Humanización de los Cuidados. Ph.D. Thesis, Universidad de Almería, Almería, Spain, 2018. [CrossRef]
36. Yon, Y.; Ramiro-Gonzalez, M.; Mikton, C.R.; Huber, M.; Sethi, D. The prevalence of elder abuse in institutional settings: A systematic review and meta-analysis. *Eur. J. Public Health* **2019**, *29*, 58–67. [CrossRef] [PubMed]
37. Kusmaul, N.; Bern-Klug, M.; Bonifas, R. Ethical Issues in Long-term Care: A Human Rights Perspective. *J. Hum. Rights Soc. Work* **2017**, *2*, 86–97. [CrossRef]
38. Rubio Acuña, M. Maltrato institucional a adultos mayores. *Gerokomos* **2012**, *23*, 169–171. [CrossRef]
39. Ruelas-González, M.G.; Pelcastre-Villafuerte, B.E.; Reyes-Morales, H. Maltrato institucional hacia el adulto mayor: Percepciones del prestador de servicios de salud y de los ancianos. *Salud Publica Mex.* **2014**, *56*, 631–637. Available online: http://www.scielo.org.mx/scielo.php?script=sci_arttext&pid=S0036-36342014000600013&lng=es (accessed on 3 January 2024). [CrossRef]
40. Reverté-Villarroya, S.; Ortega, L.; Raigal-Aran, L.; Sauras-Colón, E.; Ricomà-Muntané, R.; Ballester-Ferrando, D.; Rascón-Hernán, C.; Botigué, T.; Lavedán, A.; González-Osorio, L.; et al. Psychological Well-Being in Nursing Students: A Multicentric, Cross-Sectional Study. *Public Health* **2021**, *18*, 3020. [CrossRef] [PubMed]
41. Osorio-Spuler, X.; Illesca-Pretty, M.; Gonzalez-Osorio, L.; Masot, O.; Fuentes-Pumarola, C.; Reverté-Villarroya, S.; Ortega, L.; Rascón-Hernán, C. Emotional exhaustion in nursing students. A multicenter study. *Rev. Esc. Enfermagem.* **2023**, *57*. [CrossRef] [PubMed]
42. Lea, E.; Marlow, A.; Bramble, M.; Andrews, S.; Eccleston, C.; Mcinerney, F.; Robinson, A. Improving student nurses' aged care understandings through a supported placement. *Int. Nurs. Rev.* **2015**, *62*, 28–35. [CrossRef] [PubMed]

43. Garbrah, W.; Kankkunen, P.; Välimäki, T. Gerontological nurse teachers' abilities and influence on students' willingness in older people nursing: A cross-sectional, correlational survey. *Nurse Educ. Today* **2020**, *90*, 104461. [CrossRef]
44. Bono-Neri, F. Pedagogical Nursing Practice: Redefining nursing practice for the academic nurse educator. *Nurse Educ. Pract.* **2019**, *37*, 105–108. [CrossRef] [PubMed]
45. Buil, I.; Hernández, B.; Sesé, F.J.; Urquizu, P. Los foros de discusión y sus beneficios en la docencia virtual: Recomendaciones para un uso eficiente. *INNOVAR Rev. Cienc. Adm. Y Soc.* **2012**, *22*, 131–143. Available online: https://revistas.unal.edu.co/index.php/innovar/article/view/35518 (accessed on 2 January 2024).
46. Chan, Z.C.Y. A systematic review of critical thinking in nursing education. *Nurse Educ. Today* **2013**, *33*, 236–240. [CrossRef]
47. Ceallaigh, T.J.Ó. Navigating the role of teacher educator in the asynchronous learning environment: Emerging questions and innovative responses. *Ir. Educ. Stud.* **2021**, *40*, 349–358. [CrossRef]
48. Osborne, D.M.; Byrne, J.H.; Massey, D.L.; Johnston, A.N.B. Use of online asynchronous discussion boards to engage students, enhance critical thinking, and foster staff-student/student-student collaboration: A mixed method study. *Nurse Educ. Today* **2018**, *70*, 40–46. [CrossRef]
49. Reverté-Villarroya, S.; Gil-Mateu, E.; Sauras-Colón, E.; Barceló-Prats, J.; Albacar-Riobóo, N.; Ortega, L. Stressor Factors for Spanish Nursing Students in a Pandemic Context: An Observational Pilot Survey. *Nurs. Rep.* **2022**, *12*, 708–716. [CrossRef]

nursing reports

MDPI

Review

Exploring the Opportunities and Challenges of Healthcare Innovation in UK Higher Education: A Narrative Review

Renske Emicke [1], Ashley Shepherd [2] and Dylan Powell [2,*]

[1] Nursing, Social Work and Therapy, University of Applied Sciences Appollon, 28359 Bremen, Germany
[2] Faculty of Health Sciences and Sport, University of Stirling, Stirling FK9 4LA, UK; ashley.shepherd@stir.ac.uk
* Correspondence: dylan.powell@stir.ac.uk

Abstract: Background: The healthcare sector is under increasing pressure due to an ageing population, rising multimorbidity, and a projected global workforce shortage of 10 million by 2030. It is becoming increasingly apparent that addressing these challenges requires more than simply increasing workforce numbers—it necessitates a shift towards innovative practices in healthcare education. Higher education (HE) plays a crucial role in preparing future healthcare professionals, yet embedding innovation within HE presents challenges such as resistance to change, resource limitations, and difficulties in interdisciplinary collaboration. This review explores the barriers and opportunities associated with fostering innovation in HE health programmes. **Methods**: This narrative review explored the recent literature on innovation in healthcare HE, examining national policies, institutional strategies, and emerging technological advancements. It describes the impact of digital learning tools, simulation-based education, artificial intelligence (AI), and interprofessional education (IPE) on student learning outcomes and workforce preparedness. **Results**: Findings suggest that while digitalisation and AI-driven innovations offer opportunities to enhance HE health programmes, their effectiveness is dependent on appropriate pedagogical integration and resource. Challenges include upskilling workforce to new more modern methods, ensuring equitable access to digital resources, and maintaining a balance between technological innovation and traditional face-to-face learning. **Conclusions**: To embed innovation effectively within healthcare HE, institutions may need to prioritise interdisciplinary collaboration, entrepreneurial thinking, and sustainable funding models. While technology is key to modernising education, it should be implemented alongside evidence-based pedagogical strategies to ensure meaningful learning outcomes and long-term workforce preparedness.

Keywords: healthcare; innovation; technology transfer; nursing education; higher education; health information technology

1. Introduction

The healthcare sector faces mounting pressures. Driven by an increasingly ageing and multimorbid population, the complexity of care continues to grow. With a projected global health workforce shortage of 10 million workers by 2030 [1,2], there is an urgent need to explore and implement innovative solutions that can address these challenges effectively. However, to meet these demands in parallel, the transformation of healthcare requires more than an increase in workforce numbers [1]. It necessitates a paradigm shift toward adopting innovative practices tailored to evolving healthcare needs. However, embedding such practices within both clinical and educational settings carries several challenges, including resistance to change and the difficulty of fostering environments conducive to innovation [3]. This underscores the importance of understanding strategies that can facilitate the adoption and integration of innovation effectively. Higher education (HE) plays an important role in the training, education, and research of many health professions. As such, promoting innovation in HE health programmes is pivotal to preparing future healthcare professionals to address these challenges. Establishing a shared understanding of innovation and recognising the barriers that organisations and individuals face when confronted with change are essential steps in this process [3,4]. Innovation is inherently complex, resource-intensive, and often met with hesitance from stakeholders [3,4]. Furthermore, it is a multifaceted phenomenon that varies in scale and scope [5].

This narrative review describes the recent literature to explore the challenges and opportunities associated with implementing innovation within higher education. It aims to provide insights into how innovation can be fostered effectively, addressing resistance, and leveraging educational environments to support change.

2. Methods

To address this complex topic, a narrative review of the recent literature was conducted to explore the challenges and opportunities associated with implementing innovation in HE. The search process was conducted in October 2023 using PUBMED. A search was performed using a Boolean search strategy, combining the keywords "Barriers" AND "Innovation" AND "Higher Education", along with relevant synonyms. Given the complexity of the topic, the inclusion criteria were peer-reviewed publications from 2020 onward, available in German, Dutch, or English, with full-text accessibility, and relevant to the fields of healthcare and education. To identify additional relevant studies, a hand search was conducted to locate materials not retrieved through the systematic search.

Duplicate studies were then removed, and the titles and abstracts of the identified studies were reviewed. Articles that did not align with the topic of interest were excluded. No software was used to sort the available articles. To resolve any uncertainty, the inclusion or exclusion of articles was confirmed through discussions among different authors.

A total of 13 articles were identified. Among these, three did not meet the inclusion criteria, and one lacked full-text availability, resulting in nine articles being included. Five additional studies were identified through the supplementary hand search and assessed as meeting the inclusion criteria, resulting in a total of fourteen included studies. Content analysis was performed using Excel, where descriptive codes were assigned. In the next step, these codes were categorised into themes, guiding the narrative of this article.

3. Background to Innovation in Higher Education

3.1. Definition of Innovation

Innovation in healthcare lacks a universally agreed-upon definition. Kelly and Young [6] attempt to define it as the combination of "invention + adoption + diffusion" (p. 121), emphasising both the creation and dissemination of new ideas. Similarly, the World Health Organization [7] describes health innovation as something either new or improved. At its core, innovation involves change, leading to ongoing debates about whether change itself is the fundamental element of innovation [8]. Given these discussions, it is essential to explore the challenges faced by both organisations and individuals when encountering change, as there is often resistance to adopting new practices.

In the context of healthcare and rapidly advancing technology, innovation must encompass the application of novel concepts to address the evolving demands of the field [9]. However, innovation is not solely dependent on large-scale advancements. Flessa and Huebner argue that innovation is a process that can vary in scale, ranging from small improvements to transformative changes [5]. Grounding the concept in healthcare, Kaya et al. [4] define innovation as "activities motivated by the desire to improve healthy person/patient care outcomes and the need to reduce costs" (p. 1674).

The COVID-19 pandemic has further highlighted the role of innovation in healthcare, with emerging research assessing its impact and effectiveness. In this context, innovation has been defined as the introduction of new methods, approaches, or processes aimed at improving public health, as well as the implementation of novel ideas that lead to meaningful change [10].

Although the literature provides varying perspectives, an initial analysis suggests that innovation in healthcare is commonly understood as "change" or "something new" in relation to methods, processes, and approaches. However, Pusic and Ellaway make an important distinction, arguing that innovation should be seen as doing something new, while change refers to doing something differently [11]. As efforts to foster innovation in healthcare HE continue, it is crucial to establish a shared understanding of what innovation entails [4,12]. This shared definition could serve as a foundation for adapting HE curricula to ensure that future healthcare professionals are equipped to meet the evolving needs of the field. However, Leary et al. caution against the dilution of the term "innovation" within health education programmes [13], further illustrating the need for further research, analysis, and harmonisation in approaches.

3.2. Current State in the United Kingdom

According to the 2023 Academic Ranking of World Universities, the United Kingdom (UK) is home to two universities ranked in the global top ten, underscoring its status as a leading destination for HE. In Scotland, the government has committed to supporting innovation, learning, and entrepreneurship in universities [14]. The Scottish National Innovation Strategy articulates Scotland's ambition to become "one of the most innovative small nations in the world" (p. 2). This aligns with the national strategy for the health and social care workforce, which aims to adapt the healthcare system to evolving needs [14]. These national strategies reflect a broader trend towards prioritising innovation within HE, which is critical for addressing the healthcare workforce challenges outlined in the introduction.

While there is no universally agreed-upon definition of innovation in higher education, it remains a central theme globally, with various concepts being actively explored. This makes consensus and comparisons difficult. Researchers argue that teaching practices must be grounded in innovative methodologies, fostering the development of competencies and problem-solving skills through cooperative work, critical thinking, and technological support [15]. Research has long advocated for the integration of social innovation activities in HE; however, they acknowledge the lack of understanding and political support for this aspect [16]. These perspectives align with the need for institutions to not only adapt to but also drive innovation in response to the evolving demands on healthcare systems, as highlighted in the introduction of this paper.

Institutional changes and new models are also being introduced as researchers explore opportunities for innovation in HE. It has been established that top management's emphasis on knowledge value and the implementation of knowledge-based rewards positively impact the speed and quality of innovation within HE institutions [17]. Additionally, the rise in digitalisation and online learning represents a shift in education. Distance learning has been established for some time, and the use of hybrid learning and e-learning has increased [18]. These developments benefit students by providing flexibility and allowing them to manage responsibilities while studying. Institutions benefit by expanding course offerings and improving student access to required courses. García-Morales et al., 2021 assert that online learning is here to stay, with the COVID-19 pandemic contributing to its permanence [19]. These developments resonate with the broader context discussed in the introduction, where the need for innovative approaches in healthcare education is increasingly urgent.

4. Challenges of Innovation in Higher Education

4.1. Legacy Impacts of COVID-19

The COVID-19 pandemic had a profound influence on education worldwide. According to research conducted during this time, there was a rapid transformation in teaching methods and platforms to facilitate e-learning, as face-to-face learning was not feasible during certain phases of the pandemic [20]. Although remote learning possibilities were already established, Anderson et al. note that the pandemic led to a further decrease in classroom attendance, further highlighting the shift to online learning [21]. While this transition was crucial in the face of the pandemic, the shift towards online learning was likely inevitable even without COVID-19. Research has emphasised the need for adequate learning opportunities in preparation for potential future pandemics [22]. Despite the swift adaptation required, the education sector encountered many challenges in integrating online learning, revealing that it was not fully equipped to handle this sudden shift.

These observations are particularly relevant to the challenges discussed in the introduction, where the integration of innovative practices within HE is recognised as essential for preparing healthcare professionals for a rapidly changing environment. The pandemic has underscored the importance of equipping students with the necessary skills to adapt to a future immersed in digital healthcare [22]. Amankwaa et al., 2022 reinforce this sentiment, stating that organisations' innovation initiatives heavily depend on employee human capital and behaviour at work and therefore may present as an opportunity for healthcare [23]. As digitalisation continues to evolve, it is evident that e-learning must play a crucial role in health science HE. Education must be adapted to new methods of learning that align with the ongoing developments in healthcare.

4.2. Ensuring Relevant and Evidence-Based Pedagogy

One of the key challenges in incorporating new innovations into education is supporting teaching staff in developing and adapting their teaching methods. Amankwaa et al. describe how staff faced considerable pedagogical challenges due to the rapid adjustments necessitated by the COVID-19 pandemic [3]. Many educators had limited experience with e-learning prior to the pandemic [20,23], and face-to-face learning from experienced professionals remains a preferred method in some cases, suggesting that it will continue to be an important component of HE.

This discussion resonates with the introduction's emphasis on the challenges of implementing innovative practices in educational settings. The concept of learning by doing, rooted in the work of early educational progressives like John Dewey, posits that students learn most effectively through hands-on, real-world experiences [24]. Despite the abundance of online educational resources, the absence of bedside teaching in health-related programmes has negatively impacted students' direct interaction with patients, compromising the development of physical examination and non-technical skills [25]. Papapanou et al. also highlight this issue, arguing that the limitation of interpersonal contact in e-learning hinders the development of essential communication and empathy skills needed for patient interaction [22]. Another challenge in e-learning is the potential for ethical issues, such as unequal access to reliable internet, which can exacerbate educational disparities [20]. Despite these challenges, the importance of preparing students in health science HE for a digital work environment remains paramount, aligning with the broader aim of fostering innovation in HE health programmes.

The integration of simulation-based learning has already been implemented in education programmes. Notably, the International Nursing Association of Clinical Simulation and Learning (INACSL) published a glossary for best practice, including digital opportunities, as early as 2016. Recent advancements in artificial intelligence (AI) may have further expanded the potential for enhancing simulation-based learning in HE [26].

4.3. Collaboration and Interdisciplinary Research

Collaboration and interdisciplinary approaches are essential in modern healthcare education and practice, yet individual disciplines often operate in silos, hindering the integration of diverse perspectives and expertise. The process of interdisciplinary collaboration ensures comprehensive treatment by integrating various resources and addressing systemic barriers, while also advocating for policy changes that benefit public health, particularly for vulnerable populations [27]. Barriers to transdisciplinary collaboration include limited time, geographical distance, and established disciplinary ways of working, which hinder an interdisciplinary approach [28]. This is supported by Ju et al. who describes differences in expertise which, along with varying levels of commitment, are considered the biggest obstacles to successful collaboration [29,30]. Similarly, Leon and Lipuma highlighted barriers to interdisciplinary research, such as varying disciplinary terminology, methodological discrepancies, and a culture of siloed disciplines. In response to these challenges, the researchers proposed strategies like fostering environments that encourage interdisciplinary dialogue, developing a common language for interdisciplinary communication, and providing transdisciplinary training, concluding that effective communication can enhance collaboration and research results. This ensures that all stakeholders can contribute effectively to advancing healthcare outcomes while bridging the gap between varied academic and professional practices.

5. The Opportunity for Innovation

While the concepts of innovation and health professions are not new, the intersection of these two domains has witnessed a dramatic acceleration in the past two decades [31–33]. This growth is a direct response to increasingly complex global health challenges, including workforce shortages, multimorbidity, and demands for more agile care delivery models. To fully harness the potential of innovation, however, the skillsets and training of health professionals must also evolve.

A seminal report, the 2019 Topol Review, highlighted the skills and technologies that clinicians will require in the digital age and how technological advances can improve the flexibility and responsiveness of training [34]. For example, immersive technologies like virtual reality (VR) can improve learning retention and clinicians' ability to conduct complex procedures. While there is no substitute for real-world clinical training involving patient interactions, innovations like VR or augmented reality may provide a reliable, convenient, and auditable solution for training undergraduates, upskilling newly qualified clinicians, and enabling more experienced staff to maintain or improve their clinical skillsets [31].

In this dynamic and ever-changing healthcare landscape, allied health education must evolve. The integration of innovation, specifically in technology, digital health, and simulation, offers a promising avenue to enhance learning experiences and skill development for health professionals.

5.1. Moving from Traditional to Digital Approaches in HE

There is a growing body of evidence supporting the integration of digital innovations within health sciences higher education, one recent example being the use of virtual and high-fidelity simulation [23]. Ethical concerns regarding patient safety have become increasingly central in teaching and medical training, prompting the widespread adoption of virtual simulation as a standard component of training [35]. A systematic review with meta-analyses demonstrated that virtual simulation can enhance clinical reasoning in nursing students, although several factors need to be considered. For instance, 2D simulations appear to have greater impact compared to 3D, and longer sessions (lasting over 30 min) are associated with more substantial positive effects on clinical reasoning [36].

While practical training remains essential, institutions are developing strategies to mitigate the limitations of reduced face-to-face teaching. For instance, Imperial College London has created a digital library of patient encounters to mitigate the impact of reduced hands-on training resulting from e-learning [37]. Other digital formats are being explored to enrich educational delivery. Dedeilia et al. highlight the value of podcasts as tools for self-paced, in-depth learning [38]. Another innovative tool is Learning Analytics. As defined by the Society for Learning Analytics Research, this approach involves collecting, measuring, analysing, and reporting data on learners and their contexts. It aims to enhance the learning process and personalise the learning experience—tracing student profiles, abilities, and learning patterns to inform adaptive teaching strategies. This new and innovative approach, facilitated by digitalisation, presents important opportunities. Furthermore, research has shown that the introduction of student information systems and virtual learning environments such as Blackboard® and Moodle® has marked a shift in medical education. The e-learning era seems to open up great possibilities for collaboration between faculties and universities. Webinars can be utilised for interdisciplinary learning [39,40]. Lecture videos, online reading materials, etc., can be integrated into a "Massive Open Online Course", which can be utilised either online or during classroom teaching [41–43]. These platforms not only support the delivery of educational content but also provide a foundation for broader pedagogical innovation and the integration of digital tools in healthcare higher education [44–46].

5.2. The Role of Organisation and Collaboration

As stated above many challenges exist for educators in the adoption digital transformation. This is also an organisational challenge that should be taken seriously. Gonsalo et al. state that to implement innovation in health systems, supportive structures are needed to manage its complexity [36]. Therefore, it should be argued that support from the institution and its stakeholders is crucial for innovation to happen. Amankwaa et al. observed that stakeholders can be inclined to make pedagogical adjustments without institutional support, highlighting a disconnect between faculty and administrators [3,23]. However, innovation within the higher education system involves a multitude of stakeholders beyond faculty, administrators, and government. Alumni and corporations can play a valuable role in the development of entrepreneurial, innovative campuses [14,47].

The financial shortfall is another organisational challenge that can hinder the progress of initiatives. Dula et al. advocate that although skills-based and in-person education is important, it requires substantial resource [48]. Underfunding issues are also being increasingly recognised, and it is proposed that education needs to focus on competencies, with interpersonal and trans-professional education requiring unified planning. Universities appear to be open to exploring funding models due to their endowment wealth [14]. Innovative funding opportunities are probably essential to empower innovation within the HE sector.

Furthermore, collaborations outside of the educational institutions should be further explored. Wells et al. report on a "Model of Collaborative Health Education, CPD [continuing professional development], Research and Innovation" [47,49]. This model allows healthcare employers to be involved in the development of education programmes.

It is suggested that employer feedback is crucial in developing programmes and that a co-production model of collaboration between the health and social care sector and universities can have advantages to all parties involved, including professionalisation; skills and academic development; research and innovation; and engagement.

The integration of technology, digital health, and simulation into allied health education has the potential to impact the student learning experience. This impact is reflected in the UKPSF (UK Professional Standards Framework) Dimensions which emphasise the importance of understanding how students learn and how to use evidence-informed approaches to enhance student learning [39].

For example, evidence shows that the use of VR simulations in training improves student engagement and the retention of complex clinical skills [50]. However, it is essential to critically assess the long-term impact of such innovations on clinical competence and patient outcomes as well as respecting the individual learning styles which may not suit everyone. This requires a robust analysis of data related to academic practice, as outlined in the UKPSF. By systematically collecting and analysing data on student performance, satisfaction, and post-graduation outcomes, there is an opportunity to demonstrate the impact of these innovations on the student learning experience and make informed adjustments to the curriculum [39].

Simulation-based education has emerged as a cornerstone of allied health training, providing a safe and controlled environment for skill development and error analysis. High-fidelity simulators have become increasingly sophisticated, replicating real-world clinical scenarios with remarkable accuracy. However, the transferability of skills from simulation to clinical practice remains a subject of ongoing research and development. This also raises the question: is it the technology itself or the human factors that are most critical in enabling learning? Additionally, the cost-effectiveness of simulation compared to traditional training methods requires further exploration [50].

5.3. The Role of Entrepreneurship

The importance of institutional policies that promote innovation among students and staff has been recognised in the UK. While collaboration between large organisations and academia is challenging and requires time and effort from both sides, it also presents substantial opportunities [46]. The Scottish government's strategy for entrepreneurial campuses highlights higher education as a key driver of innovation and economic development. This strategy emphasises the need to inspire young people to engage in entrepreneurial thinking, which necessitates adjustments to the curriculum, as well as leveraging extracurricular resources and external expertise [14].

The goal is that fostering an innovative and entrepreneurial approach within higher education can contribute to economic growth and development. According to Rubens et al. (2017) [38], universities are increasingly shifting from their traditional roles of teaching and research to embrace entrepreneurship, community engagement, and sustainable development [47,51]. These sustainable developments include not only economic growth but also contributions to environmental changes and social cohesion [52,53]. Research suggests that the presence of human capital—skills, knowledge, and expertise within a community—and institutional intellectual capital—collective knowledge, policies, and practices within institutions—correlates with increased economic growth and development [36]. Therefore, innovation in higher education could be a crucial factor in driving economic and societal progress.

5.4. *Artificial Intelligence*

The rapid growth and acceleration of AI present both substantial opportunities and potential barriers to innovation in health science higher education. AI is progressively reshaping how individuals engage, communicate, learn, and work. Chiu et al. describe the influence of AI on student learning, teaching, and assessment; in particular, the emergence of tools like ChatGPT has sparked widespread discussions, marking a substantive shift in public attitudes towards AI [22]. However, the deployment in education also raises concerns, including issues of data privacy, security, bias, and the evolving nature of teacher–student relationships [49]. Addressing these concerns is essential to ensure the responsible and ethical integration of AI in educational settings. It is not enough for students to merely become proficient in using AI; they must also understand that the nature of the work they are preparing for is undergoing changes due to its advancements. Universities have a responsibility to adequately prepare students for this shift, which requires a deep understanding of its implications both in education and within health science professions. By embracing these opportunities, higher education institutions can equip students with the necessary skills and knowledge to thrive in a rapidly evolving digital landscape [54]. AI is poised to revolutionise healthcare professions, enhancing efficiency and quality of care. These developments will shape the future roles of healthcare professionals and require new and adaptive competencies.

6. Challenges and Considerations

Despite the potential benefits of technological innovations in allied health education, several challenges must be addressed. The integration of technology into the curriculum requires substantial investment in infrastructure, faculty training, and ongoing support with linkage to pedagogy [55]. There are also concerns about the accessibility of technology for all students and those from diverse learning communities [56]. Moreover, the rapid pace of technological advancement necessitates continuous curriculum updates to ensure that students are learning relevant and contemporary skills [57]. This presents further technical challenges for staff to ensure that they understand and can adapt to the implications of quality assurance in particular within healthcare professional training and its regulation [23].

Another consideration is the potential impact of technology on the students' expectations of healthcare and communication. While online learning and digital tools can facilitate independent learning, they may also lead to undesirable effects including a sense of isolation and a diminished capacity for empathic engagement—a key component of clinical practice [6,53,54]. It is crucial to maintain a balance between digital and face-to-face interactions to preserve the human element of education, with many aspects of care still face to face. Moving forward, ethical considerations also play a role in the adoption of technology in healthcare education [22]. The use of patient data in digital health tools raises questions about privacy, consent, and data security [31,32]. Finally, it is important to recognise that innovation is not synonymous with clinical improvement and/or patient outcomes; therefore, the core aims of healthcare must also be considered [55–57].

7. Conclusions

This narrative review has explored the multifaceted challenges and opportunities associated with fostering innovation in health science higher education. The increasing complexity of healthcare demands a dynamic and adaptive workforce, making it imperative for educational institutions to embrace interdisciplinary collaboration, innovative teaching methodologies, and new technologies. However, these technical advancements are not without their challenges, as traditional academic silos, varying regulatory environments, and the rapid pace of technological change can create barriers to effective implementation.

The role of entrepreneurship within HE is particularly crucial in driving innovation and economic development. By fostering an entrepreneurial mindset among students and staff, and by leveraging collaboration with external stakeholders, higher education institutions can become key contributors to societal progress. Furthermore, the integration of AI into education presents a transformative opportunity, albeit one that requires careful consideration of ethical implications and the evolving nature of professional roles.

As digital healthcare continues to evolve, it is crucial to equip students with the necessary skills to navigate and adapt to this transformation. The integration of technology in healthcare will not only reshape the roles of healthcare professionals but also demand new competencies in data management, telemedicine, and digital tools. By preparing students today, we ensure they are ready to meet the challenges and opportunities of a future driven by digital innovation, ultimately improving patient care and healthcare efficiency [22].

While new technologies and approaches can offer exciting possibilities, they must be rigorously evaluated to ensure that they are effective and beneficial in their own context. The adoption of innovation should be guided by evidence-based practices and a commitment to continuous improvement. The importance of considering the wider context of contemporary issues in higher education and how they impact teaching and assessment practices should also be emphasised.

Ultimately, for health science HE to respond to the demands of a rapidly changing world, it must continue to innovate and adapt. This will require not only the adoption of new technologies and pedagogies, but also the cultivation of a collaborative, interdisciplinary, and research-informed culture. Through this, higher education can play a pivotal role in preparing the next generation of healthcare professionals to meet future challenges with creativity, resilience, and a commitment to excellence.

Author Contributions: R.E. developed the initial concept and first draft. D.P. and A.S. provided project supervision and writing and reviewing support. All authors have read and agreed to the published version of the manuscript.

Funding: This research received no external funding.

Institutional Review Board Statement: Not applicable.

Informed Consent Statement: Not applicable.

Data Availability Statement: No new data were created.

Public Involvement Statement: No public involvement in any aspect of this research.

Guidelines and Standards Statement: Not applicable.

Use of Artificial Intelligence: AI-assisted tools were used for language editing and grammar in drafting aspects of this manuscript.

Conflicts of Interest: D.P. and R.E. declare no conflicts of interest. A.S. is a Guest Editor in the Special Issue of *Nursing Reports* and played no role in the internal review or decision to publish the article.

References

1. Boniol, M.; Kunjumen, T.; Nair, T.S.; Siyam, A.; Campbell, J.; Diallo, K. The global health workforce stock and distribution in 2020 and 2030: A threat to equity and 'universal' health coverage? *BMJ Glob. Health* **2022**, *7*, e009316. [CrossRef] [PubMed]
2. Health Workforce. Available online: https://www.who.int/health-topics/health-workforce#tab=tab_1 (accessed on 30 December 2024).

3. Amankwaa, I.; Boateng, D.; Quansah, D.Y.; Akuoko, C.P.; Desu, A.P.B.; Hales, C. Innovations in Nursing Education in Response to the COVID-19 Pandemic: A Scoping Review. *Nurs. Prax. Aotearoa N. Z.* **2022**, *38*, 2022. [CrossRef]
4. Kaya, N.; Turan, N.; Aydın, G.Ö. A Concept Analysis of Innovation in Nursing. *Procedia Soc. Behav. Sci.* **2015**, *195*, 1674–1678. [CrossRef]
5. Flessa, S.; Huebner, C. Innovations in Health Care-A Conceptual Framework. *Int. J. Environ. Res. Public Health* **2021**, *18*, 10026. [CrossRef]
6. Kelly, C.J.; Young, A.J. Promoting innovation in healthcare. *Future Healthc. J.* **2017**, *4*, 121–125. [CrossRef]
7. WHO Innovation Hub. Available online: https://www.who.int/teams/digital-health-and-innovation/who-innovation-hub (accessed on 10 April 2025).
8. Mcsherry, R.; Douglas, M. Innovation in nursing practice: A means to tackling the global challenges facing nurses, midwives and nurse leaders and managers in the future. *J. Nurs. Manag.* **2011**, *19*, 165–169. [CrossRef]
9. Weintraub, P.; McKee, M. Leadership for Innovation in Healthcare: An Exploration. *Int. J. Health Policy Manag.* **2018**, *8*, 138–144. [CrossRef]
10. Elden, N.M.K.; Mandil, A.M.A.; Hegazy, A.A.; Nagy, N.; Mabry, R.M.; Khairy, W.A. Health innovations in response to the COVID-19 pandemic: Perspectives from the Eastern Mediterranean Region. *J. Public Health* **2023**, *45*, 470–480. [CrossRef]
11. Pusic, M.V.; Ellaway, R.H. Researching models of innovation and adoption in health professions education. *Med. Educ.* **2024**, *58*, 164–170. [CrossRef]
12. Wu, T.C.; Ho, C.T.B. A Narrative Review of Innovative Responses During the COVID-19 Pandemic in 2020. *Int. J. Public Health* **2022**, *67*, 1604652. [CrossRef]
13. Leary, M.; Villarruel, A.M.; Richmond, T.S. Creating an innovation infrastructure in academic nursing. *J. Prof. Nurs.* **2022**, *38*, 83–88. [CrossRef]
14. Scottish Government. Entrepreneurial Campus: Report. 27 June 2023. Available online: https://www.gov.scot/publications/entrepreneurial-campus-higher-education-sector-driving-force-entrepreneurial-ecosystem/ (accessed on 15 March 2025).
15. Suyo-Vega, J.A.; Fernández-Bedoya, V.H.; Meneses-La-Riva, M.E. Beyond traditional teaching: A systematic review of innovative pedagogical practices in higher education. *F1000Research* **2024**, *13*, 22. [CrossRef]
16. Monteiro, S.; Isusi-Fagoaga, R.; Almeida, L.; García-Aracil, A. Contribution of Higher Education Institutions to Social Innovation: Practices in Two Southern European Universities. *Sustainability* **2021**, *13*, 3594. [CrossRef]
17. Iqbal, A. Innovation speed and quality in higher education institutions: The role of knowledge management enablers and knowledge sharing process. *J. Knowl. Manag.* **2021**, *25*, 2334–2360. [CrossRef]
18. Simonson, M. Research in Distance Education: A Summary. *Q. Rev. Distance Educ.* **2019**, *20*, 31–43.
19. García-Morales, V.J.; Garrido-Moreno, A.; Martín-Rojas, R. The Transformation of Higher Education After the COVID Disruption: Emerging Challenges in an Online Learning Scenario. *Front. Psychol.* **2021**, *12*, 616059. [CrossRef] [PubMed]
20. Etando, A.; Amu, A.A.; Haque, M.; Schellack, N.; Kurdi, A.; Alrasheedy, A.A.; Timoney, A.; Mwita, J.C.; Rwegerera, G.M.; Patrick, O.; et al. Challenges and innovations brought about by the covid-19 pandemic regarding medical and pharmacy education especially in africa and implications for the future. *Healthcare* **2021**, *9*, 1722. [CrossRef] [PubMed]
21. Anderson, M.L.; Turbow, S.; Willgerodt, M.A.; Ruhnke, G.W. Education in a Crisis: The Opportunity of Our Lives. *J. Hosp. Med.* **2020**, *15*, 287–289. [CrossRef]
22. Dedeilia, A.; Papapanou, M.; Papadopoulos, A.N.; Karela, N.R.; Androutsou, A.; Mitsopoulou, D.; Nikolakea, M.; Konstantinidis, C.; Papageorgakopoulou, M.; Sideris, M.; et al. Health worker education during the COVID-19 pandemic: Global disruption, responses and lessons for the future—A systematic review and meta-analysis. *Hum. Resour. Health* **2023**, *21*, 13. [CrossRef]
23. Amankwaa, A.; Susomrith, P.; Seet, P.S. Innovative behavior among service workers and the importance of leadership: Evidence from an emerging economy. *J. Technol. Transf.* **2022**, *47*, 506–530. [CrossRef]
24. Mclaughlin, E. The "Real-World" Experience: Students' Perspectives on Service-Learning Projects. *Am. J. Bus. Educ.* **2010**, *3*, 109–118. [CrossRef]
25. Peddle, M.; Mckenna, L.; Bearman, M.; Nestel, D. Development of non-technical skills through virtual patients for undergraduate nursing students: An exploratory study. *Nurse Educ. Today* **2019**, *73*, 94–101. [CrossRef]
26. INACSL Standards Committee. INACSL Standards of Best Practice: Simulation^{SM} Simulation Glossary. *Clin. Simul. Nurs.* **2016**, *12*, S39–S47. [CrossRef]
27. Dai, C.P.; Ke, F. Educational applications of artificial intelligence in simulation-based learning: A systematic mapping review. *Comput. Educ. Artif. Intell.* **2022**, *3*, 100087. [CrossRef]
28. Pannell, J.L.; Dencer-Brown, A.M.; Greening, S.S.; Hume, E.A.; Jarvis, R.M.; Mathieu, C.; Mugford, J.; Runghen, R. An early career perspective on encouraging collaborative and interdisciplinary research in ecology. *Ecosphere* **2019**, *10*, e02899. [CrossRef]
29. Zumstein, M.; Mscn, S.; Grace, P.J.; Zumstein-Shaha, M. Competency frameworks, nursing perspectives, and interdisciplinary collaborations for good patient care: Delineating boundaries. *Nurs. Philos.* **2023**, *24*, e12402. [CrossRef] [PubMed]

30. Ju, B.; Stewart, J.B.; Jin, T. "A bit hard for us to explain": Barriers to creating new information in scientific collaboration. *Libr. Inf. Sci. Res.* **2022**, *44*, 101173. [CrossRef]
31. Powell, D. How Digital Technology Is Changing Healthcare: A Physiotherapists Perspective—Thoughts from the Centre | Deloitte UK. 2022. Available online: https://blogs.deloitte.co.uk/health/2022/01/how-digital-technology-is-changing-healthcare-a-physiotherapists-perspective.html (accessed on 15 August 2022).
32. Powell, D.; Hannah, A. The dichotomy of diagnostics: Exploring the value for consumers, clinicians and care pathways. *npj Digit. Med.* **2024**, *7*, 101. [CrossRef]
33. Powell, D.; Godfrey, A. Considerations for integrating wearables into the everyday healthcare practice. *npj Digit. Med.* **2023**, *6*, 70. [CrossRef]
34. Topol, E. The Topol Review. Preparing the Healthcare Workforce to Deliver the Digital Future. 2019. Available online: https://topol.hee.nhs.uk/the-topol-review/ (accessed on 7 May 2024).
35. Parsons, T.D. Ethical Challenges of Using Virtual Environments in the Assessment and Treatment of Psychopathological Disorders. *J. Clin. Med.* **2021**, *10*, 378. [CrossRef]
36. Sim, J.J.M.; Bin Rusli, K.D.; Seah, B.; Levett-Jones, T.; Lau, Y.; Liaw, S.Y. Virtual Simulation to Enhance Clinical Reasoning in Nursing: A Systematic Review and Meta-analysis. *Clin. Simul. Nurs.* **2022**, *69*, 26–39. [CrossRef]
37. Elevating Healthcare Education: Imperial Introduces Cutting-Edge XR Course | Imperial News | Imperial College London. Available online: https://www.imperial.ac.uk/news/247113/elevating-healthcare-education-imperial-introduces-cutting-edge/ (accessed on 30 December 2024).
38. Rubens, A.; Spigarelli, F.; Cavicchi, A.; Rinaldi, C. Universities' third mission and the entrepreneurial university and the challenges they bring to higher education institutions. *J. Enterprising Communities People Places Glob. Econ.* **2017**, *11*, 354–372. [CrossRef]
39. Dedeilia, A.; Sotiropoulos, M.G.; Hanrahan, J.G.; Janga, D.; Dedeilias, P.; Sideris, M. Medical and Surgical Education Challenges and Innovations in the COVID-19 Era: A Systematic Review. *In Vivo* **2020**, *34*, 1603. [CrossRef] [PubMed]
40. Gamage, S.H.P.W.; Ayres, J.R.; Behrend, M.B. A systematic review on trends in using Moodle for teaching and learning. *Int. J. STEM Educ.* **2022**, *9*, 9. [CrossRef]
41. Aljawarneh, S.A. Reviewing and exploring innovative ubiquitous learning tools in higher education. *J. Comput. High. Educ.* **2020**, *32*, 57–73. [CrossRef]
42. Jeong, S.; Hwang, H. Do we need Moodle in medical education? A review of its impact and utility. *Kosin Med. J.* **2023**, *38*, 159–168. [CrossRef]
43. Fascia, M.; Brodie, J. Structural barriers to implementing open innovation in healthcare. *Br. J. Health Manag.* **2017**, *23*, 338–343. [CrossRef]
44. Dula, C.A.C.; Porter, A.L. Addressing Challenges in Skills-based Education Through Innovation and Collaboration. *Am. J. Pharm. Educ.* **2021**, *85*, 8788. [CrossRef]
45. Wells, I.; Ware, A.; Dearing, W. Wales Institute of Digital Information (WIDI): A Model of Collaborative Health Education, CPD, Research and Innovation. *Stud. Health Technol. Inform.* **2022**, *298*, 78–81. [CrossRef]
46. Filho, W.L.; Sierra, J.; Price, E.; Eustachio, J.H.P.P.; Novikau, A.; Kirrane, M.; Dinis, M.A.P.; Salvia, A.L. The role of universities in accelerating the sustainable development goals in Europe. *Sci. Rep.* **2024**, *14*, 15464. [CrossRef]
47. Pottle, J. Virtual reality and the transformation of medical education. *Future Healthc. J.* **2019**, *6*, 181–185. [CrossRef]
48. Baniasadi, T.; Ayyoubzadeh, S.M.; Mohammadzadeh, N. Challenges and Practical Considerations in Applying Virtual Reality in Medical Education and Treatment. *Oman Med. J.* **2020**, *35*, e125. [CrossRef] [PubMed]
49. Guimarães, B.; Ferreira, M.A. Is Medical Education Changing? Five Challenges for the Near Future. *Acta Med. Port.* **2020**, *33*, 365–366. [CrossRef] [PubMed]
50. Ojelabi, A.O.; Ling, J.; Roberts, D.; Hawkins, C. Does interprofessional education support integration of care services? A systematic review. *J. Interprofessional Educ. Pract.* **2022**, *28*, 100534. [CrossRef]
51. Pink-Harper, S.A. Educational Attainment. *Econ. Dev. Q.* **2015**, *29*, 167–179. [CrossRef]
52. Chiu, T.K.F. The impact of Generative AI (GenAI) on practices, policies and research direction in education: A case of ChatGPT and Midjourney. *Interact. Learn. Environ.* **2024**, *32*, 6187–6203. [CrossRef]
53. Kamalov, F.; Santandreu Calonge, D.; Gurrib, I. New Era of Artificial Intelligence in Education: Towards a Sustainable Multifaceted Revolution. *Sustainability* **2023**, *15*, 12451. [CrossRef]
54. Wiljer, D.; Hakim, Z. Developing an Artificial Intelligence-Enabled Health Care Practice: Rewiring Health Care Professions for Better Care. *J. Med. Imaging Radiat. Sci.* **2019**, *50*, S8–S14. [CrossRef] [PubMed]
55. Toohey, S.; Wray, A.; Hunter, J.; Waldrop, I.; Saadat, S.; Boysen-Osborn, M.; Sudario, G.; Smart, J.; Wiechmann, W.; Pressman, S.D. Comparing the Psychological Effects of Manikin-Based and Augmented Reality–Based Simulation Training: Within-Subjects Crossover Study. *JMIR Med. Educ.* **2022**, *8*, e36447. [CrossRef]

56. Anine, M.; Kari, R.; Monica, Ø.; Hilde, S.S. Health professional students' self-reported emotions during simulation-based education: An interpretive descriptive study. *Nurse Educ. Pract.* **2022**, *63*, 103353. [CrossRef]
57. Tilwani, R.; Awasthi, A.; Maheshwari, M.; Tilwani, K.; Deep, A. Impact of online teaching on mental health and quality of life among medical teachers during COVID-19 pandemic—A cross-sectional study. *Ann. Indian Psychiatry* **2022**, *6*, 320. [CrossRef]

nursing reports

MDPI

Protocol

Artificial Intelligence in Wound Care Education: Protocol for a Scoping Review

Rúben Encarnação [1,2,*], Tânia Manuel [1,3], Hélder Palheira [1,4,5], João Neves-Amado [1] and Paulo Alves [1]

1 Centre for Interdisciplinary Research in Health, Faculty of Health Sciences and Nursing, Universidade Católica Portuguesa, 4169-005 Porto, Portugal; tscarvalho@ucp.pt (T.M.); helder.palheira@hc-healthcare.com (H.P.); jamado@ucp.pt (J.N.-A.); pjalves@ucp.pt (P.A.)
2 Cardiology ICU, São João University Hospital Center, 4200-319 Porto, Portugal
3 Prove.pt, Grupo Saúde Nuno Mendes, 4560-164 Penafiel, Portugal
4 HC Healthcare & Innovation, 4445-176 Alfena, Portugal
5 Cardiothoracic Center, São João University Hospital Center, 4200-319 Porto, Portugal
* Correspondence: rcencarnacao@ucp.pt

Abstract: As healthcare continues evolving in the age of digital technology, the integration of artificial intelligence has emerged as a powerful force, particularly in wound care. The education of healthcare professionals in wound care is crucial for ensuring they acquire the necessary knowledge and skills, optimizing patient outcomes. This paper outlines the protocol for a scoping review with the goal of mapping and analyzing the current scientific evidence regarding the potential impact of artificial intelligence in wound care education. The current protocol follows the JBI methodological framework. The search was conducted in December 2023 in the following databases: CINAHL Complete (via EBSCOhost), MEDLINE (via PubMed), Cochrane Library, Academic Search Complete, Scientific Electronic Library Online (Scielo), Scopus, and Web of Science. Electronics searches were conducted in the Scientific Open Access Scientific Repositories of Portugal (RCAAP) and ProQuest Dissertations and Theses, OpenAIRE, and Open Dissertations databases to access gray literature. Additionally, searches were performed on Google Scholar and specific journals such as the International Wound Journal, Skin Research and Technology, Journal of Wound Care, and Wound Repair and Regeneration. The initial database searches retrieved a total of 11,323 studies. After removing duplicates, a total of 6450 studies were submitted for screening. Currently, 15 studies are included in this review, and data charting and analysis are underway. The findings of this scoping review will likely provide insights into the application of artificial intelligence in wound care education.

Keywords: artificial intelligence; wound; education; scoping review

1. Introduction

Wound care is an essential field of healthcare that involves the proper management and treatment of wounds to promote complete and timely healing and prevent complications that may lead to amputation, infection, and other potentially life-threatening outcomes. Traditionally, wound care has involved standard protocols, often relying on primary dressings and routine procedures. In recent years, innovative technologies, such as artificial intelligence (AI), have revolutionized wound care, providing more effective and efficient solutions for acute and chronic injuries.

The exact definition of AI remains a point of ongoing discussion. The term, created by John McCarthy in 1955, refers to the creation of computer systems able to perform tasks and solve problems that usually require human intelligence, such as image recognition, decision-making, and natural language processing [1–4]. It can be broadly defined as the incorporation of human intelligence into machines.

With the integration of AI-based technologies in daily life, applying such technologies will be indispensable for every organization. AI stands out as a highly promising technology within the healthcare sector. There is great optimism that these technologies have the potential to provide significant improvements in all healthcare domains [5–10]. Several AI functionalities are applied in the health sector, such as decision-making support, patient monitoring, early diagnosis, workflow improvement, information sharing, security, remote surgery, virtual patients, and virtual assistants [4–9,11].

Furthermore, AI has significantly transformed the training and education of professional healthcare personnel, offering numerous benefits. AI in education includes intelligent tutoring systems, chatbots, robots, and automated assessment tools integrated into digitized materials that improve education [4]. These advancements provide students with personalized, efficient, and immersive learning experiences, enhancing teachers' understanding of students' learning processes and enabling machine-supported queries at any time [4,12–14].

A significant feature of incorporating AI into medical education is its adaptive learning ability to analyze and offer instant feedback and assessment, allowing students to monitor their knowledge gaps, recognize weaknesses, and receive immediate guidance for improvement [4]. AI has the capability to tailor the learning experience based on each student's individual needs, knowledge level, and preferred learning style, ensuring the delivery of relevant and efficient educational materials [12]. Educators can also gain advantages from analytics generated by AI, which offer assistance in recognizing trends and patterns in student performance, adapting teaching approaches as needed, and enhancing the overall learning experience. This can contribute to enhanced working efficiency and teaching competence.

Generative AI is defined as a form or subset of AI that uses machine learning and deep learning techniques to create new data. A crucial element of generative AI is the capability of understanding potential data distributions and producing new data that mirror the original set. This technology diverges from traditional AI tasks like classification or regression, as it is capable of autonomously generating new content, including images and text. Its applications extend to different areas; in image generation, Generative Adversarial Networks (GANs) are often used, while Recurrent Neural Networks (RNNs) and transformer networks are employed in natural language processing to produce novel textual content. This technology is also recognized for its potential to transform medical education [15,16].

The application of AI in education has drawn worldwide interest across numerous areas of healthcare professional education. Physicians and nurses have increasingly incorporated AI technology to enrich students' learning experiences with more realistic, sophisticated, complex, and immersive simulations [17–19]. This enables students and healthcare professionals to refine their clinical skills within a secure and controlled learning environment [12]. The potential of generative AI in medical education can significantly enhance wound care training and practice. It offers innovative methods for personalized learning, cased-based learning and simulation-based training, continuous education, and research assistance [16].

Despite the various benefits and the potential of AI in medical education, some areas still require further investigation. These include clarifying the long-term implications of AI-driven learning methodologies for student performance, instructor–student interactions, and the ethical implications of AI [4,6,7,10,17,20,21].

Despite ongoing improvements in the wound care field, AI provides valuable contributions to early detection, risk factor analysis, risk stratification, prediction, diagnosis, intelligent treatment, outcome prediction, and prognosis evaluation [8,11,22–26]. From innovative dressings embedded with sensors to advanced imaging techniques, this technology is improving the healing process and supplying healthcare professionals with real-time data for decision-making support and predictive risk assessment related to wounds. This technology is transforming wound care from prevention to treatment, and wound care must adjust to this changing world to improve patient care [11,26].

Treating wounds is often a significant challenge for healthcare professionals, as the multitude of treatment criteria, care products, patient conditions, and responses complicate the healing process and results. To maximize patient outcomes in wound care, it is recommended that those involved possess the appropriate knowledge and skills [27,28]. Wound care education contributes significantly to patient well-being and healthcare efficiency.

While specific studies directly addressing the role of AI in wound care education are limited, emerging technologies are making significant progress in this area. For instance, the use of metaverse technology, including virtual reality (VR) simulations, provides immersive learning and training experiences that closely resemble real-life surgical scenarios, while also being more efficient in the use of resources [29,30]. Another advancement is the integration of Augmented Reality (AR) with machine learning (ML) algorithms, which facilitates real-time interventions and diagnostic information [29,30]. These developments in medical education highlight the growing integration of AI technologies, offering students realistic and immersive scenarios, especially in surgical fields, and this approach can be extended to wound care education [29,30]. The potential of combining these technologies with machine learning and AI indicates a promising future for more effective, personalized, and interactive learning experiences in healthcare education.

Using generative AI to create personalized quizzes or images of detailed and varied different wound types would enhance personalized and case-based learning, allowing students to diagnose and plan treatment for a wide range of wound conditions, and learning materials and feedback can be tailored specifically to wound care [31]. This approach would allow educators to address individual students' strengths and weaknesses in wound care techniques, pathology, and patient management, for example.

The challenge lies in ensuring the academic integrity and validity of AI-generated research [31]. The impact on scholarly communication is profound, as it necessitates new methods for peer review and verification to maintain the credibility of the scientific process [31]. This emerging scenario presents both opportunities and challenges for academic communities.

In 1947, Alan Turing, a pioneering figure in computer science, delivered one of the earliest public lectures about computer intelligence, saying "What we want is a machine that can learn from experience" and the "possibility of letting the machine alter its own instructions provides the mechanism for this". Integrating AI literacy into medical education curricula and rethinking assessment methods considering AI's capabilities are essential for the rapid evolution of AI.

A preliminary search in the CINAHL Complete, MEDLINE (PubMed), Cochrane Database of Systematic Reviews, PROSPERO, and Open Science Framework (OSF) databases indicates that, at present, there are no published or ongoing scoping reviews or systematic reviews concerning the use of AI in wound care education. The literature refers to a considerable number of AI applications for wound care. However, the integration of AI into wound care education remains uncertain. Thus, the authors conducted a scoping review to map and analyze the existing scientific literature on the potential impact of AI in wound care education.

2. Methods

Given the limited knowledge about AI applications in wound care education and the emerging nature of this topic, a scoping review approach was determined to be the most appropriate method, given its purpose in mapping the evidence [32,33]. In addition, it emerged as the starting point for subsequent research [33,34]. Given their exploratory nature, scoping reviews are particularly useful when the goal is to map the existing literature on a broad topic, identify key concepts, and provide an overview of the available evidence [33–35].

Furthermore, unlike systematic reviews, scoping reviews provide greater flexibility in study selection, enabling a more expansive exploration of the literature [34,35]. This adaptability proves especially valuable in emerging fields with evolving evidence, where research questions may be less defined [34,35]. It aids researchers in understanding the current knowledge landscape, clarifying concepts, and shaping future research directions [35].

This exploratory approach makes them valuable for gaining a comprehensive understanding and mapping out this research area. This mapping can provide a detailed description of the available information on AI applications in wound care education, identifying possible gaps in knowledge, offering conclusions about the current state of research activity in this area, and making recommendations for future research.

This review protocol was registered in the Open Science Framework (OSF) platform (https://doi.org/10.17605/OSF.IO/MTGDX, accessed on 30 November 2023).

The scoping review follows the Joanna Briggs Institute's (JBI) methodology for scoping reviews [33,36] and the Guidance for Conducting Systematic Scoping Reviews [33]. Results will be presented following the Preferred Reporting Items for Systematic and Meta-Analyses extension for Scoping Reviews (PRISMA-ScR) [32] guidelines.

2.1. Research Questions

It is suggested that scoping review questions should have a broad scope [37]. This involves delineating the concept, specifying the target population, and identifying health outcomes of interest to bring clarity to the scoping study's focus and develop a robust search strategy [37]. The research questions were formulated through collaborative discussions with the research team and relevant stakeholders. A panel of experts, including advanced practice nurses, nurse researchers, and educators in the fields of digital health technologies and health education, were consulted to shape the research questions aligning with the objective of this review.

To achieve this study's aims, the following research question was identified according to JBI recommendations in the PCC mnemonic guide: what evidence currently exists regarding the application of AI in wound care education?

Additionally, this review aims to answer the following sub-questions:

- How is AI integrated into wound care education?
- How is AI being used to educate healthcare students about wound assessment and management?
- How does AI contribute to the education of healthcare professionals in wound assessment and management, particularly in clinical and academic settings?
- What evidence currently exists regarding the use of machine learning and simulation technologies in AI-driven wound care education?
- What evidence currently exists regarding the application of AI in formal wound care educational programs and training?
- What are the benefits of AI application in wound care education for healthcare practitioners, students, and educators?
- What experiences and perceptions do healthcare practitioners, students, and educators have regarding AI in wound care education?
- What learning outcomes result from integrating AI technology in wound care education?
- What are the barriers to and facilitators of applying AI technology in wound care education?

2.2. Inclusion Criteria

To determine the main subjects under investigation and formulate the eligibility criteria, the PCC (Population, Concept, Context) framework was used:

- Participants: this study will encompass all literature that discussed participants as healthcare practitioners, students, and educators.
- Concept: this review will include literature that analyzes AI and its influence on wound care education.
- Context: education. To expand the scope of the review, the context will be broad and involve any educational settings without geographic restrictions.

The scope of the literature reviewed will include any quantitative, qualitative, and mixed-method studies. Additionally, gray literature (conference abstracts, theses, government reports, clinical practice guidelines, editorial and opinion papers) will be included as well. Provided they meet the eligibility criteria, this analysis may also include additional relevant manuscripts. Studies that do not explore AI in wound care education will be excluded.

Literature sources were limited to English, Portuguese, and Spanish, based on the authors' language proficiency, without imposing geographical or cultural restrictions.

2.3. Search Strategy

We used the PCC method and field knowledge to identify relevant keywords concerning this topic. As recommended by JBI scoping review methodology [38], we performed preliminary research using keywords (artificial intelligence, wound, and education) on two databases relevant to the topic of interest: Medical Literature Analysis and Retrieval System Online (MEDLINE via PubMed) and the Cumulative Index to Nursing and Allied Health Literature (CINAHL via EBSCOhost). The titles, abstracts, and index terms of the identified studies were reviewed to extract the MeSH thesaurus and CINAHL Subject Headings used to describe the literature. Subsequently, in collaboration with a health sciences librarian, two reviewers developed the search strategy, which was peer-reviewed by the third expert reviewer based on the Peer Review of Electronic Search Strategies (PRESS) [32]. The MEDLINE (via Pubmed) search strategy can be found in Appendix A. The search strategy, including all identified keywords and index terms, was customized for each literature source. When available, subject headings such as MeSH and Emtree terms were used.

As experts in the development of scoping review protocols, team members reviewed the search terms, Boolean operators, and results to edit and enhance the search strategy.

Article reference lists were sourced for additional articles. This step aims to check for additional studies not previously identified. Establishing contact with the authors of the identified studies might be useful for potential clarifications or obtaining references.

The whole search was carried out in the following databases: CINAHL Complete (via EBSCOhost), MEDLINE (via PubMed), Cochrane Library, Academic Search Complete, Scientific Electronic Library Online (Scielo), Scopus, and Web of Science. Electronic searches were also conducted in the Scientific Open Access Scientific Repositories of Portugal (RCAAP) and ProQuest Dissertations and Theses, OpenAIRE, and Open Dissertations databases to access gray literature. Additionally, searches were performed on Google Scholar and specific journals such as the International Wound Journal, Skin Research and Technology, Journal of Wound Care, and Wound Repair and Regeneration. The selection of these databases was performed in collaboration with the health sciences librarian to guarantee comprehensive coverage of the key concepts (artificial intelligence, wounds, and education).

The searches were carried out on 1 December 2023, and all results were imported into Endnote vX20 (Clarivate Analytics, Philadelphia, PA, USA). Duplicated studies were subsequently removed.

2.4. Evidence Screening and Study Selection

In the first phase, article titles and abstracts were screened independently by two reviewers for eligibility criteria using the Rayyan QCR platform. In the second phase, potentially relevant records were obtained in full through institutional access or by emailing authors. The full text of potentially relevant evidence was screened according to the inclusion criteria by two independent reviewers.

To systematize the review and minimize research bias, two independent reviewers were involved in each selection phase. Any disagreements were addressed and resolved by reaching a consensus with a third reviewer until complete agreement was achieved. The review team conducted a pilot test of this process and held regular meetings to ensure consistency in the application of the eligibility criteria. During this process, 10% of the records were screened, and the results were compared and discussed with the team. Inclusion criteria were modified as needed.

The final scoping review will document the reasons for excluding studies that do not meet the inclusion criteria.

The methodological quality of the included studies will not be assessed. Scoping reviews, in contrast to systematic reviews, do not require the same degree of evidence since they do not synthesize results from sources through a formal appraisal process but instead aim to provide an overview of the literature [34].

The decision not to assess the methodological quality of the included studies is deliberate as it will allow us to conduct a comprehensive review that includes a broad range of relevant studies to address the research question and achieve the primary study objective. In scoping reviews, assessing critical appraisal or risk of bias is generally not recommended because the aim is to map the available evidence rather than provide a synthesized and clinically meaningful answer to a question [33,34]. Due to the diverse spectrum of study methods and interventions and the inclusion of both gray and published literature, conducting a critical appraisal was not feasible. Given the emerging nature of this topic, performing a methodological quality appraisal and subsequently excluding studies based on this evaluation may result in the rejection of relevant research. The decision not to conduct a quality assessment promotes transparency and rigor.

The research results will be fully described in the final review, and, at this stage, they are presented in a PRISMA-ScR flow diagram [39] (Figure 1).

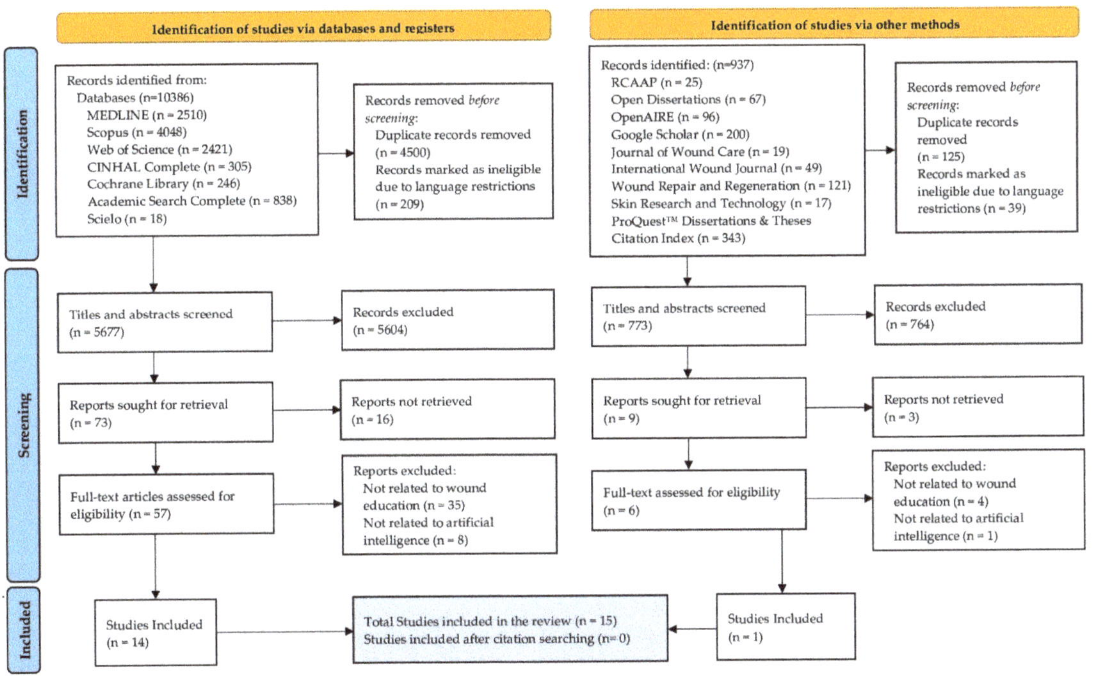

Figure 1. PRISMA (Preferred Reporting Items for Systematic Reviews and Meta-Analyses) 2020 flow diagram.

2.5. Data Charting

Following the JBI methodology, data will be extracted from included records by two independent reviewers using a data extraction tool created by the review team based on the JBI instrument for extracting study details, characteristics, and results [33,34]. The authors will develop a pilot test of this form to ensure the appropriate capture of all relevant data. The initial three records extracted will be discussed and extracted data compared to assess any conflicts. Any disagreements between the reviewers will be resolved through discussion or with a third reviewer.

The extracted data contain specific details about the population (wounds), concept (artificial intelligence), context (education), and critical findings relevant to the review question and objective (Appendix B). This includes the title, author, year of publication, country of origin, research design, research purpose, participant details, wound specifics, AI characteristics, and education program details.

Participant details indicate the role (health student, health educator, or health practitioner). Regarding AI characteristics, the data include AI technology, tools, equipment, main functions, and other details (adaptive learning, interactive engagement, visual recognition, diagnostic assistance, feedback mechanism, continuous monitoring, and real-time updates). The data presented also encompass details of the education program, specifically the educational setting where it takes place (hospital, universities, and non-university settings), education level (undergraduate or post-graduate), and the outcomes measured.

It should be highlighted that adjustments to the data extraction tool could be carried out during the review stage. If there is any missing information in the included records, the respective authors will be contacted to request it.

2.6. Data Analysis

Data will be presented in a table and in narrative form to describe how the tabulated results relate to the review's objective and question.

The same reviewers involved in the previous step will independently carry out this procedure. A third reviewer may be consulted to gain consensus on the differences found.

3. Results

A cohort of 15 studies has been earmarked for intricate data charting and analytical review. This selection follows a preliminary scrutiny of 6450 studies, distilled from an exhaustive retrieval of 11,323 potential studies.

The included papers were published between 2006 and 2023, encompassing a variety of study types, including conference papers, experimental studies, editorial papers, and other original articles. The majority of studies included in the review address various types of wounds, with some focusing specifically on certain types, such as pressure ulcers or diabetic foot ulcers.

The integration of AI in wound care education, as evidenced by these studies, marks a pivotal shift towards enhancing clinical decision support and e-learning platforms. This evolution is illuminated by these studies, which showcase AI's capacity to transform healthcare education by offering tailored and engaging learning experiences. Moreover, these papers collectively underline the importance of evidence-based, personalized learning approaches facilitated by AI.

Several of these studies underscore the pivotal role of AI in fostering active learning and hands-on experiences. This is achieved through the development of e-learning scenarios that draw upon real-world experiences, thereby enriching the educational process with practical, applicable knowledge and insights.

The integration of AI paradigms, such as Bayesian Inference, Case-Based Reasoning, and Intelligent Agents, into e-learning platforms exemplifies a forward-thinking approach to medical education. This approach enables participants to analyze wound images based on color and texture, helping them to understand wound healing barriers such as non-viable tissue, infection, inflammation, and moisture imbalance.

Images entirely generated by AI to facilitate pattern recognition and clinical case discussions are also presented as a promising strategy to improve medical education. These AI-created visuals, not being real, carry the added benefit of preserving patient privacy while providing an innovative tool for educational purposes.

Other papers suggest employing smartphone-based AI applications for pressure injury assessment and utilizing case-based reasoning as educational tools. These methods enable learners to practice and enhance their knowledge and evidence levels, thereby maximizing their motivation and performance.

Large language models like ChatGPT are also presented as potential tools in providing personalized, accessible, and up-to-date educational content for healthcare professionals. This perspective underscores the flexibility and scalability of AI technologies in improving educational practices within the domain of wound care. It acknowledges, however, the necessity to address challenges pertaining to data privacy and the accuracy of the content provided.

In conclusion, the included studies indicate a promising future for AI in wound care education, pointing to the need for ongoing development, validation, and testing. Its relevance and pertinence to the research question are undeniable.

The comprehensive review will collate and present the outcomes within the main conceptual frameworks identified in this study. The authors will discuss and cross-validate the findings to ensure validity and credibility. They will also address the implications for future research, clinical practice, and policy while critically evaluating the significance of the findings concerning the study's primary objective.

4. Discussion

As the World Health Organization (WHO) acknowledges, the use of AI in medical education presents a paradigm shift, offering unprecedented personalization and decision-making enhancements [40]. However, it also brings ethical dilemmas, such as ensuring patient privacy, fairness in AI-driven decisions, and legal accountability [40].

The WHO document on AI in health outlines several advantages and ethical pitfalls of AI in medical education. Some advantages are related to Enhanced Management and Diagnostics: AI aids in managing complex cases and streamlining routine diagnoses, enhancing the educational process with practical applications; Reduced Administrative Burden: AI reduces the workload on healthcare providers by handling clerical tasks, allowing more focus on education; Novel Insights from Data: AI provides new insights from health data, enriching educational content with advanced knowledge; and Support in Education and Research: AI tools support medical and nursing education and research, improving the understanding of medical conditions [40].

Despite this, we have as Potential Ethical Pitfalls the Quality of Education: AI inaccuracies could negatively impact medical education quality; the Additional Burden on Healthcare Workers: AI integration may require additional training for healthcare professionals not yet skilled in digital technologies; Bias and Privacy Concerns: AI in education raises issues of bias, privacy breaches, and accessibility, necessitating fairness and data protection; and Skills Degradation and Moral De-skilling: over-reliance on AI might erode clinicians' skills and confidence in making independent decisions and moral judgments [40].

As emphasized by Drabiak et al., while AI and machine learning bring significant promise to education, particularly in personalizing learning experiences and enhancing educational efficiency, they also raise critical ethical concerns [41]. These concerns include issues related to data privacy, the responsibility of AI decision-making, trustworthiness of AI systems, and ensuring fairness in educational outcomes [41]. This perspective highlights the need for a balanced approach in AI implementation, ensuring that the technological advancements contribute positively to the educational landscape while conscientiously addressing ethical implications [41].

Incorporating AI into wound care education demands careful consideration of ethical aspects. The effectiveness of AI is also deeply influenced by the quality of the data it processes. For wound care education, it is essential to use high-quality, diverse, and representative data to avoid biases in AI algorithms. These biases can arise from both the data and human input, potentially distorting educational outcomes. Consequently, special attention to data selection and algorithm design is crucial for equitable and accurate educational experiences [41].

Furthermore, ethical aspects of AI, such as interpretability, accountability, and bias, are critical and need to be addressed carefully. Recent research has identified a need for better understandability of machine learning algorithms and predictions [42]. This includes clarifying AI's role in decision-making, advocating for transparency, reducing algorithmic bias, and enhancing trust among stakeholders [42].

The integration of AI in wound care education should be ruled by robust ethical oversight. This involves establishing committees for the ethical review of AI applications, ensuring alignment with ethical principles, and respecting learner rights. Continuous assessment of the risks and benefits of AI in education is vital for maintaining integrity and trustworthiness.

Balancing the benefits of data sharing with the protection of individual privacy is a critical ethical challenge. Rigorous data security measures and transparent data usage tracking mechanisms are elemental. This approach helps maintain trust while leveraging AI's educational advantages.

Transparency in AI operations and decision-making processes is also crucial in education. On the practical side, the implementation of AI faces technical and pedagogical hurdles. The cross-disciplinary nature of AI necessitates joint consideration of technical and legal aspects, especially in sensitive areas such as data cleaning in medical AI [19]. Instructors' technological skills are instrumental but not sufficient for integrating AI in classrooms, further complicating the issue [19].

By addressing these ethical considerations, AI can be used in wound care education effectively, while also being ethically rigorous and responsible [43]. This approach enhances the educational experience while safeguarding the interests and rights of all involved stakeholders [43].

5. Limitations

We acknowledge potential limitations of the scoping review, particularly its restriction to studies published in English, Portuguese, and Spanish. However, no studies will be excluded based on country. Potentially relevant studies will be listed in a supplement of the final review.

The inclusion of diverse sources, with various study designs, may challenge the validity of the results. Variability in how AI and wound care education are defined and measured across studies may also affect construct validity.

While scoping reviews typically do not appraise the quality of included articles, and explicit reasons for not conducting such appraisals in this review are provided, this is acknowledged as another potential limitation of the scoping review. The lack of critical appraisal may limit the scoping review's ability to provide concrete recommendations for practice or policy, as the quality of the included studies is not systematically evaluated. Despite these limitations, given that scoping reviews are considered a precursor to a systematic review [34], critical appraisal could be implemented if the conditions for conducting a systematic review are met.

Scoping reviews aim to offer a comprehensive overview rather than specific recommendations, limiting the ability to draw detailed conclusions and generalize findings. The applicability of results to various educational settings or populations might be constrained by the specific focus on AI in wound care education. Additionally, findings may not be directly transferable to different healthcare systems, educational institutions, or regions with distinct practices and resources.

We will consider the impact of these limitations and address any additional limitations that may arise when reporting our results.

6. Conclusions

AI plays a significant role in the future of healthcare education. Therefore, embracing AI and related technologies is not merely an option but a transformative trend that organizations must acknowledge and leverage for competitive advantage. While AI tools have been employed to assess wound care, efforts are needed to enhance their potential impact on wound care education. Integrating AI into health education, specifically wound care, represents a paradigm shift in how educational content is delivered and processed. This transformation goes beyond traditional methods to provide a more personalized, efficient, and interactive learning experience. AI-driven tools can adapt to individual learning styles and provide tailored teaching materials and simulations. This adaptability improves the learning process, making it more engaging and efficient for students and professionals alike. With AI's ability to analyze and interpret complex medical data, students and physicians can gain insights into wound care from remote locations, breaking down geographic barriers in education. This is especially important in the current global situation, where distance learning and telemedicine are becoming increasingly important. We hope that integrating AI into wound care education will not only revolutionize the delivery of knowledge but also directly improve patient outcomes. By more effectively training healthcare professionals in wound care, AI can help better diagnose, treat, and manage wounds, ultimately improving the quality of patient care. This is consistent with the broader goals of health education, which focus on improving health outcomes and the standards of patient care.

As this scoping review will illustrate, harnessing the potential of AI in wound care education requires not only a thorough understanding of its capabilities but also a commitment to addressing the ethical and practical challenges associated with its implementation. A careful exploration of the ethical aspects surrounding artificial intelligence in wound care education is essential. As AI shapes the educational landscape, addressing issues like data privacy and bias is crucial for a responsible integration that ensures both educational excellence and ethical approval.

As far as we know, this is the first review to explore the influence of AI in the context of wound care education. The findings of this scoping review will likely provide insights into the application of AI in wound care education, identify research gaps in the literature, and promote further research initiatives. Hopefully, it will also be relevant for educators, students, policymakers, health and education organizations, and researchers in healthcare sciences and engineering.

The results will be disseminated through presentations at health education meetings and conferences and publication in a peer-reviewed health education journal.

Author Contributions: Conceptualization, R.E., T.M., H.P., J.N.-A. and P.A.; methodology, R.E.; validation, T.M., J.N.-A. and P.A.; investigation, R.E., T.M., J.N.-A. and P.A.; resources, R.E., T.M., J.N.-A. and P.A.; writing—original draft preparation, R.E.; writing—review and editing, R.E., T.M., H.P., J.N.-A. and P.A.; visualization, R.E.; supervision, P.A.; project administration, R.E. All authors have read and agreed to the published version of the manuscript.

Funding: This research was supported by national funds through FCT within the scope of the Centre for Interdisciplinary Research in Health (UIDB/04279/2020).

Data Availability Statement: For data supporting reported results, please contact the authors of this review.

Public Involvement Statement: There was no public involvement in any aspect of this research.

Guidelines and Standards Statement: This scoping review follows the Joanna Briggs Institute's (JBI) methodology for scoping reviews.

Acknowledgments: The authors express their gratitude to Maria Perdigão from the Library Services at the Catholic University of Portugal for her support in developing the search strategy.

Conflicts of Interest: Author Tânia Manuel was employed by the company Prove.pt, Grupo Saúde Nuno Mendes. This company was not involved in the study design, collection, analysis, interpretation of data, the writing of this article or the decision to submit it for publication. Author Hélder Palheira was employed by the company HC Healthcare & Innovation. This company was not involved in the study design, collection, analysis, interpretation of data, the writing of this article or the decision to submit it for publication. The remaining authors declare that the research was conducted in the absence of any commercial or financial relationships that could be construed as a potential conflict of interest.

Appendix A. Search Strategy Used for MEDLINE (via PubMed) Database

Search	Query	Results
#1	"wound*"[Title/Abstract] OR "ulcer*"[Title/Abstract] OR "bed sore*"[Title/Abstract] OR "bedsore*"[Title/Abstract] OR "pressure sore*"[Title/Abstract] OR "diabetic feet"[Title/Abstract] OR "diabetic foot"[Title/Abstract] OR "surgical dressing*"[Title/Abstract] OR "injury"[Title/Abstract] OR "injuries"[Title/Abstract] OR "pressure ulcer"[MeSH Terms] OR "wounds and injuries"[MeSH Terms] OR "surgical wound"[MeSH Terms] OR "wound healing"[MeSH Terms] OR "wound infection"[MeSH Terms] OR "varicose ulcer"[MeSH Terms] OR "ulcer"[MeSH Terms] OR "leg ulcer"[MeSH Terms] OR "skin ulcer"[MeSH Terms] OR "foot ulcer"[MeSH Terms] OR "diabetic foot"[MeSH Terms]	2,127,690
#2	"artificial Intelligence"[Title/Abstract] OR "AI"[Title/Abstract] OR "chatgtp"[Title/Abstract] OR "expert system*"[Title/Abstract] OR "computational intelligence"[Title/Abstract] OR "computer reasoning"[Title/Abstract] OR "computer vision"[Title/Abstract] OR "machine intelligence"[Title/Abstract] OR "machine learning"[Title/Abstract] OR "deep learning"[Title/Abstract] OR "natural language processing"[Title/Abstract] OR "neural network*"[Title/Abstract] OR "artificial Intelligence"[MeSH Terms] OR "Expert Systems"[MeSH Terms] OR "machine learning"[MeSH Terms] OR "deep learning"[MeSH Terms] OR "natural language processing"[MeSH Terms] OR "neural networks, computer"[MeSH Terms]	362,875
#3	"educat*"[Title/Abstract] OR "teach*"[Title/Abstract] OR "student*"[Title/Abstract] OR "training"[Title/Abstract] OR "instruction*"[Title/Abstract] OR "simulat*"[Title/Abstract] OR "interactive learning"[Title/Abstract] OR "gamification"[Title/Abstract] OR "game*"[Title/Abstract] OR "health education"[MeSH Terms] OR "teaching"[MeSH Terms] OR "learning"[MeSH Terms] OR "education"[MeSH Terms] OR "educational technology"[MeSH Terms] OR "simulation training"[MeSH Terms] OR "high fidelity simulation training"[MeSH Terms] OR "students"[MeSH Terms] OR "students, health occupations"[MeSH Terms] OR "students, medical"[MeSH Terms] OR "students, nursing"[MeSH Terms] OR "students, nursing"[MeSH Terms] OR "education, medical"[MeSH Terms] OR "education, medical, graduate"[MeSH Terms] OR "education, medical, undergraduate"[MeSH Terms] OR "education, graduate"[MeSH Terms] OR "education, medical, continuing"[MeSH Terms] OR "education, professional"[MeSH Terms] OR "health educators"[MeSH Terms] OR "educational personnel"[MeSH Terms] OR "faculty, medical"[MeSH Terms] OR "faculty, nursing"[MeSH Terms] OR "education, nursing"[MeSH Terms] OR "education, nursing, graduate"[MeSH Terms] OR "education, nursing, continuing"[MeSH Terms] OR "education, nursing, baccalaureate"[MeSH Terms] OR "education, continuing"[MeSH Terms]	3,242,478
#4	#1 AND #2 AND #3	2510

* includes truncated words in PUBMED.

Appendix B. Preliminary Data Charting Tool

Study characteristics	Extracted data
	Title
	Author(s)
	Publication year
	Country of origin
	Research purpose
	Research design
	Participants details (health practitioner, student, or educator)
Population	Type of wounds
Artificial intelligence characteristics	Technology (deep learning, expert system, machine learning)
	Tools, equipment and main functions
	AI details (adaptive learning, interactive engagement, visual recognition, diagnostic assistance, feedback mechanism, continuous monitoring, real-time updates, user-friendly interface, others)
	Evaluation metrics (to describe how the performance of AI technologies was measured)
Education program details	Domain (administration, assessment, learning, teaching)
	Educational level (undergraduate or post-graduate)
	Curricular structure and duration (to provide context regarding the scope and depth of the evaluated education programs)
	Outcomes of students
	Outcomes of teachers
Key findings	Relevant key findings
Clinical implications	To report how findings may influence real-life practice
Study limitations	To provide transparency and critical context

References

1. Wang, P. On Defining Artificial Intelligence. *J. Artif. Gen. Intell.* **2019**, *10*, 1–37. [CrossRef]
2. Jakhar, D.; Kaur, I. Artificial intelligence, machine learning and deep learning: Definitions and differences. *Clin. Exp. Dermatol.* **2020**, *45*, 131–132. [CrossRef]
3. Helm, J.M.; Swiergosz, A.M.; Haeberle, H.S.; Karnuta, J.M.; Schaffer, J.L.; Krebs, V.E.; Spitzer, A.I.; Ramkumar, P.N. Machine Learning and Artificial Intelligence: Definitions, Applications, and Future Directions. *Curr. Rev. Musculoskelet. Med.* **2020**, *13*, 69–76. [CrossRef]
4. Chiu, T.K.F.; Xia, Q.; Zhou, X.; Chai, C.S.; Cheng, M. Systematic literature review on opportunities, challenges, and future research recommendations of artificial intelligence in education. *Comput. Educ. Artif. Intell.* **2023**, *4*, 100118. [CrossRef]
5. Bohr, A.; Memarzadeh, K. The rise of artificial intelligence in healthcare applications. In *Artificial Intelligence in Healthcare*; Academic Press: Cambridge, MA, USA, 2020; pp. 25–60. [CrossRef]
6. Lee, D.; Yoon, S.N. Application of artificial intelligence-based technologies in the healthcare industry: Opportunities and challenges. *Int. J. Environ. Res. Public Health* **2021**, *18*, 271. [CrossRef]
7. Ali, O.; Abdelbaki, W.; Shrestha, A.; Elbasi, E.; Alryalat, M.A.A.; Dwivedi, Y.K. A systematic literature review of artificial intelligence in the healthcare sector: Benefits, challenges, methodologies, and functionalities. *J. Innov. Knowl.* **2023**, *8*, 100333. [CrossRef]
8. Jiang, F.; Jiang, Y.; Zhi, H.; Dong, Y.; Li, H.; Ma, S.; Wang, Y.; Dong, Q.; Shen, H.; Wang, Y. Artificial intelligence in healthcare: Past, present and future. *Stroke Vasc. Neurol.* **2017**, *2*, 230–243. [CrossRef] [PubMed]
9. Loh, H.W.; Ooi, C.P.; Seoni, S.; Barua, P.D.; Molinari, F.; Acharya, U.R. Application of explainable artificial intelligence for healthcare: A systematic review of the last decade (2011–2022). *Comput. Methods Programs Biomed.* **2022**, *226*, 107161. [CrossRef] [PubMed]
10. Davenport, T.; Kalakota, R. The potential for artificial intelligence in healthcare. *Future Healthc. J.* **2019**, *6*, 94–98. [CrossRef] [PubMed]

11. Queen, D.; Harding, K. Data-driven specialisation of wound care through artificial intelligence. *Int. Wound. J.* **2019**, *16*, 879–880. [CrossRef]
12. De Gagne, J.C. The State of Artificial Intelligence in Nursing Education: Past, Present, and Future Directions. *Int. J. Environ. Res. Public Health* **2023**, *20*, 4884. [CrossRef] [PubMed]
13. Ouyang, F.; Zheng, L.; Jiao, P. Artificial intelligence in online higher education: A systematic review of empirical research from 2011 to 2020. *Educ. Inf. Technol.* **2022**, *27*, 7893–7925. [CrossRef]
14. Chan, K.S.; Zary, N. Applications and Challenges of Implementing Artificial Intelligence in Medical Education: Integrative Review. *JMIR Med. Educ.* **2019**, *5*, e13930. [CrossRef] [PubMed]
15. Yu, H.; Guo, Y. Generative artificial intelligence empowers educational reform: Current status, issues, and prospects. *Front. Educ.* **2023**, *8*, 1183162. [CrossRef]
16. Preiksaitis, C.; Rose, C. Opportunities, Challenges, and Future Directions of Generative Artificial Intelligence in Medical Education: Scoping Review. *JMIR Med. Educ.* **2023**, *9*, e48785. [CrossRef] [PubMed]
17. Mirchi, N.; Bissonnette, V.; Yilmaz, R.; Ledwos, N.; Winkler-Schwartz, A.; Del Maestro, R.F. The virtual operative assistant: An explainable artificial intelligence tool for simulation-based training in surgery and medicine. *PLoS ONE* **2020**, *15*, e0229596. [CrossRef]
18. Shorey, S.; Ang, E.; Yap, J.; Ng, E.D.; Lau, S.T.; Chui, C.K. A virtual counseling application using artificial intelligence for communication skills training in nursing education: Development study. *J. Med. Internet Res.* **2019**, *21*, e14658. [CrossRef]
19. Harmon, J.; Pitt, V.; Summons, P.; Inder, K.J. Use of artificial intelligence and virtual reality within clinical simulation for nursing pain education: A scoping review. *Nurse Educ. Today* **2021**, *97*, 104700. [CrossRef]
20. King, M.R. A Conversation on Artificial Intelligence, Chatbots, and Plagiarism in Higher Education. *Cell Mol. Bioeng.* **2023**, *16*, 1–2. [CrossRef]
21. Mohammad Amini, M.; Jesus, M.; Fanaei Sheikholeslami, D.; Alves, P.; Hassanzadeh Benam, A.; Hariri, F. Artificial Intelligence Ethics and Challenges in Healthcare Applications: A Comprehensive Review in the Context of the European GDPR Mandate. *Mach. Learn Knowl. Extr.* **2023**, *5*, 1023–1035. [CrossRef]
22. Sarp, S.; Kuzlu, M.; Wilson, E.; Cali, U.; Guler, O. The enlightening role of explainable artificial intelligence in chronic wound classification. *Electronics* **2021**, *10*, 1406. [CrossRef]
23. Chan, K.S.; Chan, Y.M.; Tan, A.H.M.; Liang, S.; Cho, Y.T.; Hong, Q.; Yong, E.; Chong, L.R.C.; Zhang, L.; Tan, G.W.L.; et al. Clinical validation of an artificial intelligence-enabled wound imaging mobile application in diabetic foot ulcers. *Int. Wound J.* **2022**, *19*, 114–124. [CrossRef] [PubMed]
24. Barakat-Johnson, M.; Jones, A.; Burger, M.; Leong, T.; Frotjold, A.; Randall, S.; Kim, B.; Fethney, J.; Coyer, F. Reshaping wound care: Evaluation of an artificial intelligence app to improve wound assessment and management amid the COVID-19 pandemic. *Int. Wound J.* **2022**, *19*, 1561–1577. [CrossRef]
25. Tehsin, S.; Kausar, S.; Jameel, A. Diabetic wounds and artificial intelligence: A mini-review. *World J. Clin. Cases* **2023**, *11*, 84–91. [CrossRef]
26. Cross, K.; Harding, K. Risk profiling in the prevention and treatment of chronic wounds using artificial intelligence. *Int. Wound J.* **2022**, *19*, 1283–1285. [CrossRef]
27. Powers, J.G.; Higham, C.; Broussard, K.; Phillips, T.J. Wound healing and treating wounds Chronic wound care and management. *J. Am. Acad. Dermatol.* **2016**, *74*, 607–625. [CrossRef]
28. Welsh, L. Wound care evidence, knowledge and education amongst nurses: A semi-systematic literature review. *Int. Wound J.* **2018**, *15*, 53–61. [CrossRef]
29. Luo, C. Unlocking Medical Potentials: An In-depth Investigation of Augmented Reality Technology in Medicine. *Commun. Humanit. Res.* **2024**, *27*, 126–130. [CrossRef]
30. Mah, E. Metaverse, AR, machine learning & AI in Orthopaedics? *J. Orthop. Surg.* **2023**, *31*. [CrossRef]
31. Mcintosh, T.R.; Susnjak, T.; Liu, T.; Watters, P.; Halgamuge, M.N. From Google Gemini to OpenAI Q* (Q-Star): A Survey of Reshaping the Generative Artificial Intelligence (AI) Research Landscape. *J. Latex Cl. Files* **2023**, *1*, 1–30. [CrossRef]
32. McGowan, J.; Sampson, M.; Salzwedel, D.M.; Cogo, E.; Foerster, V.; Lefebvre, C. PRESS Peer Review of Electronic Search Strategies: 2015 Guideline Statement. *J. Clin. Epidemiol.* **2016**, *75*, 40–46. [CrossRef]
33. Peters, M.D.; Marnie, C.; Tricco, A.C.; Pollock, D.; Munn, Z.; Alexander, L.; McInerney, P.; Godfrey, C.M.; Khalil, H. Updated methodological guidance for the conduct of scoping reviews. *JBI Evid. Synth.* **2020**, *18*, 2119–2126. [CrossRef] [PubMed]
34. Aromataris, E.; Munn, Z. (Eds.) *JBI Manual for Evidence Synthesis*; JBI: Adelaide, Australia, 2020. [CrossRef]
35. Munn, Z.; Peters, M.D.J.; Stern, C.; Tufanaru, C.; McArthur, A.; Aromataris, E. Systematic review or scoping review? Guidance for authors when choosing between a systematic or scoping review approach. *BMC Med. Res. Methodol.* **2018**, *18*, 143. [CrossRef]
36. Tricco, A.C.; Lillie, E.; Zarin, W.; O'Brien, K.K.; Colquhoun, H.; Levac, D.; Moher, D.; Peters, M.D.; Horsley, T.; Weeks, L.; et al. PRISMA Extension for Scoping Reviews (PRISMA-ScR): Checklist and Explanation. *Ann. Intern. Med.* **2018**, *169*, 467–473. [CrossRef]
37. Levac, D.; Colquhoun, H.; O'Brien, K.K. Scoping studies: Advancing the methodology. *Implement. Sci.* **2010**, *5*, 69. [CrossRef]
38. Peters, M.D.J.; Godfrey, C.M.; Khalil, H.; McInerney, P.; Parker, D.; Soares, C.B. Guidance for conducting systematic scoping reviews. *Int. J. Evid. Based Healthc.* **2015**, *13*, 141–146. [CrossRef] [PubMed]

39. Page, M.J.; McKenzie, J.E.; Bossuyt, P.M.; Boutron, I.; Hoffmann, T.C.; Mulrow, C.D.; Shamseer, L.; Tetzlaff, J.M.; Akl, E.A.; Brennan, S.E.; et al. The PRISMA 2020 statement: An updated guideline for reporting systematic reviews. *BMJ* **2021**, *372*, 105906. [CrossRef]
40. World Health Organization. Ethics and Governance of Artificial Intelligence for Health. Ethics and Governance of Artificial Intelligence for Health: Who Guidance. 2021. Available online: https://iris.who.int/bitstream/handle/10665/341996/9789240029200-eng.pdf?sequence=1 (accessed on 10 February 2024).
41. Drabiak, K.; Kyzer, S.; Nemov, V.; El Naqa, I. AI and machine learning ethics, law, diversity, and global impact. *Br. J. Radiol.* **2023**, *96*, 1150. [CrossRef] [PubMed]
42. Balasubramaniam, N.; Kauppinen, M.; Rannisto, A.; Hiekkanen, K.; Kujala, S. Transparency and explainability of AI systems: From ethical guidelines to requirements. *Inf. Softw. Technol.* **2023**, *159*, 107197. [CrossRef]
43. Zhang, J.; Zhang, Z. Ethics and governance of trustworthy medical artificial intelligence. *BMC Med. Inform. Decis. Mak.* **2023**, *23*, 7. [CrossRef]

MDPI AG
Grosspeteranlage 5
4052 Basel
Switzerland
Tel.: +41 61 683 77 34

Nursing Reports Editorial Office
E-mail: nursrep@mdpi.com
www.mdpi.com/journal/nursrep

www.ingramcontent.com/pod-product-compliance
Lightning Source LLC
Chambersburg PA
CBHW061510210926
51850CB00008B/1867
9783725866564